Clinical Transplantation
Current Practice and Future Prospects

IMMUNOLOGY AND MEDICINE SERIES

Immunology of Endocrine Diseases
Editor: A. M. McGregor

Clinical Transplantation: Current Practice and Future Prospects
Editor: G. R. D. Catto

Complement in Health and Disease
Editor: K. Whaley

Immunological Aspects of Oral Diseases
Editor: L. Ivanyi

Immunoglobulins in Health and Disease
Editor: M. A. H. French

Immunology of Malignant Diseases
Editors: V. S. Byers and R. W. Baldwin

Lymphoproliferative Diseases
Editors: D. B. Jones and D. H. Wright

Phagocytes and Disease
Editors: M. S. Klempner, B. Styrt and J. Ho

HLA and Disease
Authors: B. Bradley, P. T. Klouda, J. Bidwell and G. Laundy

Lymphocytes in Health and Disease
Editors: G. Janossy and P. L. Amlot

Mast Cells, Mediators and Disease
Editor: S. T. Holgate

Immunodeficiency and Disease
Editor: A. D. B. Webster

Immunology of Pregnancy and its Disorders
Editor: C. Stern

Immunotherapy of Disease
Editor: T. J. Hamblin

Immunology of Sexually Transmitted Diseases
Editor: D. J. M. Wright

IMMUNOLOGY
· SERIES · SERIES · SERIES · SERIES **AND** SERIES · SERIES · SERIES · SERIES ·
MEDICINE

Clinical Transplantation
Current Practice and Future Prospects

Edited by
G. R. D. Catto
Department of Medicine
Aberdeen Royal Infirmary
Foresterhill, Aberdeen

Series Editor: Professor W. G. Reeves

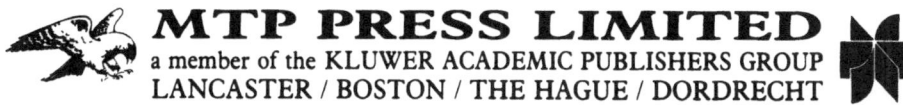

MTP PRESS LIMITED
a member of the KLUWER ACADEMIC PUBLISHERS GROUP
LANCASTER / BOSTON / THE HAGUE / DORDRECHT

Published in the UK and Europe by
MTP Press Limited
Falcon House
Lancaster, England

British Library Cataloguing in Publication Data

Clinical transplantation: current practice and future prospects.—
    (Immunology and medicine series).
    1. Transplantation of organs, tissues, etc.
    I. Catto, Graeme R. D.   II. Series
    617'.95   RD120.7

    ISBN-13: 978-94-010-7944-0   e-ISBN-13: 978-94-009-3217-3
    DOI: 10.1007/978-94-009-3217-3

Published in the USA by
MTP Press
A division of Kluwer Academic Publishers
101 Philip Drive
Norwell, MA 02061, USA

Library of Congress Cataloging in Publication Data

Clinical transplantation.

    (Immunology and medicine series)
    Includes bibliographies and index.
    1. Transplantation of organs, tissues, etc.
I. Catto, Graeme R. D.   II. Series.
[DNLM: 1. Kidney—transplantation.   2. Transplantation.   WO 660 C641]
RD120.7.C58   1987   617'.95   87-2938

Typeset by Lasertext Ltd, Manchester

Contents

Preface

This volume has been written specifically for the practising clinician. All aspects of clinical transplantation have expanded enormously in recent years, but many of the doctors involved have received little or no tuition in immunology as medical students. The various chapters, written by physicians, surgeons, pathologists and immunologists present many of the currently important issues in transplantation and demonstrate that a basic undertaking of immunology is now essential in many areas of clinical practice. Perhaps this book will not only produce an increasing awareness of immunological technique but also and, more importantly, stimulate an abiding interest in this clinically relevant topic.

Graeme R. Catto
Aberdeen Royal Infirmary

Series Editor's Note

The modern clinician is expected to be the fount of all wisdom concerning conventional diagnosis and management relevant to his sphere of practice. In addition, he or she has the daunting task of comprehending and keeping pace with advances in basic science relevant to the pathogenesis of disease and ways in which these processes can be regulated or prevented. Immunology has grown from the era of antitoxins and serum sickness to a state where the study of many diverse cells and molecules has become integrated into a coherent scientific discipline with major implications for many common and crippling diseases prevalent throughout the world.

Many of today's practitioners received little or no specific training in immunology and what was taught is very likely to have been overtaken by subsequent developments. This series of titles on IMMUNOLOGY AND MEDICINE is designed to rectify this deficiency in the form of distilled packages of information which the busy clinician, pathologist or other health care professional will be able to open and enjoy.

Professor W. G. Reeves, FRCP, FRCPath
Department of Immunology
University Hospital, Queen's Medical Centre
Nottingham

List of Contributors

J. M. BURTON
Royal Liverpool Hospital
Liverpool

A. K. BURNETT
The Walton Unit
Department of Haematology
Glasgow Royal Infirmary
Castle Street
Glasgow G4 0SF

G. R. D. CATTO
Department of Medicine
University of Aberdeen
Foresterhill
Aberdeen

J. ENGESET
Department of Surgery
University of Aberdeen
Foresterhill
Aberdeen

G. GALEA
Aberdeen and North East Scotland
  Blood Transfusion Service
Aberdeen Royal Infirmary
Foresterhill
Aberdeen

S. GLOVER
Ham Green Hospital
Bristol

B. K. GUNSON
University of Birmingham
Queen Elizabeth Hospital
Birmingham

A. N. HILLIS
Royal Liverpool Hospital
Liverpool

I. V. HUTCHINSON
Nuffield Department of Surgery
University of Oxford
John Radcliffe Hospital
Oxford

R. W. G. JOHNSON
University Department of Surgery
The Royal Infirmary
Oxford Road
Manchester M13 9WL

R. M. KIRBY
University of Birmingham
Queen Elizabeth Hospital
Birmingham

ix

G. A. McDONALD
The Walton Unit
Department of Haematology
Glasgow Royal Infirmary
Castle Street
Glasgow G4 0SF

C. G. A. McGREGOR
Department of Cardiothoracic Surgery
Freeman Hospital
Freeman Road
Newcastle upon Tyne NE7 7DN

A. M. MacLEOD
Department of Medicine
University of Aberdeen
Foresterhill
Aberdeen

P. McMASTER
University of Birmingham
Queen Elizabeth Hospital
Birmingham

K. ROLLES
Department of Surgery
University of Cambridge
Addenbrooke's Hospital
Cambridge

H. F. SEWELL
Immunopathology Laboratory
Department of Pathology
University of Aberdeen
Foresterhill
Aberdeen AB9 2ZD

A. W. THOMSON
Immunopathology Laboratory
Department of Pathology
University of Aberdeen
Foresterhill
Aberdeen AB9 2ZD

S. J. URBIANAK
Aberdeen and North East Scotland
   Blood Transfusion Service
Foresterhill
Aberdeen

G. G. YOUNGSON
Department of Surgery
University of Aberdeen
Foresterhill
Aberdeen AB9 2ZB

1
Medical Aspects of Renal Transplantation

A. M. MacLEOD AND G. R. D. CATTO

INTRODUCTION

Kidney transplantation is now well established as an acceptable and even desirable form of treatment for patients in terminal renal failure. If successful it offers a return to near normal health free from the restrictions of chronic dialysis, and provides the most economical and effective form of treatment for end-stage renal disease[1]. Some remain wary of suggesting increasing numbers of their patients as candidates for transplants, fearing the mortality to be unacceptably high. This is reflected in the data submitted to the European Dialysis and Transplant Registry[2,3] which show that, despite a four-fold increase in their numbers over the past decade, the proportion of patients with functioning grafts has remained static at around 20% of those requiring replacement therapy (Table 1.1). The use of the available modes of therapy for end-stage renal disease varies from country to country, however,

Table 1.1 Patients with functioning transplants as a proportion of those requiring treatment for end-stage renal disease (ESRD) in Europe*

	Total number	Patients per million population	Patients with functioning transplants	Percentage of total with functioning transplants
Patients on treatment for ESRD at 31st December 1974 (27 centres)	22 305	45.9	4 378	19.6
Patients on treatment for ESRD at 31st December 1983 (32 centres)	85 188	146.3	16 315	19.2

*Data from European Dialysis and Transplant Association Registry

1

and recent analyses[4] show that the survival of patients in countries favouring transplantation is the same as in those where over 80% are treated by dialysis (Figure 1.1).

Although there has been some improvement in allograft survival over the past ten years[3], between 15% and 40% of renal transplants fail within one year largely as a result of immunological rejection. Greater flexibility in patient care can be achieved by linking dialysis and transplantation services. Over the past decade the gradual adoption of such an integrated approach to treatment in the United Kingdom has not only increased the proportion of patients with functioning transplants from 34% to 45%[2,3], but has also improved the quality of life for many of those with end-stage renal disease.

PATIENT SELECTION

The criteria used to select recipients for renal transplants are becoming increasingly liberal. Patients previously labelled as high risk are being reconsidered and now, with few exceptions, those accepted for chronic dialysis are suitable candidates for renal transplantation. The patient's age and the nature of the renal disease must however be taken into account.

Age

As early as 1974 data collected by the Registry of the European Dialysis and Transplant Association showed that transplantation played a greater part in the treatment of children compared to adults in end-stage renal failure[5]. Recent figures[6] show that 46% of such children aged under 15 years have functioning transplants, and allograft survival in this age group is as good as that in adults (Table 1.2). Very few of these children were under five years

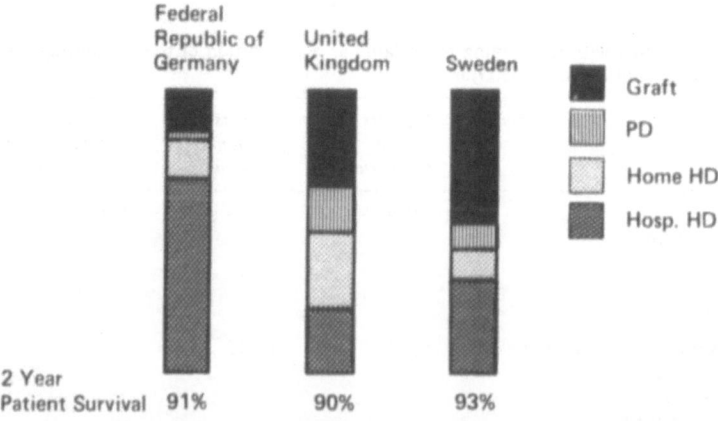

Figure 1.1 Data from 3 countries showing the proportional contribution of different therapies for end-stage renal disease and patient survival at 2 years. (Patients starting treatment 1981–1983, age 15–45, diabetes excluded)[3]. Data from European Dialysis and Transplant Registry

2

old, however, and transplantation below this age remains controversial. Some recent studies[7,8,9] show promising results particularly for living related transplants, but the technical problems are greater and mortality in this age group is higher than for older children. Transplantation has been performed successfully in infants under a year old[10,11] but in general both graft and patient survival are poor.

It was hoped that the restoration of relatively normal renal function after transplantation would improve the retarded growth seen in children with terminal renal disease. Recent figures[12] do show that growth is better in

transplanted children under 11 years old compared with those on dialysis. Reports on children whose bone age is over 12 years[12,13] provides less convincing evidence for a beneficial effect of transplantation on growth.

At the other end of the age spectrum both patient and graft survival decline. Two-year patient survival in those aged 45–54 years is 66% compared to 86% in the 35–44-year-old group, but the mortality of the older age group on haemodialysis is also high – 68% at 2 years[14]. Others have also reported similar survival rates on the two modes of therapy for those over 60[15]. The incidence of steroid-related complications is higher in older patients and death results principally from cardiovascular disease and infection.

The number of those older than 55 years accepted for renal replacement therapy has more than doubled in the past eight years[3]. Graft survival data therefore require frequent recalculation to determine the current place of transplantation for those older patients, particularly as immunosuppressive regimes change and steroid dosages are reduced.

Renal disease

Glomerulonephritis

Transplantation is no longer restricted to patients with primary renal diseases but is now also performed in those whose kidney failure results from multisystem and metabolic diseases.

Glomerulonephritis in its various forms, however, remains the commonest cause of terminal renal failure and in almost all types of this condition transplantation is a successful form of treatment. Antibodies to the glomerular basement membrane in anti-GBM nephritis can damage the transplanted kidney[16], but there is evidence to suggest that these antibodies occur

Table 1.2 Renal transplant survival in children

Age (years)	Author	Number of transplants performed	% Allograft survival LRT*	% Allograft survival CTD†	Follow up period (months)
<15	EDTA Registry 1983[16]	423	88.9	73.9	12
<5	Rizzoni et al. 1980[7]	31	75	26	24
<6	Arbus et al. 1983[8]	39	—	48	mean 40 months

*LRT: Living related donor transplant
†CDT: Cadaver donor transplant

3

transiently and that transplantation may be carried out successfully in their absence[17]. Glomerulonephritis may recur in the allografted kidney and one series reported a biopsy-proven recurrence rate of 16%[18]. In particular, the dense deposits of Type II mesangiocapillary glomerulonephritis were noted in the basement membranes of up to 88% of kidneys transplanted into patients whose end-stage renal diseases resulted from this form of glomerulonephritis[19]. In only 10% of cases, however, did the recurrent nephritis contribute to graft failure. Transplantation is not contraindicated in any form of glomerulonephritis as the risk of graft loss from recurrent disease is extremely low.

Pyelonephritis and polycystic diseases of the kidneys

Chronic pyelonephritis is another common cause of end-stage renal disease but in the absence of obstruction, recurrent urinary tract infections at this late stage of the disease are unusual. Bilateral nephrectomy prior to transplantation is thus only undertaken when marked hydronephrosis and reflux might result in infection in an immunosuppressed patient. Polycystic kidneys associated with reflux and frequent infection may also require removal. Patients who have undergone bilateral nephrectomy have fewer urinary infections after transplantation than those whose kidneys remain *in situ*[20].

Metabolic diseases

Patients with *diabetes mellitus* in terminal renal failure are increasingly being accepted for long-term dialysis and transplantation, although the proportion of diabetic patients in the transplant programmes of individual countries varies widely. In Finland diabetics comprised 27% of recipients transplanted in 1983 whereas comparable figures for the United Kingdom and the Federal Republic of Germany were 4% and 0% respectively. The known variation in the incidence of diabetic nephropathy cannot fully account for these differences[21]. The peroperative management of diabetic transplant recipients is more complex than that of the non-diabetic, and diabetic recipients have a higher incidence of myocardial infarction, stroke and infection in the post-transplant period[22]. Despite these problems, allograft and particularly patient survival have improved markedly since the mid-1970s (Figure 1.2). In addition there is some evidence that the extrarenal manifestations of diabetes may progress more slowly in transplanted patients than in those treated by dialysis[23].

Transplantation has a more limited role in some of the rarer metabolic causes of end-stage renal disease. The survival of patients who have undergone transplantation for *renal amyloidosis* has improved in recent years[24]. Although the disease may recur in the graft, this is less likely in secondary amyloidosis when the precipitating conditions has become inactive[25]. Renal failure in *oxalosis* results from the deposition of oxalate in the kidney. Transplantation is not generally recommended for such patients as there is a high recurrence rate in the graft, and patient survival is about 50% at one year after transplant and 64% after three years on haemodialysis[14]. Similarly

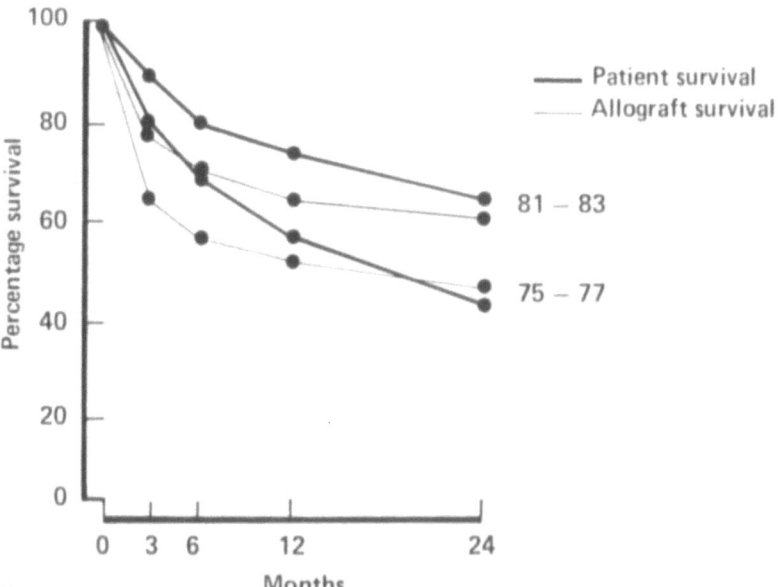

Figure 1.2 Comparison of patient and transplant survival after first cadaver grafts performed between 1974–1977 and 1981–83[3] in diabetic renal allograft recipients

transplantation in *Fabry's disease* is unsuccessful: sepsis occurs frequently and there is no relief of the recurrent pain suffered by these patients[26]. In contrast transplantation is the treatment of choice in children in whom *cystinosis* has caused end-stage renal failure: mortality in this group is less than in children transplanted for other causes of renal failure[27].

Collagen disease

Transplantation may be a useful form of treatment for end-stage renal disease resulting from systemic lupus erythematosis. The risk of recurrence of nephropathy although present[28] is small[29], and the extra renal complications tend to remain quiescent – possibly because of the immunosuppressive therapy[30]. Few patients with *polyarteritis nodosa* or *Wegener's granulomatosis* have undergone transplantation as there is a risk of haemorrhage and of neuropathy occurring in the post-transplant period: cases of successful transplantation have, however, been reported in such patients[31].

ASSESSMENT OF THE POTENTIAL TRANSPLANT RECIPIENT

Patients undergoing chronic dialysis frequently have pathology in organs other than the kidney. If these conditions are likely to progress after transplantation, particularly as a result of immunosuppressive therapy, they should be investigated and treated prior to surgery.

5

Gastrointestinal system

Peptic ulceration occurs in up to 48% of dialysis patients[32] and both gastric acid secretion[33] and plasma gastrin levels[32] are raised. Haemorrhage or perforation may follow transplantation and the reported incidence of upper gastrointestinal haemorrhage in the post-transplant period varies from 1–12%[34,35] with a mortality of up to 65%[36]. In those with a history of ulcer disease there is a 70% incidence of endoscopic abnormality in the post-transplant period, but this figure drops by two-thirds if the ulcer is treated with cimetidine prior to transplantation[37]. Peptic ulcer should therefore be confirmed before transplantation and treated with an H_2 antagonist: surgery should be considered if this therapy fails or if the ulcer recurs. Inflammation and ulceration of the upper gastrointestinal tract occur more commonly in recipients treated with high doses of corticosteroids as part of their immunosuppressive regime[37]. Over the past eight years most centres have reduced post-transplant steroid therapy in line with the original evidence that such a reduction does not affect graft survival adversely[38].

Cardiovascular system

Hypertension occurs commonly in patients with renal failure about to start dialysis, and prevalance rates of 80–100% have been reported[39,40]. In the vast majority, hypertension is due to sodium and water retention and generally responds so well to fluid removal during haemodialysis that drug treatment is not required[40]. In the few patients unresponsive to saline depletion it is suggested[41] that the renin released as a consequence of sodium loss is inappropriately high and that this leads to a rise in blood pressure. Drug treatment or even bilateral nephrectomy may be necessary to control this form of hypertension. However, since the angiotensin I-converting enzyme inhibitors have become available, removal of the patient's own kidneys is less commonly required[42].

Hypertension along with anaemia and fluid overload contribute to the high incidence of left ventricular failure in patients on dialysis. There is also an increase in occlusive arterial disease relative to the normal population. Clinical studies suggest that arteriosclerosis is not accelerated by dialysis[43], however, and this is confirmed by a report[44] showing that the severity of post-mortem vascular changes is unrelated to the length of time on dialysis. Investigation and treatment of both peripheral and cardiovascular diseases may therefore be necessary in the potential transplant recipient, and indeed some have required operative intervention including coronary artery surgery[45].

Bone disease

Metabolic bone disease occurs in patients with chronic renal failure probably as a result of both phosphate retention and failure of production of the vitamin D metabolite, 1,25-dihydroxycholecalciferol, by the diseased kidneys. Renal osteodystrophy is a complex disease entity including, to varying degrees, features of osteitis fibrosa, osteomalacia and osteoporosis. At present the most effective treatment appears to be vitamin D therapy with either 1,25-dihydroxycholecalciferol (calcitriol) or its synthetic analogue, 1α-hydroxycholecalciferol (alfacalcidol), and calcium supplementation. Phosphate binding agents such as aluminium hydroxide have been used to control hyperphosphataemia but aluminium toxicity is now known to cause a severe form of fracturing bone disease[46]. Perhaps the best available treatment at present is oral calcium carbonate (2 g/day) which not only provides supplementary calcium but also binds phosphate in the gastrointestinal tract and helps to buffer the uraemic acidosis.

In some patients hypercalcaemia occurs and, if it persists after cessation of treatment with vitamin D and calcium supplements, parathyroidectomy may be necessary[47]. Total parathyroidectomy with implantation of fragments of the parathyroid glands into muscles of the forearm may be the operation of choice as it permits (1) ready diagnosis of recurrent secondary hyperparathyroidism by measuring parathyroid hormone concentration in blood obtained from a forearm vein, and (2) uncomplicated surgical correction of the condition. It is, however, useful to retain some functioning parathyroid tissue in patients with end-stage renal failure so that normal calcium homeostasis may be restored in the event of a subsequent successful renal transplant secreting both 1,25- and 24,25-dihydroxycholecalciferol. Parathyroidectomy is also considered if there is radiological and bone biopsy evidence of progressive osteitis fibrosa with an elevated plasma parathyroid hormone concentration which is unresponsive to vitamin D therapy[48]. Hyperparathyroidism may also contribute to the bone necrosis seen after transplantation[49] in as many as 20–30% of patients[50,51].

Infection

Infection is one of the principal problems in the immunosuppressed transplant recipient. Foci of infection, particularly those in the respiratory and urinary tract, should therefore be sought and treated prior to transplantation. A search for evidence of active disease is required in those with a previous history of tuberculosis, but screening of uraemic patients by tuberculin testing is unreliable as false negative results frequently occur[52].

Peritoneal fluid from patients on CAPD should be sent for regular bacteriological examination and any catheter exit site infection treated promptly. Sera from all potential transplant recipients should be screened for hepatitis B-associated antigen because of the risk of transmitting serum hepatitis to other patients and to staff.

Cytomegalovirus (CMV) infection is a cause of morbidity after transplantation and may prove fatal. Primary infection in a previously seronegative patient is generally more severe than secondary infection resulting from either reactivation of latent virus or from reinfection[53]. CMV titres can be estimated prior to transplantation and severe CMV infection avoided by transplanting seronegative recipients with kidneys from seronegative donors. Another more practical approach would be to immunize potential transplant recipients with CMV vaccine. One study[54] showed that infection only with the particular vaccine strain was prevented, but that CMV antibody titres

7

increased. The object of a vaccination programme is therefore to obtain a reduction in the incidence of severe primary infection after transplantation[55]. To date such vaccination programmes have not been widely adopted.

PREPARATION OF THE RECIPIENT

As discussed above, the patient's general health should be optimal before transplantation is undertaken. In addition, certain investigations and procedures can be carried out in the period prior to transplantation in an attempt to improve the survival of the allograft.

Bilateral nephrectomy

Ten years ago it was claimed that nephrectomized patients had increased renal allograft survival rates[56]. However, this observation has not been confirmed[57] and apparent benefit may have resulted from the increased number of blood transfusions these patients received while on dialysis.

It was also suggested that bilateral nephrectomy reduced anti-glomerular basement membrane (GBM) antibody levels in patients with anti-GBM glomerulonephritis[58]. A recent review[19], however, indicated that this operation has no effect on such antibody levels and hence is no longer justified.

The main indications at present for pre-transplant bilateral nephrectomy therefore are:

(1) Hypertension resistant to medical therapy;
(2) Reflux nephropathy with frequent urinary tract infections;
(3) Polycystic kidneys which are:
    (a) The source of persistent infection, or
    (b) Too large to permit implantation of a transplanted kidney.

Splenectomy

The effect of splenectomy on renal allograft survival remains controversial. Initial enthusiasm diminished when a large study[59] showed no beneficial effect on transplant outcome and when increased mortality and morbidity from infection were reported[60]. More recently two centres in the USA have shown improved allograft survival without any increased mortality[61,62]. The one-year allograft survival rates of splenectomized patients at these centres were 61% and 65% respectively. Many units achieve similar results without performing splenectomy prior to transplantation, and although this procedure may be helpful in permitting transplantation of leukopenic patients, it is not now generally undertaken.

Blood grouping and tissue typing

Blood is tested for ABO grouping in all patients awaiting transplantation. Organ transplantation follows the rules of blood transfusion with blood group O being the universal donor. If a transplant is performed across a major ABO barrier an aggressive hyperacute or accelerated rejection results[63]. Since Rh antigens are not expressed in the graft[64], matching for this system is not necessary for successful renal transplantation.

Prospective transplant recipients are also typed for the A, B, C and DR antigens coded for by the corresponding gene loci of the HLA system. These genes are co-dominant and two alleles are expressed at each locus: the group of A, B, C and DR alleles inherited from each patient is known as a haplotype. The HLA system is the principal factor in determining acceptance or rejection of foreign tissue and is the human major histocompatibility complex.

Tissue typing in living related transplantation

Transplant survival rates vary directly with the number of haplotypes shared by donor and recipient. Where two haplotypes are shared (an HLA identical transplant) transplant survival is over 90% at one year[65] and where there is no haplotype in common it is around 60%[66]; one haplotype mismatched transplants have survival rates between these two figures. The excellent correlation between the number of haplotypes shared and transplant outcome established beyond doubt that the HLA system is the major histocompatibility complex in man. Prior to living related transplantation, therefore, members of the patient's family wishing to donate a kidney are tissue typed and, in the absence of any other contraindication, an HLA identical sibling is selected as the donor.

Tissue typing in cadaver donor transplantation

Unfortunately the relationship of HLA matching with graft outcome in the larger group of cadaver donor renal transplants is less convincing. Certain large studies have failed to show an overall benefit of HLA-A and B matching on transplant outcome[67] although other groups have demonstrated a slight effect[68]. The evidence for HLA-DR matching is stronger[69] and since there are fewer alleles at this locus a good match is easier to obtain. Centres therefore vary in the emphasis they place on tissue matching when selecting a recipient for a particular cadaver donor. This subject is more fully discussed in Chapter 3.

Blood transfusion

It is generally accepted that blood transfusions given prior to cadaver donor renal transplantation improve graft outcome. There is a risk, however, that the patient will develop antibodies deleterious to a proportion – sometimes over 90% – of potential grafts. This is a particular problem in women who have had previous pregnancies and in patients with a previous failed transplant[70,71]. This topic will be discussed fully in Chapter 4, but at a practical level most units deliberately give all potential transplant recipients between one and five units of blood in the pre-transplant period. Some centres modify their transfusion practices for parous women (F. Hendricks, A. Ting, personal communication) and some give transfusions of donor blood to potential recipients of a one haplotype mismatched living related transplant and have shown improved survival of these grafts[72].

Other immunosuppressive measures

(1) Thymectomy is no longer undertaken as it has no beneficial effect on allograft survival[73].

(2) Depletion of T lymphocytes by drainage of the thoracic duct has been shown to improve transplant outcome[74,75]. Subsequent infection is a major problem, however, and few centres use this form of immunosuppression.

(3) Whole body irradiation is no longer used to prevent transplant rejection because of its toxic effects. Preliminary experience with total lymphoid irradiation[76], similar to that used to treat Hodgkin's disease, has yielded promising results.

IMMEDIATE PRE-TRANSPLANT MANAGEMENT

Most transplant units have a routine protocol which is carried out immediately prior to cadaver donor renal transplant (Table 1.3). Blood from the donor is assayed for the presence of hepatitis B-associated antigens and more recently units have begun to screen potential donors for antibodies to the HTLV III virus. If either of these tests proves positive the kidneys are not used for transplantation.

General physical examinations

It is important to note any intercurrent illness in the potential recipient which might preclude general anaesthesia or surgery. The peritoneal effluent from patients on CAPD should be clear (and subsequently shown to be sterile) and the catheter exit site free from infection. The amount of urine normally passed by the patient is noted as this helps in interpreting the significance of urine output after transplantation.

Table 1.3 Pre-operative management of the renal transplant recipient

(1) General physical examination

(2) Investigations:
  weight
  serum biochemistry
  grouping and crossmatch for 4 units of blood
  chest X-ray
  electrocardiogram
  baseline viral titres
  lymphocytotoxic crossmatch test

(3) Additional measures in patients with diabetes mellitus

(4) Haemodialysis

(5) Initial immunosuppression

Investigations

Certain investigations are required in addition to those normally carried out before a surgical procedure. Base line viral titres, particularly levels of anti-CMV antibody, allow designation of viral illness in the post-transplant period as primary or secondary.

The cytotoxic crossmatch test is performed in all patients prior to transplantation. If recipient serum kills donor lymphocytes in a positive crossmatch test, transplantation is generally contraindicated as hyperacute rejection commonly results[77,78]. This is more likely to occur if a patient has developed antibodies to a high proportion of lymphocyte panel members while on dialysis: those showing over 90% reactivity are known as highly sensitized patients. In recent years two exceptions to this general ruling have emerged:

(1) Non-damaging cytotoxic antibodies have been described which react with the patient's own lymphocytes and characteristically with lymphocytes from 100% of normal panel members. They are therefore seen most often in highly sensitized patients and may be directed against both B and T lymphocytes or against B lymphocytes alone. Several studies report that transplantation may be safely undertaken where a positive crossmatch is caused by such autoantibodies[79,80,81].

(2) Preliminary evidence suggests that graft outcome may not be adversely affected if a positive crossmatch occurs with a serum obtained months or years before transplant and not with the serum obtained on the day of operation[82]. Further evaluation of this phenomenon is required, however, before transplantation under these circumstances can be advocated for all transplant centres.

Additional measures in patients with diabetes mellitus

Diabetic patients in terminal renal failure are frequently treated by CAPD prior to renal transplantation. This is convenient as insulin can be added to the peritoneal dialysate before it is drained into the peritoneum. Blood glucose should be maintained at optimal levels, an estimation made immediately prior to transplantation and the peritoneal catheter sealed before the patient goes to theatre. In diabetic patients treated by CAPD or haemodialysis an intravenous line should be established pre-operatively for the administration of dextrose and insulin.

Haemodialysis

Haemodialysis patients are likely to require an extra treatment pre-operatively if they have not undergone dialysis in the previous 24 hours. This is also necessary if the serum potassium is high or there is evidence of fluid overload. Care should be taken, however, not to cause fluid depletion such that adequate perfusion of the transplanted kidney is jeopardized.

Initial immunosuppression

The final decision to undertake transplantation is made when the crossmatch test is reported as negative and all other investigations indicate that the patient is fit for surgery. The first dose of immunosuppressive therapy is then given and this is usually before the patient leaves for theatre.

IMMUNOSUPPRESSION

Rejection of the allografted kidney is the major problem after renal transplantation. All patients receive routine prophylatic immunosuppressive therapy although the types of drugs used and the treatment regimes vary between transplant units. As all these drugs cause non-specific depression of the recipient's immune system, infection is a major cause of morbidity and mortality in the transplant recipient.

Prednisolone and azathioprine

Prednisolone and azathioprine have been the mainstay of immunosuppressive therapy since this combination of drugs was first used in clinical practice in 1962[83]. Corticosteroids are powerful immunosuppressive drugs although their precise mode of action is unclear. In addition, they have anti-inflammatory effects which may also play a part in the suppression of the imune response[84]. Azathioprine is a derivative of 6-mercaptopurine and acts by inhibiting DNA and RNA synthesis, thus impeding cell proliferation including the lymphocyte response to antigen: antibody production is thus inhibited[85]. Both drugs have troublesome side effects, particularly the corticosteroids (Table 1.4), and the transplant recipient requires careful monitoring.

The many dosage regimes can be divided into two main groups: azathioprine combined with either high or low doses of corticosteroid. In the 'high

Table 1.4 Complications associated with corticosteroid and azathioprine therapy

Corticosteroids	Azathioprine
Growth retardation	Bone marrow depression
Impaired wound healing	Megaloblastic anaemia
Cushingoid appearance	Hepatic dysfunction
Osteoporosis and myopathy	Hair loss
Hirsutism	Effect potentiated by allopurinol
Acne	Malignancy
Cataracts	Increased risk of infection
Diabetes mellitus	
Peptic ulceration	
Hypertension	
Pancreatitis	
Colonic perforation	
Malignancy	
Increased risk of infection	

dose' steroid regimes (Table 1.5) large doses are given initially and then gradually tapered over the first few weeks[86]. Steroid complications are inevitable and in 1977 the Belfast group[38,87] pioneered the use of azathioprine with only 20 mg of prednisolone from the first post-operative day. They achieved a transplant survival rate of 78% at one year for first grafts and a considerable reduction in steroid side effects. A subsequent prospective controlled trial[88] of high and low dose prednisolone therapy showed convincingly that the lower doses were as effective in preventing rejection and markedly reduced both the infective and non-infective complications of corticosteroid therapy. Other groups have now confirmed these observations[89,90]. The dose of azathioprine, however, assumes a greater importance when low dose corticosteroid therapy is given. An Australian study[91] showed that under 60% of kidneys transplanted are functioning at one year if the recipient is given less than 1.75 mg/kg azathioprine per day along with low doses of prednisolone: those given higher doses of azathioprine have one year allograft survival approaching 80%.

In adults, one daily dose of prednisolone is usually given in the morning in an attempt to spare the adrenal pituitary axis[92]. Giving corticosteroids on alternative days has been advocated as the risks of infection[93] and growth retardation in children[94] are less. The effect on subsequent renal function is unclear: some centres have reported no differences in graft loss, renal function or rejection episodes[93] but others have shown a decline in glomerular filtration rate of 20% which is reversed on re-establishing daily prednisolone treatment[95]. Since this has not been evaluated for patients in 'low dose' steroid regimes, once-daily prednisolone has been suggested for adults and alternative day treatment for children with well-functioning transplants[96].

Table 1.5 Immunosuppression with azathioprine and prednisolone

High dose steroid regime[85]		Low dose steroid regime[56]	
Methylprednisolone, then prednisolone	20 mg/kg/day for 3 days 2 mg/kg/day tapering to 0.5 mg/kg/day in the first month	Hydrocortisone Azathioprine Hydrocortisone	200 mg ⎫ immediately prior 5 mg/kg ⎭ to operation 200 mg IV 6-hourly until 18 h after transplant

ALG	20–30 mg/kg/day for 2 weeks after transplant	If no significant function:
		  azathioprine
		  prednisolone
			
			1.5 mg/kg/day
			20 mg/day

Azathioprine	5 mg/kg/day tapering to 2.5 mg/kg/day in the first week	Creatinine clearance >30 ml/min:
		  azathioprine
		  prednisolone
			
			3 mg/kg/day
			20 mg/day
			for 6 months reducing to 10 mg daily is no sign of rejection

Cyclosporin A

Cyclosporin A is a new immunosuppressive drug which is challenging azathioprine and prednisolone as the major prophylactic anti-rejection therapy. It is a fungal derivative first isolated in 1976[97] and exerts its principal action against T helper lymphocytes[98] by preventing the production of T cell growth factors[99]. In turn cytotoxic T cell proliferation is inhibited and an increase in T suppressor cells[100] permitted.

Cyclosporin was first used in clinical trials in 1978[101,102]. Although it was found to be a powerful immunosuppressive drug, nephrotoxicity, a high incidence of infection and the development of lymphomas were noted when it was administered along with other agents. When cyclosporin was used alone as initial therapy a graft survival of 82% at one year was reported[103] although infection remained a problem.

Since then many centres have used cyclosporin and large multicentre trials[104,105] have shown improved allograft survival with cyclosporin when compared with azathioprine and prednisolone. Since nephrotoxicity remained a serious side effect with long-term therapy, a controlled study[106] of short-term (three months) treatment with cyclosporin and subsequent conversion to azathioprine and prednisolone was compared to treatment with azathioprine and prednisolone alone. Transplant outcome was significantly better in the cyclosporin-treated group, although the improvement in survival of first grafts did not achieve statistical significance. The loss of only one graft could be clearly attributed to conversion from cyclosporin A to azathioprine and prednisolone, but rejection episodes occurred after conversion in about 30% of patients: others[107] have confirmed these figures. A lower incidence of rejection has been reported when azathioprine and prednisolone are added as the cyclosporin dose is reduced[108].

Nephrotoxicity has emerged as the principal complication of cyclosporin therapy and this has been noted in recipients of bone marrow[109], liver[110] and heart[111] allografts. In certain cases renal damage was such that recipients of cardiac transplants required dialysis for terminal renal failure. Levels of cyclosporin can be measured in whole blood or plasma, but investigators disagree about the relationship between such levels and either the adequacy of immunosuppression or the toxicity[111,112]. There is however a consensus view that very low or markedly elevated levels are helpful in distinguishing rejection from toxicity in a recipient with a rising creatinine[113]. One group[114] has recently shown that with time there is a gradual increase in cyclosporin blood level with a decrease in clearance and a lengthening of half-life. They suggest that in most patients the same immunosuppressive effect can therefore be achieved by both a reduction in the cyclosporin A dose and a lengthening of the dosage interval during therapy. Long-term nephrotoxic effects may also be dose-related. One study noted progressive pathological changes only in patients receiving high doses of cyclosporin A in the six months immediately following transplantation[115]. Long-term clinical studies are few and necessarily refer to patients given high doses of cyclosporin initially. Calne[116] showed significantly higher creatinine levels after three years of treatment with cyclosporin compared to azathioprine and prednisolone: the mean creatinine of the cyclosporin-treated group was, however, 213 μmol/L, consistent with good clinical graft function.

The dosage of cyclosporin varies between transplant units: in several published studies[103,104,105,106] the initial dose was at least 17 mg/kg/day and this was tapered over several months. There was general agreement, however, at a recent meeting[117] that a maximum of 14 mg/kg/day should be given as a starting dose and this should be reduced to 6–8 mg/kg/day by 6 days and 5–6 mg/kg/day by 180 days after transplantation. As well as nephrotoxicity cyclosporin may cause hepatic damage, gum hyperplasia and hypertrichosis which is particularly distressing to female patients. Cyclosporin is also extremely expensive: maintenance therapy of 5 mg/kg/day costs over £2000 per patient per year compared to around £200 for azathioprine and prednisolone. Short-term cyclosporin A therapy with conversion to conventional therapy at three months may be one way to cut costs and avoid chronic nephrotoxicity. Another approach is to use triple therapy with low doses of cyclosporin along with prednisolone and azathioprine. Preliminary results suggest that nephrotoxicity may be reduced without increased graft loss[118] although some report an increase in infective complications[119].

Anti-lymphocyte globulin

Anti-lymphocyte globulin (ALG) is prepared by immunizing an animal with human lymphoid cells. The IgG fraction of the animal serum is a powerful immunosuppressive agent and acts by decreasing markedly the number of T lymphocytes and preventing their subsequent proliferation by the induction of suppressor cells[120].

ALG is administered intravenously and therapy is started along with azathioprine and prednisolone at the time of transplantation. It is mainly used in the USA and several trials have been performed, some showing a significant benefit[121,122] and others not[123,124]. It is infrequently used in Europe principally because it is expensive and acceptable allograft survival can be achieved with azathioprine and prednisolone or cyclosporin[125].

REJECTION

Rejection is the single most common cause of allograft loss and its diagnosis and management constitute the major clinical problem in the post-transplant period. It results from the host's response to foreign histocompatibility antigens in the donor tissue. Chapter 6 is directed to the discussion of the immunological aspects of rejection.

Clinically, rejection may be divided into three main types:

(1) *Hyperacute rejection:* This form of rejection occurs within hours of transplantation and is mediated by preformed lymphocytotoxic antibodies in the recipient serum directed towards donor histocompatibility antigens. Such antibodies should be detected in the crossmatch test: since this test was described in 1969[77] hyperacute rejection has become a rare event although it can still occur despite a negative

crossmatch[126]. Unfortunately no treatment is effective and the transplanted kidney must be removed. Pathological examination reveals a polymorphonuclear cell infiltrate in glomerular and peritubular capillaries with widespread vascular necrosis and tissue infarction.

(2) *Acute rejection:* Acute rejection episodes occur in almost all recipients of a cadaveric renal transplant. The term may be used for any rejection in the first 3 months or even as late as 5 years in a transplant with stable function[127]. It commonly occurs, however, between 4 and 30 days after operation. Sensitized T lymphocytes attach to the glomerular capillary endothelium and cause swelling, fibrinoid necrosis and thrombosis.

(3) *Chronic rejection:* Often the only clinical feature of this insidious form of rejection, which occurs more than 3 months after transplantation, is a slowly rising serum creatinine. The patient may be hypertensive but fever and graft tenderness are usually absent. Proteinuria may occur and chronic rejection is the commonest cause of post-transplant nephrotic syndrome[128]. Treatment is generally ineffective and the patient returns eventually to dialysis therapy.

The diagnosis of rejection

The diagnosis of rejection may be difficult to establish, particularly as many patients have an initial period of delayed graft function due to acute tubular necrosis. Accurate diagnosis is important in order to prevent unnecessary administration of high doses of corticosteroids or ALG. A slight delay in the treatment of rejection in humans and in animal models does not seem to affect graft outcome adversely[57].

Non-immmunological methods

The classical features of acute rejection are a swollen, tender graft, pyrexia, and a fall in urine output with a rise in blood pressure and weight. The blood urea and serum creatinine concentrations generally rise, although rejection should also be suspected by a reduction in the rate of their decline in a patient whose renal function was previously improving[129]. These clinical features of rejection may be very much less marked in patients on cyclosporin therapy in whom a rising serum creatinine may be due to nephrotoxicity. The clinical diagnosis of rejection is therefore more difficult in these patients.

A decrease in urinary sodium concentration, widely accepted as a feature of acute rejection, is a most unreliable sign but an increase in the enzyme N-acetyl-β-D-glucosaminidase may be of clinical value[130]. Isotope renography is a non-invasive technique which provides information on changes in renal blood flow. It is of value in excluding renal artery thrombosis and ureteric obstruction as causes of anuria[131]. Renal biopsy is helpful in demonstrating the pathological features and the severity of rejection. It has been suggested that the findings on biopsy may indicate whether response to treatment will be effective[132], but it has proved difficult to correlate the severity of the histopathological features with graft outcome: recovery of function may occur despite severe pathological changes of rejection[133]. The appearance of marked interstitial fibrosis, atrophy of nephrons and glomerulosclerosis may suggest that renal damage has been caused by cyclosporin although such changes are also seen in rejecting kidneys[134,135].

Immunological methods

It has long been hoped that monitoring of the patient's immune response in the post-transplant period might result in the early diagnosis of rejection. The development in recipient serum of donor specific lymphocytoxic antibodies[136], the failure of recipient lymphocytes to suppress the mixed lymphocyte response[137] and an increase in cell-mediated lympholysis[138] are all associated with acute rejection. A sample of the cells infiltrating the transplanted kidney can be obtained by fine needle aspiration biopsy with minimal trauma. Characteristic cell patterns[139] and changes in cell populations have been shown to correlate with rejection[140]. As yet, however, these tests have not found a definite role in clinical renal transplantation.

Treatment of rejection

An increase in corticosteroid therapy is the standard method used to treat acute rejection. One gram of methylprednisolone (or 0.5 g) can be given intravenously on three occasions at 12 or 24 h intervals[141]. An increase in oral steroid dosage has also been found effective: 200 mg prednisolone are given for three days followed by a gradual reduction in doses to maintenance levels[57]. ALG has been successfully used to treat rejection in some North American centres[142,143] but the recipient is at risk from viral and fungal infections[144] and the preparations are likely to be of varying efficacy.

In an attempt to find more specific and less toxic means of immunosuppression at the time of rejection, anti-lymphocyte monoclonal antibodies have been studied. Such antibodies have only become available since the advent of hybridoma technology. Cultured lymphocytes from an animal immunized with a given antigen produce specific antibodies but the cells' life span is short. When they are hybridized to myeloma cell lines, however, the malignant cells' property of perpetual replication can be combined with specific antibody production. Monoclonal antibodies have thus been obtained against various populations of T lymphocytes. OKT3 is a pan-T cell antibody which has been used successfully in uncontrolled studies to treat rejection in human kidney transplant recipients[145,146]. Further rejection episodes occurred after treatment, however, and some infective complications were noted along with development of anti-OKT3 antibodies. A recent controlled trial[147] showed that OKT3 reversed acute rejection in 94% of cases whereas conventional steroid therapy was successful in only 75% of cases: subsequent rejection episodes and infectious complications were similar in the two groups. Evaluation of this form of anti-rejection therapy continues. Plasma exchange has been tried in an attempt to reverse rejection episodes but has been unsuccessful[148,149].

MEDICAL ASPECTS OF POST-TRANSPLANT MANAGEMENT

In many transplant units the management of patients at ward level is undertaken by a combined team of surgeons and physicians. The surgeons take care of technical complications after transplantation and this is described elsewhere.

Immediate transplant function occurs in nearly all recipients of a living related graft but in only 50%–60% of those who receive a cadaver donor kidney. Acute tubular necrosis is the most common cause of such early non-function but whether this does[150] or does not[57] harm graft survival in the long term is not clear. As renal function improves, haemoglobin concentration rises with the consequent relief of angina, neuropathy and bone disease improve, and sexual function returns to normal. Pregnancy, rare in patients on dialysis, is possible and over 300 babies born to women with a functioning transplant had been reported to the European Dialysis and Transplant Registry by 1982[3] although the rate of fetal abnormality was higher than in the general population. Rehabilitation is in general excellent with more than 63% of European[151] and more than 80% of British recipients[152] capable of working full time.

Complications

Gastrointestinal system

With the reduction in dosage of corticosteroid given after transplantation the incidence of severe gastrointestinal haemorrhage has declined[32]. Prophylactic therapy with H_2 antagonists has been advocated by some for all transplant recipients[153]: others, however, feel that if low dose prednisolone is used, cimetidine or ranitidine is required only for those patients with a previous history of peptic ulcer[37,154].

Cardiovascular system

Hypertension occurs commonly after renal transplantation. McHugh and colleagues[155] showed that non-nephrectomized subjects who had hypertension while on dialysis were likely to remain hypertensive after transplantation. Others[156], however, have found that those hypertensive prior to transplant have no greater incidence of hypertension in the post-transplant period. Acute rejection is commonly associated with hypertension related to both increased plasma renin activity[157] and fluid retention. Steroid therapy may also result in hypertension although this is less marked in those on low dose prednisolone maintenance therapy[158]. Hypertension in the post-transplant period may respond to fluid restriction and treatment of rejection but drugs such as diuretics, β-blockers and vasodilators may be required. Captopril may be used successfully when hypertension is resistant to all other therapy[159] although very low doses should be given to those with impaired renal function and the white blood cell count should be monitored frequently. Resistant hypertension may arise from disease in the host's native kidneys and nephrectomy[160] or bilateral renal artery embolisation[161] may lead to a significant reduction in blood pressure. A further cause of particularly severe hypertension is stenosis of the transplant renal artery which may present as a sharp decline in renal function on treatment with angiotension I-converting enzyme inhibitors[162]: surgical repair or balloon angioplasty may be necessary.

Cardiovascular complications are the second most common cause of death in patients with a functioning graft. Pre-existing vascular disease, hypertension and lipid abnormalities[43] may contribute to this problem. The risk of these complications increases significantly after the age of 50 years and is particularly high immediately after transplantation[163].

Bone disease

Effective treatment of renal osteodystrophy prior to transplantation should decrease the incidence of disabling bone disease which affects 14% of those with functioning renal allografts[164]. Avascular necrosis occurs particularly in those given high dose prednisolone[87] for the routine prophylaxis of rejection. Recent findings confirm this [165] but show that neither the maximum nor the accumulative dose of steroid was greater in the group of recipients who developed avascular necrosis compared to those who did not. The femoral head is the site most frequently affected and total hip replacement is successful in 94% of cases[164].

Infection

Although infectious complications have decreased markedly since lower doses of corticosteroid have been used for immunosuppression, they still cause death in recipients with functioning transplants. Infection is particularly common in hyperglycaemic transplant recipients[166], those who have undergone splenectomy[167] and in the elderly[15]. Common pathogens cause the majority of infections but overwhelming oppportunistic infections can occur. CMV is the commonest viral infection[168] and may be completely asymptomatic or cause death from pneumonitis. Infections in immunocompromized patients will be fully discussed in Chapter 12. Antibiotics need to be selected with care in renal transplant recipients who may have impaired renal function, and dose adjustment with blood level monitoring may be necessary. In particular certain drugs are known to potentiate the nephrotoxicity of cyclosporin A: these include the aminoglycosides[169] and trimethoprim[170].

Malignant disease

Penn[171] has shown that the recipient of a transplant from a donor who died of cancer may develop the malignancy both in the graft and systemically. Evidence of tumour is thus sought at the time of donor nephrectomy. Cancer may develop *de novo* after transplantation although rates vary from 1.6% in Europe[14] to 24% in Australia[172], the latter being accounted for mainly by skin cancers. Malignant lymphomas are also relatively common in transplant recipients and contribute 30% of non-skin malignancies[173]. Although Calne and colleagues[102] reported a high incidence of lymphoma

19

when cyclosporin A was first used clinically, a subsequent study[174] has reported only 13 cases in 1400 cyclosporin-treated recipients, and only one case in a patient who had received cyclosporin as the sole immunosuppressive agent. Certain other cancers were thought to occur less frequently in transplant recipients[171] but as more data is amassed[172] malignancies of all types appear to occur more frequently in transplant recipients than in the general population.

RESULTS OF RENAL TRANSPLANTATION

Transplant survival is best in recipients of a kidney from a monozygotic twin, and patient survival of these recipients is 94% at 8 years[164]. In general the outcome of transplants from living related donors is better than those from cadavers, although no improvement in transplant survival has been seen in the former group over the past ten years despite the use of donor specific transfusion[3].

Cadaveric graft survival has improved since 1975. European data[3] show that one-year transplant survival of first grafts performed between 1981 and 1983 is 65%, i.e. 10% higher than those carried out between 1975 and 1977: the increase in patient survival during this period is even greater. There has been considerable study of the factors which could account for these improvements: most have been discussed earlier in this chapter but are summarized here:

(1) *HLA matching:* The beneficial effect of HLA-A and B matching on allograft survival is disputed but large studies[67] suggest that it is not marked. Matching for the HLA-DR antigens has a more powerful effect on graft outcome[69] and there is evidence that further improvement can be gained by matching at both HLA-B and DR loci[68].

(2) *Blood transfusions:* It is now generally accepted that blood transfusions given prior to renal transplantation improve graft outcome. In 1982 a large study[67] reported a one-year allograft survival of 43% in untransfused recipients compared to 70% in those given between 5 and 10 units of blood. These results are characteristic of those obtained in most individual transplant centres.

(3) *Immunosuppression:* Recipient mortality decreased and transplant outcome remained unaltered when drug regimes incorporating low doses of corticosteroids were introduced in the late 1970s. More recently, several centres have reported improved transplant survival when cyclosporin A is given either alone or along with corticosteroid therapy. The side effects of this drug, however, especially its nephrotoxicity, require evaluation in the long term.

(4) *Centre effect:* Many countries show differences in graft and patient survival rates between transplant units[175,176,177]. This may reflect differences in selection policies, treatment regimes and possibly clinical experience.

It is encouraging that the overall improvement in results has occurred despite the acceptance for transplantation of more high risk patients. These include older patients, those with multisystem diseases including diabetes and those requiring a second or third transplant.

CONCLUSIONS

Currently the major issues in renal transplantation which will affect future practice include the following:

(1) Transplantation is now indicated for all but a minority of patients accepted for dialysis therapy. The age range of potential recipients has widened and most diseases causing terminal renal failure are considered suitable for treatment by transplantation.

(2) Transplant survival rates have improved since a policy of pre-transplant blood transfusion has been widely practised.

(3) HLA-DR matching consistently correlates with better transplant outcome and is being adopted by more transplant centres.

(4) Patient survival has improved as (a) dialysis and transplantation have become integrated, and (b) the dose of corticosteroid immunosuppressive therapy has been reduced.

(5) As more patients receive second and third transplants the management of patients with high levels of cytotoxic antibodies becomes an important clinical problem.

(6) Cyclosporin A has become established as a major new immunosuppressive agent.

References

1. Pincherle, G. (1979). Kidney transplantation and dialysis. In Rainsbury R. (ed.) *Topics of our Time. Vol. 2: Kidney Transplants and Dialysis*, (HMSO: London)
2. Brunner, F. P., Giesecke, B., Gurland, H. J., Jacobs, C., Parsons, F. M., Scharer, K., Seyfart, G., Spees, G. and Wing, A. J. (1975). Combined report on regular dialysis and transplantation in Europe. V, 1974. In *Proceedings of the European Dialysis and Transplant Association*. Vol. 12, p. 3. (Tunbridge Wells: Pitman Medical Press)
3. Kramer, P., Broyer, M., Brunner, F. P., Brynger, H., Challah, S., Oules, R., Rizzioni, G., Selwood, N. H., Wing, A. J. and Balas, E. A. (1984). Combined report on regular dialysis and transplantation in Europe. XIV, 1983. In *Proceedings of the European Dialysis and Transplant Association*. Vol. 21, p. 5. (London: Pitman Medical Press)
4. Brunner, F. P., Broyer, M., Brynger, A., Challah, S., Fassbinder, W., Oules, R., Rizzioni, G., Selwood, N. H., and Wing, A. J. (1985). Combined report on regular dialysis and transplantation in Europe. XV, 1984. In *Proceedings of the European Dialysis and Transplant Association – European Renal Association*. Vol. 22, p. 3. (London: Baillière Tindall)
5. Scharer, K., Chantler, C., Brunner, F. P., Gurland, H. J. and Wing, A. J. (1974). Combined report on regular dialysis and transplantation of children in Europe, 1973. In *Proceedings of the European Dialysis and Transplant Association*. Vol. 12, p. 65. (Tunbridge Wells: Pitman Medical Press)

6. Rizzoni, G., Broyer, M., Brunner, F. P., Brynger, H., Challah, S., Kramer, P., Oules, R., Selwood, N. H., Wing, A. J. and Balas, E. A. (1984). Combined report on regular dialysis and transplantation of children in Europe. XIII, 1983. In *Proceedings of the European Dialysis and Transplant Association–European Renal Association*. Vol. 21, p. 69. (London: Pitman Medical Press)

7. Rizzoni, G., Molezadeh, M. H., Pennisi, A. J., Ettenger, R. B., Uittenbogaart, C. H. and Fine, R. F. (1980). Renal transplantation in children less than 5 years of age. *Arch. Dis. Child.*, **55**, 532–6

8. Arbus, G. S., Hardy, B. E., Williamson-Balfe, J., Churchill, B. M., Steele, B. T. and Curtis, R. N. (1983). Cadaveric renal transplants in children under 6 years of age. *Kidney Int.*, (Suppl.), 15, S-111-S-115

9. Trompeter, R. S., Haycock, G. B., Bewick, M. and Chantler, C. (1983). Renal transplantation in very young children. *Lancet*, **1**, 373–5

10. Cerilli, C. J., Nelson, C. and Dorfman, L. (1972). Renal transplantation in infants and children with the haemolytic uremic syndrome. *Surgery*, **71**, 61–77

11. Miller, L. C., Bock, G. H., Lum, C. T. and Mauer, S. M. (1982). Transplantation of the adult kidney into the very small child: longterm outcome. *J. Paediatr.*, **100**, 680

12. Merrin, J. J. (1983). Management of children with progressive renal failure. *Ann. Rev. Med.*, **34**, 21–34

13. Griskin, C. M. and Fine, R. N. (1973). Growth in children following renal transplantation. *Am. J. Dis. Child.*, **125**, 514–6

14. Jacobs, C., Broyer, M., Brunner, F. P., Brynger, H., Donckerwolcke, R. A., Kramer, P., Selwood, N. H., Wing, A. J. and Blake, P. H. (1981). Combined report on regular dialysis and transplantation in Europe. XI, 1980. In *Proceedings of the European Dialysis and Transplant Association*. Vol. 18, p. 4. (London: Pitman Books)

15. Ost, L., Groth, C-G., Lindholm, B., Lungren, G., Magnusson, G. and Tillegard, A. (1980). Cadaveric renal transplantation in patients of 60 years and above. *Transplantation*, **30**, 339–40

16. Porter, K. A., Dosseter, J. B., Marchioro, T. L., Peart, W. E., Rendell, J. J. M., Starzl, T. E. and Trasaki, P. I. (1967). Human renal transplants. I Glomerular changes. *Lab. Invest.*, **16**, 153–81

17. Lockwood, C. M. and Peters, D. K. (1980). Plasma exchange in glomerulonephritis and related vasculitides. *Ann. Rev. Med.*, **31**, 167–79

18. Cameron, J. S. (1983). Effect of the recipient's disease on the results of transplantation. *Kidney Int.*, **23**, (Suppl.), 14, S-24-S-33

19. Cameron, J. S. (1982). Glomerulonephritis in renal transplants. *Transplantation*, **34**, 237–45

20. Douglas, J. F., Clarke, S., Kennedy, J., McEvoy, J. and McGeown, M. G. (1974). Late urinary tract infection after renal transplantation. *Lancet*, **2**, 1015

21. Jacobs, C., Brunner, F. P., Brynger, H., Challah, S., Kramer, P., Selwood, N. H. and Wing, D. M. (1981). The first five thousand diabetics treated by dialysis and transplantation in Europe. *Diab. Nephrop.*, **2**, 12–6

22. Friedman, E. A. (1983). Clinical imperatives in diabetic nephropathy, *Kidney Int.*, **23**, (Suppl.), 14, S-16-S-19

23. Ramsay, R. C., Cantrill, H. L., Knobloch, W. H., Goetz, F. C., Sutherland, D. E. R. and Najarian, J. S. (1983). Visual parameters in diabetic patients following renal transplantation. *Diab. Nephrop.*, **2**, 26–9

24. Jones, N. F. (1976). Renal amyloidosis: pathogenesis and therapy. *Clin. Nephrol.*, **6**, 459–64

25. Jacob, E. T. Siegal, B., Bar-Nathan, N. and Gafni, J. (1982). Improved outlook for renal transplantation in amyloid nephropathy. *Transplant. Proc.*, **14**, 41–5

26. Maizel, S. E., Simmons, R. L., Kjellstrand, C. and Fryd, D. S. (1981). Ten year experience in renal transplantation for Fabry's disease. *Transplant. Proc.*, **13**, 57–9

27. Broyer, M., Donckerwolcke, R. A., Brunner, F. P., Selwood, N. H., Wing, A. J. and Blake, P. H. (1981). Combined report on regular dialysis and transplantation of children in Europe, 1980. In *Proceedings of the European Dialysis and Transplant Association*. Vol. 18, p. 60. (London: Pitman Books)

28. Amend, W. J. C., Vincenti, F., Feduska, N. J., Salvatierra, O., Johnston, W. H. and Burnwell, E. L. (1981). Recurrent systemic lupus erythematosis involving renal allografts.

Ann. Inter. Med., **94**, 444–8

29. Advisory Committee to the Renal Transplant Registry (1975). Renal transplantation in congenital and metabolic diseases. A report from the ASC/NIH Renal Transplant Registry. *J. Am. Med. Assoc.*, **232**, 148–53

30. Ziff, M., and Helderman, J. H. (1983). Dialysis and transplantation in end-stage lupus nephritis. *N. Engl. J. Med.*, **308**, 218–9

31. Fauci, A. S., Braun, R., Chazan, J., Steinman, T., Sahyoun, A. I., Monaco, A. P. and Wolff, S. M. (1976). Successful renal transplantation in Wegener's granulomatosis. *Am. J. Med.*, **60**, 437–40

32. Doherty, C. C., O'Connor, F. A., Buchanan, K. D., Sloan, J. M., Douglas, J. F. and McGeown, M. G. (1977). Treatment of peptic ulcer in renal failure. In *Proceedings of the European Dialysis and Transplant Association.* Vol. 14, p. 386. (Tunbridge Wells: Pitman Medical Press)

33. Shepherd, A. M., Stewart, W. K. and Wormsley, K. G. (1973). Peptic ulceration in chronic failure. *Lancet*, **1**, 1357–9

34. Burleson, R. L., Kronhaus, R. J., Marbarger, P. D. and Jones, D. M. (1982). Cimetidine, post-transplant peptic ulcer complications and renal allograft survival. *Arch. Surg.*, **117**, 933–5

35. Hadjiyannakis, E. J., Evans, D. B., Smellie, W. A. B. and Calne, R. Y. (1971). Gastrointestinal complications after renal transplantation. *Lancet*, **2**, 781–5

36. Chisholm, G. D., Mee, A. D., Williams, G., Castro, J. E. and Baron, J. H. (1977). Peptic ulceration, gastric secretion and renal transplantation. *Br. Med. J.*, **1**, 1630–2

37. McWhinnie, D. L., Murray, W. R., Moffat, L. E. F. and Briggs, J. D. (1983). A five year review of upper gastrointestinal endoscopy following renal transplantation. *Br. J. Surg.*, **70**, 301–2

38. McGeown, M. G., Kennedy, J. A., Loughbridge, V. G. G., Douglas, J., Alexander, J. A., Clarke, S. D., McEvoy, J. and Hewitt, J. C. (1977). One hundred kidney transplants in the Belfast City Hospital. *Lancet*, **2**, 648–51

39. Curtis, J. R., Eastwood, J. B., Smith, E. K. M., Storey, J. M., Verroust, P. J., de Wardener, M. E., Wing, A. J. and Wolfson, E. M. (1969). Maintenance haemodialysis. *Q. J. Med.*, **38**, 49–89

40. Schupak, E., Sullivan, J. F. and Lee, D. Y. (1967). Chronic haemodialysis in 'unselected' patients. *Ann. Intern. Med.*, **67**, 708–17

41. Brown, J. J., Dusterdieck, G., Fraser, R., Lever, A. F., Robertson, J. I. S., Tree, M. and Weir, R. J. (1971). Hypertension and chronic renal failure. *Br. Med. Bull.*, **27**, 128–35

42. Briggs, J. D. (1984). The recipient of a renal transplant. In: Morris, P. J. (ed.) *Kidney Transplantation, Principles and Practice*, pp. 59–79. (London: Grune and Stratton)

43. Nicholls, A. J., Catto, G. R. D., Edward, N., Engeset, J. and MacLeod, M. (1980). Accelerated atherosclerosis in long term dialysis and renal transplant recipients: fact or fiction? *Lancet*, **1**, 276–8

44. Vincenti, F., Amend, W. J., Abele, J., Feduska, N. J. and Salvatierra, O. (1980). The role of hypertension in haemodialysis – associated atherosclerosis. *Am. J. Med.*, **68**, 363–9

45. McGeown, M. G. Clinical renal transplantation and immunosuppression. In Salaman, J. R. (ed.) *Immunosuppressive Therapy.* pp. 143–176. (Lancaster: MTP)

46. Cannata, J. B., Briggs, J. D. Junor, B. J. R. and Fell, G. S. (1983). Aluminium hydroxide intake: real risk of aluminium toxicity. *Br. Med. J.*, **286**, 1937–8

47. Catto, G. R. D. and MacLeod, M. (1976). The investigation and treatment of renal bone disease. *Am. J. Med.*, **61**, 64–73

48. de Francisco, A. M., Ellis, H. A., Owen, J. P., Cassidy, M. J. D., Farndon, J. R., Wood, M. K. and Kerr, D. N. S. (1985). Parathyroidectomy in chronic renal failure. *Q. J. Med.*, **55**, 289–315

49. Woo, K. T. Junor, B. J. R., Vikramin, P. and d'Apice, A. J. F. (1979). Serum alkaline phosphatase as predictor of avascular necrosis of bone in renal transplant recipients. *Lancet*, **1**, 620–1

50. Boyle, I. T. (1974). Vitamin D and the kidney. In *Proceedings of the European Dialysis and Transplant Association.* Vol. 12, p. 113 (Tunbridge Wells: Pitman Medical Press)

51. Cruess, R. L., Blennerhassett, J., McDonald, F. R., McLean, L. D. and Dosseter, J. (1968). Aseptic necrosis following renal transplantation. *J. Bone Joint Surg.*, **52A**, 1577–90

23

52. Monaco, A. P., Williams, G. M., Braf, Z., Codish, S. D. (1975). Control of infection in transplantation patients. *Transplant. Proc.*, **7**, 903–6
53. Betts, R. F., Freeman, R. B., Douglas, R. G., Talley, T. E. and Rundell, B. (1975). Transmission of cytomegalovirus infection with renal allograft. *Kidney Int.*, **8**, 385–92
54. Marker, S. C., Simmons, R. L. and Balfour, H. H. (1981). Cytomegalovirus vaccine in renal allograft recipients. *Transplant. Proc.*, **13**, 117–8
55. Winearls, C. G., Lane, D. J. and Kurtz, J. (1984). Infectious complications after renal transplantation. In Morris, P. J. (ed.) *Kidney Transplantation: Principles and Practice*, pp. 427–467. (London: Grune and Stratton)
56. Advisory Committee on the Renal Transplant Registry (1975). Renal transplantation in congenital and metabolic diseases. *J. Am. Med. Assoc.*, **232**, 148–53
57. McGeown, M. (1985). Renal replacement therapy. In Marsh, F. P. (ed.) *Postgraduate Nephrology*. pp. 606–626 (London: William Heinneman)
58. Wilson, C. B. and Dixon, F. J. (1979). Renal injury from immune reactions involving antigens in or of the kidney. In Wilson, C. B., Brenner, B. H., Stein, J. H. (eds.) *Immunologic Mechanisms of Renal Disease*, pp. 35–36 (Edinburgh: Churchill Livingstone)
59. Opelz, G. and Terasaki, P. I. (1973). Effect of splenectomy on human renal transplants. *Transplantation*, **15**, 605–9
60. UK Transplant 1980. *Annual Report* (1979–1980). (Bristol, England)
61. Mozes, M. F., Spigos, D. G., Thomas, P. A., Nishikawa, R. A., Cohen, C. and Jonasson, O. (1983). Antilymphocyte globulin (ALG) and splenectomy or partial splenic embolisation (PSE): evidence for a synergistic beneficial effect on cadaver renal allograft survival. *Transplant. Proc.*, **15**, 613–6
62. Fryd, O. S., Sutherland, D. E. R., Simmons, R. L., Ferguson, R. M., Kjellstrand, C. M. and Najarian, J. S. (1981). Results of a prospective randomised study on the effect of splenectomy vs. no splenectomy in renal transplant patients. *Transplant. Proc.*, **13**, 48–56
63. Sheil, A. G. R., Stewart, J. H., Tiller, D. J. and May, J. (1969). ABO blood group incompatibility in renal transplantation. *Transplantation*, **8**, 299–300
64. Carpenter, C. B. (1979). Immunological monitoring before transplantation. In Morris, P. J. (ed.) *Kidney Transplantation, Principles and Practice*, pp. 127–144 (London: Academic Press)
65. Solheim, B. G., Engebretsen, T. E., Flatmark, A., Jervell, J., Enger, E. and Thorsby, E. (1977). The influence of HLA-A, -B, -C and -D matching on kidney graft survival. *Scand. J. Urol. Nephrol.* (Suppl.), **42**, 28–31
66. Simmons, R. L., van Hook, E. J., Yunis, E. J., Noreen, H., Kjellstrand, C. M., Condie, R. M., Mauer, S. M., Baselmeier, T. and Najarian, J. S. (1977). 100 sibling transplants followed for 2 to $7\frac{1}{2}$ years. A multi-factorial analysis. *Ann. Surg.*, **185**, 196–204
67. Opelz, G. and Terasaki, P. I. (1982). International study of histocompatibility in renal transplantation. *Transplantation*, **33**, 87–95
68. Opelz, G. (1985). Effect of HLA matching blood transfusions and presensitisation in cyclosporine-treated kidney transplant recipients. *Transplant. Proc.*, **17**, 2179–83
69. Ting, A. and Morris, P. J. (1980). Powerful effects of HLA-DR matching on survival of cadaveric renal allografts. *Lancet*, **2**, 282–5
70. Opelz, G., Graver, B., Mickey, M. R. and Terasaki, P. I. (1982). Lymphocytotoxic antibody responses to transfusions in potential kidney transplant recipients. *Transplantation*, **32**, 177–83
71. Ting, A. (1984). HLA and renal transplantation. In Morris, P. J. (ed.) *Kidney Transplantation: Principles and Practice*, pp. 159–180. (London: Grune and Stratton)
72. Hillis, A. N., Sells, R. A., Bone, J. M., Evans, C. M., Duguid, J., Roberts, F., Evans, P., Kenton, P. and Barnes, R. M. R. (1985). A prospective clinical trial of cyclosporine and donor-specific transfusion versus donor-specific transfusion alone in living related allograft recipients. *Transplant. Proc.*, **17**, 1242–3
73. Starzl, T. E., Parker, K. A., Andres, G., Grath, C. G., Putman, C. W., Penn, I., Halgrimson, C. G., Starkie, S. J. and Brettschneider, L. (1970). Thymectomy and renal homo-transplantation. *Clin. Exp. Immunol.*, **6**, 803–14
74. Starzl, T. E., Iwatsuk, S., Klintmalm, G., Schrorer, G. P. J., Koep, L. J., Iwaki, Y., Terasaki, P. I. amd Porter, M. D. (1984). The use of cyclosporin A and prednisolone in cadaver kidney transplantation. *Surg. Gynec. Obstet.*, **151**, 17–26

75. Touraine, J. L., Malik, M. C. and Traeger, J. (1981). Anti-lymphocyte globulin and thoracic duct drainage in renal transplantation. In Salaman, J. (ed.) *Immunosuppressive Therapy*, pp. 55–73. (Lancaster: MTP)
76. Sampson, D., Levin, B. S., Hoppe, R. T., Bieber, C. P., Miller, E., Waer, M., Kaplan, H. S., Collins, G. and Strober, S. (1985). Preliminary observations on the use of total lymphoid irradiation, rabbit antithymocyte globulin and low dose prednisolone in human cadaver renal transplantation. *Transplant. Proc.*, **17**, 1299–303
77. Kissmeyer-Nielsen, F., Olsen, S., Peterson, V. P. and Fjeldberg, O. (1966). Hyperacute rejection of kidney allografts associated with pre-existing humoral antibodies against donor cells. *Lancet*, **2**, 648–51
78. Mario, P. J., Williams, G. M., Hume, D. M., Mickey, M. R. and Terasaki, P. I. (1968). Serotyping for homotransplantation XII. Occurrence of cytotoxic antibodies following kidney transplantation in man. *Transplantation*, **6**, 392–9
79. Cross, D. E., Greiner, R. and Whittier, F. C. (1976). Importance of autocontrol crossmatch in human renal transplantation. *Transplantation*, **21**, 307–10
80. Ettenger, R. B., Jordan, S. C. and Fine, R. N. (1983). Cadaver renal transplant outcome in recipients with autolymphocytotoxic antibodies. *Transplantation*, **35**, 429–31
81. Ting, A. (1983). The lymphocytotoxic cross-match test in clinical renal transplantation. *Transplantation*, **35**, 403–7
82. Cardella, C. J., Falk, J. A., Halloran, P. F., Robinette, M. A., Arbus, G. S. and Bear, R. A. (1985). Risk factors in renal transplant recipients with a positive cross-match on non-current sera. *Transplant. Proc.*, **17**, 2446–8
83. Murray, J. E., Merrill, J. P., Damin, G. J., Dealy, J. B., Alexandre, G. W. and Harrison, J. H. (1962). Kidney transplantation in modified recipients. *Ann. Surg.*, **156**, 337–55
84. Wood, R. F. M. (1983). *Renal Transplantation – A Clinical Handbook*, p. 98. (Eastbourne: Bailliére Tindall)
85. Bach, J. F. (1975). *The Mode of Action of Immunosuppressive Agents*, Chap. 3. (Oxford: North Holland)
86. Simmons, R. L., Matas, A. J., Rattazi, C. C., Balfour, H. H., Havard, R. J. and Najarian, J. S. (1977). Clinical characteristics of the lethal cytomegalovirus infection following renal transplantation. *Surgery*, **82**, 537–46
87. McGeown, M. G., Douglas, J. F., Brown, W. A., Donaldson, R. A., Kennedy, J. A., Loughridge, W. G., Mehta, S., Nelson, S. D., Doherty, C. C., Johnstone, R., Todd, G. and Hill, C. M. (1980). Advantages of low dose steroid from the day after renal transplantation. *Transplantation*, **29**, 287–9
88. Morris, P. J., Chan, L., French, M. E. and Ting, A. (1982). Low dose oral prednisolone in renal transplantation. *Lancet*, **1**, 525–7
89. Glass, N. R., Miller, D. T., Sollinger, H. W. and Belzer, F. O. (1983). A comparative study of steroids and heterologous antiserum in the treatment of renal allograft rejection. *Transplant. Proc.*, **15**, 617–21
90. Salaman, J. R., Griffin, P. J. A. and Price, K. (1983). High or low dose steroids for immunosuppression. *Transplant. Proc.*, **15**, 1086
91. D'Apice, A. J. F., Becker, G. J., Kincaid-Smith, P., Mathew, T. H., Ng, J., Hardie, I. R., Petrie, J. J. B., Rigby, R. J., Dauborn, J., Heale, W. F. and Miach, P. J. (1984). A prospective randomised controlled trial of low dose versus high dose steroids in cadaveric renal transplantation. *Transplantation*, **37**, 373–7
92. Grant, S. D., Forsham, P. H. and Di Raimondo, V. C. (1965). Suppression of 17-hydroxycorticosteroids in plasma and urine by single and divided doses of triamciolone. *N. Engl. J. Med.*, **273**, 1115–8
93. Dumler, F., Levin, N. W., Szego, G., Vulpetti, A. T. and Preuss, L. E. (1982). Longterm alternate day steroid therapy in renal transplantation. *Transplantation*, **34**, 78–82
94. Soyka, L. F. and Saxena, K. M. (1965). Alternate-day steroid therapy for nephrotic children. *J. Am. Med. Assoc.*, **192**, 225–30
95. Breitenfield, R. V., Hebert, L. A., Lemann, J., Piering, W. F., Kauffman, H. M., Sampson, D., Kalbfleisch, J. and Beres, J. A. (1980). Stability of renal transplant function with alternate day corticosteroid therapy. *J. Am. Med. Ass.*, **244**, 151–9
96. D'Apice, A. J. F. (1984). Non-specific immunosuppression: azathioprine and steroids. In Morris, P. J. (ed.) *Kidney Transplantation – Principles and Practice*, pp. 239–259. (London: Grune and Stratton)

97. Borel, J. F., Feurer, C., Magnee, C. and Stahelin, H. (1976). Effects of new anti-lymphocytic peptide cyclosporin A in animals. *Immunology*, **32**, 1017–25
98. Borel, J. F. (1981). Cyclosporin A – present experimental status. *Transplant. Proc.*, **13**, 344–8
99. Larsson, E-L. (1980). Cyclosporin A and dexamethasome suppress T cell responses by selectively acting at distinct sites of the triggering process. *J. Immunol.*, **124**, 2828–33
100. Leapman, S.B., Filo, R. S., Smith, E. J. and Smith, P. G. (1981). Differential effects of cyclosporin A on lymphocyte subpopulations. *Transplant. Proc.*, **13**, 405–9
101. Calne, R. Y., White, D. J. G., Thiru, S., Evans, D. B., McMaster, P., Dunn, D. C., Craddock, G. N., Pentlaw, B. D. and Rolles, K. (1978). Cyclosporin A in patients receiving renal allografts from cadaver donors. *Lancet*, **2**, 1323–7
102. Calne, R. Y., Rolles, K., White, D. J. G., Thiru, S., Evans, G. N., Henderson, R. G., Azziz, S. and Lewis, P. (1979). Cyclosporin A initially as the only immunosuppressant in 34 recipients of cadaveric organs: 32 kidneys, 2 pancreases and 2 livers. *Lancet*, **2**, 1033–6
103. Calne, R. Y. and White, D. J. (1982). The use of cyclosporin A in clinical organ grafting. *Ann. Surg.*, **196**, 330–7
104. European Multicentre Trial Group (1983). Cyclosporin in cadaveric renal transplantation: one year follow up of a multicentre trial. *Lancet*, **2**, 986–9
105. The Canadian Multicentre Transplant Study Group (1983). A randomised clinical trial of cyclosporine in cadaveric renal transplantation. *N. Engl. J. Med.*, **309**, 809–15
106. Chapman, J. R. and Morris, P. J. (1985). Cyclosporine nephrotoxicity and the consequences of conversion of azathioprine. *Transplant. Proc.*, **17**, (Suppl.) 4, 254–60
107. Carpenter, C. B., Milford, E. L., Strom, T. B., Lazarus, J. M. and Tilney, N. L. (1985). Stability of renal allograft recipients after conversion from cyclosporine to azathioprine. *Transplant. Proc.*, **17**, (Suppl.), 4, 261–5
108. Lorber, M. I., Flechner, S. M., Van Buren, C. T., Kerman, R. H. and Kahan, B. D. (1985). Cyclosporine, azathioprine and prednisolone as treatment for cyclosporine-induced nephrotoxicity on renal transplant recipients. *Transplant. Proc.*, **17**, (Suppl.) 1, 282–5
109. Yee, G. C., Kennedy, M. S., Deeg, H. J., Leonard, T. M., Thomas, E. D. and Storb, R. (1985). Cyclosporine-associated renal dysfunction in marrow transplant recipients. *Transplant. Proc.*, **17**, (Suppl.), 1, 196–201
110. Iwatsuki, S., Esquivel, C. O., Klintmalm, G. B. G., Shaw, G. B. W. and Starzl, T. E. (1985). Nephrotoxicity of cyclosporine in liver transplantation. *Transplant. Proc.*, **17**, (Suppl.), 1, 191–5
111. Myers, B. D., Ross, J., Newton, L., Leutscher, L., Perlroth, M. (1984). Cyclosporine-associated chronic nephropathy. *N. Engl. J. Med.*, **311**, 699–705
112. Keown, P. A., Stiller, C. B. and Ulan, R. A. (1981). Immunological and pharmacological monitoring in the clinical use of cyclosporin A. *Lancet*, **1**, 686–9
113. Kahan, B. D. (1985). Discussion IV. Diagnosis, incidence and severity of cyclosporine nephrotoxicity. *Transplant. Proc.*, **17**, (Suppl.) 1, 261–5
114. Henny, F. C., Kleinbloesem, C. H., Moolenaar, A. J., Paul, L. C., Breimer, D. D. and Van Es, L. A. (1985). Pharmacokinetics and nephrotoxicity of cyclosporine in renal transplant recipients. *Transplantation*, **40**, 261–5
115. Klintmalm, G., Bohman, S. O., Sundelin, B. and Wilczek, H. (1984). Interstitial fibrosis in renal allografts after 12–46 months of cyclosporin treatment: beneficial effect of low doses in early post-transplantation period. *Lancet*, **2**, 950–4
116. Calne, R. Y. and Wood, A. J. (1985). Cyclosporin in cadaveric renal transplantation: 3 year follow-up of a European Multicentre Trial. *Lancet*, **2**, 549
117. Kahan, B. D. (1985). Clinical summation. An algorithm for the management of patients with cyclosporine-induced renal dysfunction. *Transplant. Proc.*, **17**, (Suppl.), 1, 303–8
118. Canafax, D. M., Sutherland, D. E. R., Simmons, R. L., Fryd, O. S., Ascher, N. L., Payne, W. D., and Najarian, J. S. (1985). Combination immunosuppression: three drugs for mismatched related and four drugs for cadaver allograft recipients. *Transplant. Proc.*, **17**, 2671–2
119. Salaman, J. R. and Griffin, P. J. A. (1985). Immunosuppression with a combination of cyclosporine azathioprine and prednisolone may be unsafe. *Lancet*, **2**, 1066–7
120. Thomas, J. M., Carver, F. M., Haisch, C. E., Fahrenbruch, G., Deepe, R. M. and Thomas, F. T. (1982). Suppressor cells in rhesus monkeys treated with antilymphocyte globulin. *Transplantation*, **34**, 83–9

121. Sheil, A. G. R., Kelly, G. E., Storey, B. G., May, J., Kalowski, S., Mears, D., Rogers, J. H., Johnson, J. R., Charlesworth, J. and Stewart, J. H. (1971). Controlled clinical trial of antilymphocyte globulin in patients with renal allograft from cadaver donors. *Lancet*, **1**, 359–63

122. Kreis, H., Mansouri, R., Descamps, J., Sandavino, R., N'Guyen, A. T., Bach, J. F. and Crosnier, J. (1981). Antilymphocyte globulin in cadaver kidney transplantation: randomised trial based on T-cell monitoring. *Kidney Int.*, **19**, 438–44

123. Wechter, W. J., Brodie, J. A., Morrell, R. M., Rafi, M. and Schultz, J. R. (1979). Antithymocyte globulin (ATGAM) in renal allograft recipients. Multicenter trials using a 14-dose regimen. *Transplantation*, **28**, 294–302

124. Bell, P. R. F., Blamey, R. W., Briggs, J. D., Castro, J. E., Hamilton, D. N. H., Knapp, M. S., Salaman, J. R., Sells, R. A., Williams, G., Gowans, J. L., Peto, R., Richards, S., Phillips, A. W., Weinberg, A. L. and Freestone, D. S. (1983). Medical Research Council trial of antilymphocyte globulin in renal transplantation. *Transplantation*, **35**, 539–44

125. Calne, R. Y. (1981). Twenty years experience of immunosuppression in organ transplantation. *Transplant. Proc.*, **14**, 91–7

126. Morris, P. J., Mickey, M. R., Singal, D. P. and Terasaki, P. I. (1969). Serotyping for homotransplantation XXII. Specificity of cytotoxic antibodies developing after renal transplantation. *Br. Med. J.*, **1**, 758–9

127. Bosch, G. J., Galvanek, E. G. and Renaldo, E. S. (1971). Human renal allografts. Analyses of lesions in long-term survivors. *Human Pathol.*, **2**, 253–98

128. Cheigh, J-S., Stenzel, K. H., Susin, M., Rubin, A. L., Riggio, R. R. and Whitsell, J. S. (1974). Kidney transplant nephrotic syndrome. *Am. J. Med.*, **57**, 730–40

129. Knapp, M. S., Blamey, R., Cove-Smith, R. and Heath, M. (1977). Monitoring of the function of renal transplants. *Lancet*, **2**, 1183

130. Whiting, P. H., Nicholls, A. J., Catto, G. R. D., Edward, N. and Engeset, J. (1980). Patterns of N-acetyl-D-glucosaminidase excretion after renal transplantation. *Clin. Chim. Acta*, **108**, 1–7

131. Hilson, A. J. W., Maisey, M. N., Brown, C. B., Ogg, C. S. and Bewick, M. S. (1978). Dynamic renal transplant imaging with Tc-99m DTPA (Sn) supplemented by a transplant perfusion index in the management of renal transplants. *J. Nucl. Med.*, **19**, 994–1000

132. Finkelstein, F. O., Siegel, N. J., Bastl, C., Forrest, J. N. and Kashgarian, M. (1976). Kidney transplant biopsies in the diagnosis and management of acute rejection reactions. *Kidney Int.*, **10**, 171–8

133. Morris, P. J. (1979). Renal transplantation. In Black, D. A. K., Jones, N. E. (eds.) *Renal Disease*, pp. 549–587 (London: Blackwell Scientific Publications)

134. Bohman, S.-O., Klintmalm, G., Ringden, O., Sundelin, B. and Wilczek, H. (1985). Interstitial fibrosis in human kidney grafts after 12 to 46 months of cyclosporine therapy. *Transplant. Proc.*, **17**, 1168–71

135. Morris, P. J., French, M. E., Dunnill, M. S., Hunnisett, A. G. W., Ting, A., Thomson, J. F. and Ward, R. F. M. (1983). A controlled trial of cyclosporin in renal transplantation with conversion to azathioprine and prednisolone after three months. *Transplantation*, **36**, 273–7

136. Stiller, C. R., Sinclair, N. R. StC., Abrahams, S., McGirr, D., Singh, H., Havson, W. T. and Ulan, R. A. Anti-donor immune responses in the prediction of transplant rejection. *New Engl. J. Med.*, **294**, 978–82

137. Charpentier, B., Bach, M. A., Lang, P. L., Martin, B. and Fries, D. (1983). Isolation and characterisation of specific suppressor cells in tolerant human kidney transplant recipients. *Transplant. Proc.*, **15**, 719–23

138. Goulmy, E., Persijn, G., Blokland, E., D'Amaro, J. and Van Rood, J. J. (1981). Cell-mediated lympholysis studies in renal allograft recipients. *Transplantation*, **31**, 210–7

139. Hayry, P., von Willebrand, E., Ahonen, J., Eklund, B. and Lautenschlarger, I. (1981). Monitoring of organ allograft rejection by transplant aspiration cytology. *Ann. Clin. Res.*, **13**, 264–87

140. Wood, R. F. M., Bolton, E. M., Thomson, J. F., Morris, P. J. and Mason, D. Y. (1983). Characterisation of cellular infiltrates in renal allografts by fine needle aspiration – a simple technique using double labelling with monoclonal antibodies. *Transplant. Proc.*, **15**, 1847–8

141. Bell, P. R. F., Calman, K. C., Wood, R. F., Briggs, J. D., Paton, A. M., McPherson, S. G. and Kyle, K. (1971). Reversal of acute clinical and experimental organ rejection using large doses of intravenous prednisolone. *Lancet*, **1**, 876–7

142. Hoitsma, A. J., Reekers, P., Kroeftenberg, J. G., Van Lier, H. J. J., Capel, P. J. and Koene, R. A. P. (1982). Treatment of acute rejection of cadaveric renal allografts with rabbit antithymocyte globulin. *Transplantation*, **33**, 12–6

143. Simonian, S. J., Lyons, P., Chivala, R., Swartz, C., Onesti, G., Jelalian, C., Moriber-Katz, S. and Bulova, S. (1983). Reversal of acute cadaveric renal allograft rejection with added ATG treatment. *Transplant. Proc.*, **15**, 604–7

144. Cosimi, A. B. (1983). The clinical usefulness of antilymphocyte antibodies. *Transplant. Proc.*, **15**, 583–9

145. Cosimi, A. B., Burton, R. C., Colvin, R. B., Goldstein, G., Delmonico, F. L., LaQuaglia, M. P., Tolkoff-Rubin, N., Rubin, R. H., Herrin, J. T. and Russell, P. S. (1981). Treatment of acute renal allograft rejection with OKT3 monoclonal antibody. *Transplantation*, **32**, 535–9

146. Norman, D. J., Barry, J. M., Hennell, K., Funnel, M. B., Goldstein, G. and Bohannon, L. (1985). Reversal of acute allograft rejection with monoclonal antibody. *Transplant. Proc.*, **17**, 39–41

147. Kreis, H. and Goldstein, G. (1985). Monoclonal antibodies for the treatment of acute rejection episodes in renal transplantation. *Transplant. Proc.*, **17**, 2751–3

148. Cardella, C. J., Sutton, D. M. C., Katz, A., Uldall, P. R., Harding, M. and deVebar, G. A. (1980). A controlled trial evaluating intensive plasma exchange in renal transplant recipients. In *Proceedings of the European Dialysis and Transplant Association*. Vol. 17, p. 429. (London: Pitman Medical)

149. Power, D. A., Nicholls, A. J., Muirhead, N., MacLeod, A. M., Engeset, J., Catto, G. R. D. and Edward, N. (1981). Plasma exchange in acute renal allograft rejection: is a controlled trial really necessary? *Transplantation*, **32**, 162–3

150. Davison, J. M., Uldall, P. R. and Taylor, R. M. (1977). Relation of immediate post-transplant renal function to long term function in cadaver kidney recipients. *Transplantation*, **23**, 310–5

151. Brunner, F. P., Brynger, H., Chantler, C., Donckerwolke, R. A., Hathaway, R. A., Jacobs, C., Selwood, N. H. and Wing, A. J. (1979). Combined report on regular dialysis and transplantation in Europe. IX, 1978. In *Proceedings of the European Dialysis and Transplant Association*. Vol. 16, p. 2. (London: Pitman Medical)

152. Wing, A. J., Brunner, F. P., Brynger, H., Chantler, C., Donckerwolke, R. A., Jacobs, C., Kramer, P., Selwood, N. H. (1980). European Dialysis and Transplant Association Analyses. *UK Transplant Service, Annual Report* (1980). (Bristol, UK)

153. van Roermund, H. P. C., Tiggeler, R. G. W. L., Berden, J. H.M., van Lier, H. J. J. and Koene, R. A. P. (1982). Cimetidine prophylaxis after renal transplantation. *Clin. Nephrol.*, **18**, 39–42

154. Doherty, C. C. and McGeown, M. G. (1978). Cimetidine and renal-allograft rejection. *Lancet*, **1**, 1048

155. McHugh, M. I., Tanboga, H., Marcen, R., Liano, F., Robson, V. and Wilkinson, R. (1980). Hypertension following renal transplantation. The role of the host's kidneys. *Q. J. Med.*, **196**, 395–403

156. Bachy, C., Alexandre, G. P. J. and van Ypersele de Strihou, C. (1976). Hypertension after renal transplantation. *Br. Med. J.*, **2**, 1287–9

157. Popovtzer, M. M., Pinnggera, W., Katz, F. H., Corman, J. L., Robinette, J., Lanois, B., Halgrinson, C. C. and Starzl, T. E. (1973). Variations in arterial blood pressure after kidney transplantation. *Circulation*, **47**, 1297–305

158. Morris, P. J., Chan, L., French, M. E. and Oliver, D. O. (1982). Low dose and oral prednisolone in renal transplantation. *Lancet*, **1**, 525–7

159. Raine, A. E. G. and Ledingham, J. G. G. (1982). Clinical experience with captopril in the treatment of severe drug-resistant hypertension. *Am. J. Cardiol.*, **49**, 1475–9

160. Curtis, J. J., Lucas, B. A., Kotchen, T. A. and Luke, R. G. (1981). Surgical therapy for persistent hypertension after renal transplantation. *Transplantation*, **31**, 125–8

161. Thompson, J. F., Fletcher, E. W. L., Chalmers, D. H. K., Wood, R. F. M. and Morris, P. J. (1983). Bilateral renal embolisation for the control of hypertension in transplant patients. *Br. J. Surg.*, **60**, 681–2

162. Curtis, J. J., Luke, R. G., Whelchel, J. D., Diethelm, A. G., Jones, P. and Dunstan, H. P. (1983). Inhibition of angiotension-converting enzyme in renal transplant recipients with hypertension. *N. Engl. J. Med.*, **308**, 377–81

163. Nicholls, A. J., Cumming, A. M., Catto, G. R. D., Edward, N. and Engeset, J. (1981). Lipid relationships in dialysis and renal transplant recipients. *Q. Med. J.*, **50**, 149–60

164. Brynger, H., Brunner, F. P., Chantler, C., Donckerwolcke, R. A., Hathaway, R. A., Jacobs, C., Kramer, P., Selwood, N. H. and Wing, A. J. (1980). Combined report on regular dialysis and transplantation in Europe. X, 1979. In *Proceedings of the European Dialysis and Transplant Association*. Vol. 17, p. 2. (London: Pitman Medical)

165. Farge, D., Parfrey, P. S., St Andre, C., Kus, Y.-L. and Guttman, R. D. (1985). Aseptic necrosis following renal transplantation – a 25 year experience. *Transplant. Proc.*, **17**, 1947–50

166. Anderson, R. J., Schafer, L. A., Olin, D. B. and Eickoff, T. C. (1973). Infectious risk factors in the immunosuppressed host. *Am. J. Med.*, **54**, 453–60

167. McEnery, P. T. and Flannagan, J. (1977). Fulminant sepsis in splenectomized children with renal allografts. *Transplantation*, **24**, 154–5

168. Merigan, T. C. and Stevens, D. A. (1971). Viral infections in man associated with acquired immunological deficiency states. *Fed. Proc.*, **30**, 1858–64

169. Whiting, P. H., Thomson, A. W., Blair, J. T. and Simpson, J. G. (1982). The toxic effects of combined administration of cyclosporin A and gentamicin. *Br. J. Exp. Pathol.*, **63**, 554–61

170. Thomson, J. F., Chalmers, D. H. K., Hunniseth, A. G. W., Wood, R. F. M. and Morris, P. J. (1983). Nephrotoxicity of trimethoprin and cotrimoxazole in renal allograft recipients treated with cyclosporine. *Transplantation*, **36**, 204–6

171. Penn, I. (1977). Developments of cancer as a complication of clinical transplantation. *Transplant. Proc.*, **9**, 1121–7

172. Sheil, A. G. R., Mahoney, J. F., Horvarth, J. S., Johnson, J. R., Tiller, D. J., Stewart, J. S. and May, J. (1981). Cancer following successful cadaveric donor renal transplantation. *Transplant. Proc.*, **13**, 733–5

173. Sheil, A. G. R. (1984). Cancer in dialysis and transplant patients. In Morris, P. J. (ed.) *Kidney Transplantation: Principles and Practice*, p. 491. (London: Grune and Stratton)

174. Beveridge, T. (1983). Cyclosporin A: an evaluation of clinical results. *Transplant. Proc.*, **15**, 433–7

175. Cicciarelli, J., Mickey, M. R. and Terasaki, P. I. (1985). Center effects and kidney transplantation. *Transplant. Proc.*, **17**, 2803–7

176. UK Transplant (1980) *Annual Report.* (Bristol, England)

177. Sirchia, S., Mercuriali, M., Scalamogna, M., Pizzi, C., Poli, F., Vabecchi, M. G., Morabito, A. and Marubini, G. Factors influencing the cadaver kidney transplant program of North Italy. *Transplant. Proc.*, **17**, 2259–64

2
Surgical Aspects of Renal Transplantation

J. ENGESET AND G. G. YOUNGSON

INTRODUCTION

The surgical technique of kidney transplantation was fully established more than 30 years ago. The subsequent success of transplantation was hindered by inadequacies in both the understanding of the immune process and the therapeutic armamentarium. Only transplants performed between identical twins were initially successful. Most of the honour for the progress in kidney transplantation, with more than 50 000 kidney transplants having been performed around the world, must therefore go to those who have increased our knowledge of tissue typing, immunology and immunosuppression.

The breakthrough for transplantation came in the early 1960s with the introduction of an immunosuppressive regime which allowed transplantation of unrelated kidneys with a success rate of about 50%. These results were sufficiently good to stimulate demand for the treatment of an increasing number of patients with end-stage renal failure. The introduction and acceptance of the concept of brain death, partly stimulated by the need for kidneys for transplantation, was a significant step towards increasing facilities for patients requiring organ transplants for survival. The recent introduction of the new immunosuppressive agent, cyclosporin, to most transplant units has further improved allograft survival rates, with the result that the indications for kidney transplantation have gradually widened to include younger children as well as patients in the seventh and even eighth decades of their lives. The success of kidney transplantation has been a stimulus to the donation of organs but the demand from an enlarging pool of patients more than outstrips the supply.

The surgical aspects of renal transplantation include problems related to kidney harvest from either a living or a cadaver donor, preparation and storage of the kidney and the transplant operation itself. It also involves those post-operative complications which require surgical correction. These aspects will all be dealt with in this chapter with the exception of kidney preservation which will be considered in detail in Chapter 7.

KIDNEY SUPPLY AND DEMAND

A basic requirement for any kidney transplant programme is the availability of donor kidneys for transplantation. Such kidneys can only come from living donors, usually living related donors, or from cadaver donors. Living related donor kidneys, particularly from tissue type identical siblings and twins, have in the past been associated with significantly better long-term results than cadaver transplants. Pre-operative blood transfusions and cyclosporin have more recently improved both patient and graft survival in cadaver kidney transplants to such an extent that the benefit of transplantation with living donor kidneys no longer alone justifies the slight risk in terms of mortality and morbidity to the donor. However, in view of the current inadequate supply of cadaver kidneys, the use of a living related donor is justified when such a willing related donor exists. The question of using non-related living donors is much more vexing. This procedure is not favoured in Britain but it is practised in some other countries where cadaver kidneys are not readily available for religious or cultural reasons.

The aim of most dialysis and transplant units is to treat patients with end-stage renal failure by a renal replacement programme which restores the patient to as normal a life as possible. For most if not all of these patients, this will ultimately require a kidney transplant. Unfortunately the number of kidneys available is insufficient to allow all new patients as well as those with failed grafts to be transplanted. In Europe in 1984 only 22 823 of the total 101 832 people alive on renal replacement therapy had a functioning kidney graft–i.e. less than 25%. In other words approximately 80 000 people in Europe are alive on one or other form of dialysis. In the UK approximately 50% of the patients alive on renal replacement therapy have a functioning kidney graft while in Norway the figure is 70%. The reasons for these differences from country to country are complex and will not be discussed further here.

The aim in our own centre in Aberdeen is to offer a transplant to every patient on our treatment list. The patients themselves make the final decision when a kidney becomes available but only rarely refuse a transplant. It is our policy to offer transplantation to all the new patients taken on to the programme, and in addition to offer kidneys to the established and often sensitized patients as suitable kidneys are found.

As we accept just over 40 new patients per million population annually to our programme we require at least that number of kidneys. In many European countries the number of new patients has been steadily increasing and has now reached more than 60 new patients per million population, and there is evidence that the same trend is taking place in the UK (Table 2.1). The aim now must be to transplant at least 40 patients per million population yearly. Table 2.2 shows this transplantation rate was reached by the

Table 2.1 New patients per million population accepted for renal replacement therapy in some European countries

Country	1982	1983	1984
Belgium	39.6	61.0	67.8
Sweden	41.3	61.4	51.2
Norway	37.3	54.1	56.6
Denmark	26.9	40.4	39.0
FRG	44.0	55.8	62.1
France	30.9	44.3	46.7
Switzerland	44.5	55.1	66.4
Netherlands	27.4	45.7	49.7
UK	19.9	33.4	35.9

From EDTA Report XV, 1984

Scandinavian countries in 1984 although not by other European countries. For the UK with a population of approximately 60 million people this would mean 2400 kidney transplants annually, and it is immediately clear that the demand for kidneys far outstrips the availability. The number of cadaver donors has slowly increased in Britain and resulted in approximately 1500 cadaver transplants in 1984.

No accurate knowledge of the potential number of donors is available, but in Aberdeen prior to starting the transplant programme in 1975, a survey was made which indicated that around 20 patients dying in hospital annually (40 such patients per million population) were medically suitable for kidney donation. Table 2.3 shows that we have never obtained more than two thirds of this number. There is still inadequate support for organ donation among some of our medical colleagues and the general public. Table 2.3 also shows clearly the influence of adverse publicity on organ donation. On the 13th October 1980 the BBC televized an unfortunate programme on brain death which led to an increase in refusals for organ donation. For about six months thereafter, permission for organ donation in the Grampian Region was repeatedly refused by the next of kin.

The Aberdeen Transplant Unit serves the dialysis units in the Grampian

Table 2.2 The total transplantation rate in patients per million population (PMP) and the number and percentage of cadaver donors and living donors in the four most actively transplanting countries in Europe and the UK

Country	PMP	Cadaver donors		Living donors	
		No.	%age	No.	%age
Sweden	41.1	274	80.4	67	19.6
Denmark	38.4	189	96.4	7	3.6
Norway	38.1	100	64.1	56	35.9
Switzerland	30.9	195	98.5	3	1.5
UK	28.3	1445	90.8	147	9.2

From EDTA Report XV, 1984

Table 2.3 Kidneys harvested in Aberdeen/
Inverness, 1975–1985

Year	Number of kidneys
1975	10
1976	16
1977	16
1978	18
1979	28
1980	24*
1981	14
1982	25
1983	22
1983	22
1984	22
1985	26

*All before 13th October 1980

and Highland regions of Scotland with a total population of around 700 000 or one ninetieth of the population of UK and Ireland. The average population served by each transplant unit in the UK is around 2 million people. If units in the rest of the country obtained the same number of cadaver kidneys per million population, more than 2000 kidneys would be available compared to the maximum of 1654 obtained in 1984. The establishment of an increased number of small transplant units would perhaps help the supply of cadaver kidneys.

Good publicity is obviously an important factor in changing society's attitude to organ donation and careless or bad publicity certainly does untold damage. The effect of the BBC television programme is still detectable in Aberdeen where we are still refused permission for organ donation more often than we were in the early 1980s. The medical profession and the health service should make a greater effort in engaging the media in an informed way to draw attention to the good results from kidney transplantation and to the discrepancy between kidneys required and available.

Other ways of improving organ supply may be learned from the Scandinavian practice (Table 2.2). Norway and to a lesser extent Sweden performed a large number of living donor transplants while Denmark performed almost entirely cadaver transplants. Why does Denmark have more cadaver kidneys available than other countries? In Denmark kidneys from patients dying from myocardial infarction after failed resuscitation have been used. It may therefore be that Denmark is able to use kidneys from a pool of potential donors unavailable in other countries. It is notable that Denmark also has as many as five transplant units for a population of approximately 5 million people.

In summary, the prospects for increasing cadaver organ donation may depend upon:

(1) Favourable publicity,
(2) Avoidance of bad publicity,

(3)   Increased awareness by clinicians in charge of potential donors,

(4)   Establishment of more transplant units, and

(5)   Identification of alternative pools of donors.

THE CADAVER DONOR

A cadaver donor in the UK is a patient who has been diagnosed as suffering irreversible cessation of brain stem function and whose relations have given permission for the organ donation. The specific cause of coma must be diagnosed e.g. cerebral haemorrhage. Permission is also required from the Coroner or, in Scotland, the Procurator Fiscal, in cases which would ordinarily be reported to him because of the circumstances of the patient's death[1].

Brain death is diagnosed by the consultant clinicians, often neurosurgeons, neurologists or anaesthetists, looking after such patients. The patient is ventilator-dependent, with fixed dilated pupils, and must not be under the influence of any drugs. The diagnosis should not be made for at least 6 hours after the onset of coma and should be confirmed by a second set of tests 12–24 hours later. Time of death is recorded as the time of the second confirmatory test and only at this stage is the transplant team contacted. Permission for organ donation may then be obtained from the next of kin and, when necessary, the Coroner or Procurator Fiscal.

In some countries such as Norway, brain death is always confirmed by the cessation of intracranial circulation as detected by cerebral angiography when organs are to be used for transplantation purposes. In other countries such as Sweden, organs can only be removed after death has been diagnosed by the irreversible cessation of respiration and heartbeat.

Who are potential donors?

Potential donors are patients who die from irreversible brain damage. There are no strict age limits for kidney donation but it is unusual in the UK to accept donors over 65 years of age. In the UK about 30% such patients die from spontaneous intracranial haemorrhage or occasionally cerebral infarction. Most of the remaining donors, 60% to 70%, are patients who have sustained head injuries resulting from road traffic or other accidents. Occasionally patients suffering brain death as a result of intracranial tumours or self-administered drug overdose are suitable donors. Patients with myocardial infarcts are rarely if ever used in the UK but may in the future represent a significant source of donor kidneys.

Assessment of potential donors

The initial assessment of a potential donor patient is made by the clinicians responsible for the care of that patient. When a patient is a suitable organ donor, contact is made with the transplant team. The patient is at this stage invariably receiving ventilatory support and often a dopamine infusion to maintain near normal blood pressure and renal perfusion. The urine output is frequently high due to diabetes insipidus. The renal function indicated by blood urea and creatinine levels should be normal. If these are elevated the patient might have previous renal impairment and be unsuitable for kidney donation. However, such increases might represent acute tubular dysfunction as a consequence of the disease or injury suffered by the donor, in which case the transplanted kidney might have a period of diminished function but ultimately work satisfactorily. In an ideal situation with enough kidneys for all, such kidneys would be discarded. If use of such a kidney is decided upon, the cold ischaemia time should be as short as possible and preferably less than 10 hours. An abnormally high blood pressure on the potential donor's admission could similarly be a consequence of the patient's injuries, but could also indicate previous hypertension and renal disease which would preclude kidney donation. The patient's previous medical history and consultation with the general practitioner might help to clarify the situation.

Patient's with significant infections, and with any malignancies except for primary intracranial malignancies, are not suitable as organ donors. Potential donors are usually in an intensive care unit where regular bacteriological examinations of tracheal aspirate, urine and other body fluids are made. Significant growth of bacteria in any specimen is undesirable but not an absolute contraindication to donation. When a patient is considered to be a suitable potential donor, the hepatitis antigen (HBsAg) and the human T cell lymphotrophic virus type III (HTLV-III) tests must be negative.

Permission for donation

Permission for organ donation in the UK must be obtained from the person lawfully in possession of the body[1]. A person designated by the relevant health authority is normally in possession of the body in a National Health Service Hospital until such time as the body is claimed by the person with a right to possession of it. This person is either the next of kin, the Coroner or Procurator Fiscal, or the executor. In practice permission has to be obtained from the next of kin whenever a next of kin can be traced. When death results from an accident involving other people or as a result of drug overdosage, permission must be obtained from the Coroner or Procurator Fiscal. Only when none of these people claim possession of the body is permission granted by the person designated by the health service.

When a potential donor carries an organ donor card or has otherwise recorded his wishes there is no legal requirement to establish lack of objection on the part of relatives, but it is common practice to seek their consent. If they object, it is probably wise to accept their views and not proceed to organ donation.

The person most suited to ask for permission is often the consultant in charge of the potential donor's case, namely the neurosurgeon. He or she has usually established good contact with the relatives and it seems appropriate that permission is sought at the time of informing them that the patient is brain dead. This is the standard practice in our unit. On occasion the relatives may seek an interview with a member of the transplant team.

In other centres it is the duty of a member of the transplant team to seek permission. It is usual that the relatives sign a form of no objection, but their lack of objection in writing is not mandatory.

Care of the donor

Any treatment or investigation carried out on a patient prior to death must be for his or her benefit and not solely to preserve the kidneys or other organs for transplantation. It is permissible though to remove blood for tissue typing at the same time as blood is taken for routine management of the patient. The appropriate care of the patient prior to death is also the best care for organs for transplantation. The care is administered by the treating surgeons or physicians until brain death is declared. Then the transplant team take over the patient management and the subsequent treatment is aimed at ensuring the best possible care of the organs to be used for transplantation.

It is not uncommon that the relatives enquire what is to happen after brain death is diagnosed and indeed sit with the body until it is removed to the operating theatre. A gentle explanation of subsequent management and of donor procedure should be offered.

Donor nephrectomy

The technique of donor nephrectomy to be used depends on the prevailing conditions. When carried out after cardiac arrest and cessation of circulation, a fast nephrectomy is performed removing each kidney separately through a midline abdominal incision. When the kidneys are removed from a brain dead patient, an en-block removal of both kidneys is usually performed. This is the method most commonly used in our unit and it will be described in detail later. Occasionally the donor is a multiple organ donor and in that situation the heart is removed first. Perfusion of the liver through the aorta with exsanguination through a caval catheter is then carried out, with the result that both kidneys are also perfused *in situ* with cold electrolyte solution. The liver and the kidneys are well mobilized prior to the perfusion. The liver is removed and the kidneys thereafter.

En-block nephrectomy from a brain dead donor is the most common procedure in the UK. The donor is taken to the operating theatre and prepared like any other surgical patient. An anaesthetist should be present to look after the patient's cardio-respiratory state to ensure that the kidneys are in the best possible condition. Some relaxation is required as there is invariably reflex spasm of the abdominal musculature. Continued support may be required during the operation.

The surgical team should consist of the surgeon and two assistants in addition to the scrub nurse and a floor nurse. The abdomen is washed with 0.5% chlorhexidine in 70% spirit or a similar antiseptic solution from the lower chest to the top of the thighs and towelled for a midline incision from xiphisternum to pubis. A transverse incision is preferred by some but we find the full length midline incision to give good and rapid access.

37

A full inspection is made of the abdominal contents. Occasionally conditions such as ruptured bowel as a consequence of trauma sustained by the patient or malignancies preclude the use of the kidneys for transplantation. Congenital abnormalities such as horseshoe kidney, pelvic kidney or even hydronephrotic or pyelonephritic kidneys may also be found, making them unsuitable for use. In cases of doubt a renal biopsy may be performed.

Exposure of the kidneys is begun by division of the peritoneal reflection from the caecum up, lateral to the ascending colon to the hepatic flexure. The base of the small bowel mesentery medially is also divided from the ileocaecal area, over the iliac vessels and the aorta, with the result that the ascending colon and small bowel with its mesentery are detached from the retroperitoneal tissues. The duodenum is also freed by dividing the ligament of Treitz and mobilising the 4th and 3rd parts towards the right. The 2nd part of the duodenum and lateral aspect of the 3rd part along with the head of the pancreas are mobilized and retracted medially. The small bowel with its mesentery and the larger bowel are retracted upwards out of the wound. As a result of this manoeuvre the right kidney is exposed from the front with its vein and ureter, as are the vena cava, the left renal vein medially and the aorta.

The left kidney may be freed in a similar way by dividing the peritoneal reflection lateral to the sigmoid and descending colon and mobilizing the colon medially, but it is more commonly our practice to divide the inferior mesenteric vein and artery and to mobilize the peritoneum overlying the kidney in a lateral direction to expose the left kidney and ureter. Superiorly the pancreas and the duodenum are mobilized forwards to expose the superior mesenteric artery for a distance of about 2 cm from its origin. This is securely ligated and divided, facilitating exposure of the aorta proximally. The kidneys may now both be mobilized by entering the perirenal fat capsule and freeing the kidneys laterally, superiorly and posteriorly so that they are only attached by their arteries, veins and ureters. The ureters are freed with their periureteric tissues well down into the pelvis. Tapes can now be applied around the vena cava above the entry of the renal veins. On the left side it is usually necessary to ligate and divide a large suprarenal vein near its termination into the left renal vein and the gonadal vein. The mobilization of the aorta at this level is helped by dividing for a short distance the crura of the diaphragm. Care must be taken not to damage high renal polar arteries which are not infrequently found. A tape is applied around the aorta.

The aorta and vena cava are divided between Satinsky clamps applied distal to all renal vessels. The proximal Satinsky clamps are used as retractors to pull the aorta and cava gently forwards exposing their posterior branches which are then divided between haemoclips. The aorta and vena cava can thus be completely mobilized up to the proximal tapes with the circulation to the kidneys still intact. Prior to clamping the aorta and cava proximally, the donor is given 10 000 units of heparin intravenously and if there is no urine flow 25 g of mannitol as a 20% solution are given. Two straight vascular clamps are applied to the aorta and a Satinsky clamp to the vena cava above the renal vessels. This is the time we record for circulatory and ventilatory arrest. The kidneys are removed after division of the aorta and the cava and both ureters low in the pelvis. Immediately both are placed into a kidney dish containing ice-cold isotonic saline or Ringer lactate, and removed to a sterile work surface for immediate perfusion with hypertonic citrate solution at approximately 4 °C. The aorta is opened longitudinally posteriorly and an infant feeding catheter of appropriate size for the renal arteries is inserted into the renal artery ostia. The kidneys are then perfused until they are uniformly pale and cold, with clear perfusion fluid coming out of the renal veins. The kidneys are thereafter prepared by excising excess fat and freeing the renal vessels sufficiently for the transplant operation. We believe that this should always be done by the harvesting centre. Only after proper dissection can the kidneys be fully assessed. A segment of the aortic and caval wall should remain attached to the renal vessels so that patches may be fashioned whenever required for the transplant operation. The kidneys which are to be used in the harvesting centre may be kept partially covered by hypertonic citrate solution in a stainless steel container which is stored in ice or in a fridge. Kidneys which are to be exported to other centres are packed in two sterile plastic bowel bags. The plastic bags containing the kidneys are placed into a third bag surrounded by ice at 0 °C and packed in an insulated cardboard box ready for dispatch to another transplant centre. It is important not to use ice cubes freshly removed out of a deep freeze compartment as these may be so cold that the kidney becomes deep frozen and damaged.

While the kidneys are being perfused and prepared, the assistant removes the spleen and lymph glands for tissue typing purposes. The lymph nodes are most easily found in the distal small bowel mesentery. The donor's wound is then closed.

THE LIVING DONOR

The results from cadaver kidney transplantation are now such that there is little justification for the use of living donors. The benefit to the recipient may no longer outweigh the risk to the donor[2]. Unfortunately the inadequate supply of cadaver kidneys forces us to accept living related donors when the donor and the recipient express this desire. The use of non-related donors is common practice in some countries where kidneys may even be bought from non-related donors. The Transplantation Society has expressed itself firmly against this practice and contemplates expulsion of members who undertake such operations[3].

Although the risk to the donor's life is small some recent long-term follow-up studies of donors have found an incidence of hypertension in 35% of all donors. These results, although not fully confirmed, are worrying and it ought to be the aim of every transplant centre to strive to increase their supply of cadaver kidneys, ultimately abolishing the need to use living donors. In our own centre only 2 out of 167 (1.2%) were living donor transplants, giving us a living donor rate approximately the same as Denmark's (3.6%) and Switzerland's (1.5%) (see Table 2.2).

Assessment of donor

The prospective donor must be in perfect health both physically and mentally. The donor must be strongly motivated towards the donation and aware of the slight risk to life and health. The following are essential investigations for the assessment:

(1) History and examination including urinalysis,
(2) Haematological screening,
(3) Biochemical screening,
(4) Bacteriological examination of urine,
(5) Blood grouping and tissue typing,
(6) Electrocardiogram,
(7) Bilateral isotope renogram,
(8) Chest X-ray, IVP and renal arteriogram.

Any abnormality in this assessment of the donor should be regarded as an absolute contraindication to donation. With the recent suggestion that more than one third of donors may subsequently develop hypertension, a blood pressure at the upper limit of normal or a family history of hypertension should be strong arguments against donation. The presence of any detectable renal abnormality would be a contraindication to donation, but kidneys with more than one renal artery may occasionally be used. The results are best when the living donor is tissue type identical and it has been our practice only to accept haplotype identical siblings as living donors. Potential donors with responsibility for young children should rarely be accepted.

Donor nephrectomy

Either kidney may be used for the donor nephrectomy. If one of the kidneys has a double vascular supply or any other minor congenital abnormality the contralateral kidney is used. When both kidneys are entirely normal the left kidney is chosen for the transplant.

The donor should be well hydrated before and during the operation[4]. The fluid balance should be carefully monitored by having a central venous pressure line in place and it is important to maintain a diuresis during the procedure. The patient is positioned in the half-lateral position over the 'kidney bridge' near the side of the table where the operator stands. Sand bags, strapping or the Vac-Pac bag (Howmedica) can be used to secure the position. It is prudent to give the donor venous thromboembolism prophylaxis in the form of 5000 units of heparin subcutaneously twice daily postoperatively and graded compression stocking support to both legs during the operation and in the early post-operative period.

The technique of donor nephrectomy varies a little from centre to centre and the following description is just one way of performing the operation. The incision used is a long incision starting from the lateral border of the sacro-spinal muscle just below the 12th rib, carried downwards and forwards parallel to the 12th rib, curving in a mild S shape down into the upper part of the iliac fossa, 2–3 cm medial to the anterior superior iliac spine. The latissimus dorsi muscle at the back and the posterior vertical fibres of the external oblique are divided and as the lateral part of the iliac fossa is entered the external oblique is divided in the direction of its fibres. At a deeper level, the internal oblique and the lower edge of the serratus posterior inferior are cut across. The transversus abdominis is seen in the floor of the wound arising from the lumbar fascia with the subcostal nerves and vessels on its surface. The lumbar fascia which is continuous with the aponeurosis of transversus is incised or split in front of the lateral border of quadratus lumborum and the division is carried into the transversus. Three fingers are usually inserted into the extraperitoneal space to separate transversus from the peritoneum prior to its division. The peritoneum is now exposed in front and the perirenal fat capsule posteriorly.

The operating table may now be flexed further and a self-retaining retractor used to increase the exposure. The renal fascia is incised along the convex surface of the kidney and the kidney surface identified. The peritoneum and retroperitoneal fat is gently pushed away from the kidney using finger and scissor dissection to expose the ureter with its periureteric tissue which is followed down into the pelvis. The renal vein is followed medially to the vena cava and on the left side it is necessary to ligate the suprarenal vein and the gonadal vein with 2.0 neurolon ligature. The upper pole of the kidney is often adherent, but there is a plane between the kidney capsule and the suprarenal gland which is best opened up by scissor dissection. The posterior aspect of the kidney is easily freed and thereafter the kidney is gently turned forwards and the renal artery is freed posteriorly to its origin from the aorta. During the whole procedure extreme care must be exercised not to damage the blood supply to the renal pelvis and the ureter by unnecessary dissection in the renal hilum. If during the dissection the kidney becomes soft and cyanosed, it should be returned to its normal position and rested until the vascular spasm has disappeared.

The kidney should now be attached only by its vascular pedicle and ureter and be ready for removal. The ureter is divided low in the pelvis and the distal end ligated. A diuresis should be evident. It is common practice to stimulate diuresis by giving 25 g of mannitol as 20% solution or frusemide at this stage and also 5000 i.u. of heparin prior to clamping the vessels. When the left kidney is removed it is desirable to remove as much of the renal artery as possible and a Satinsky clamp applied to the wall of the aorta assures maximum length of renal artery. When the right kidney is used the renal vein is short and maximum length is obtained by applying the clamp to the side wall of the cava. The left renal vein and the right renal artery are both long and there is no difficulty in leaving enough vessel cuff to obtain secure clamping and closure. As the donor vessels are healthy and soft a 5.0 Prolene suture on a 16 mm needle is usually adequate for closure of the aorta and cava.

After the vessels are divided, the kidney is immediately removed to a container with ice-cold electrolyte solution and flushed out with hyperosmolar citrate solution or Collins solution and stored in an appropriate container until the recipient is ready for the implantation operation. The wound is closed in layers with absorbable suture such as monofilament PDS vicryl or dexon after haemostasis is secure without drains.

41

In the post-operative period the most significant risk to the donor is venous embolism. The few donors who have died as a direct result of the operation have succumbed as a result of pulmonary embolism. The main emphasis in the post-operative period should therefore be to reduce the risk of this complication. Subcutaneous heparin given in a dose of 5000 units twice daily, the wearing of graded compression stockings and early mobilization should be routine. Physiotherapy to prevent chest complications in the form of ateteclasis and pneumonia is also important. Pneumothorax is a potential hazard when the 12th rib is removed. Wound and urinary tract infections may occur, and in the long term the donors should be checked for development of hypertension. In view of the possible risk of hypertension long-term surveillance of the donors is recommended.

RECIPIENT OPERATION

Patients taken on to renal replacement programmes now include young children as well as elderly patients often with concomitant disease. These include patients with diabetes, severe atherosclerosis with myocardial ischaemia, peripheral vascular disease, long-standing hypertension and even minor strokes. The surgical challenge is therefore greater than in the past. These patients require utmost surgical care because poor wound healing results from their anaemia. They are also susceptibie to infection because of both their inherent immunosuppressed state secondary to their renal failure and the additional immunosuppressive drugs they require post-operatively. Haemostasis may also be impaired because of pre-operative haemodialysis. Meticulous attention to surgical technique and pre- and post-operative care is essential.

Anaesthesia

The complexity of the anaesthesia required by patients receiving a transplant is beyond the scope of this chapter and the reader is referred to specialized anaesthetic tests[5]. Suffice to say that the anaesthetist requires an understanding of the pathophysiology and biochemistry of uraemia and its effect on the pharmocokinetics and the metabolism of the drugs used.

Pre-operative preparation

Treatment of patients on renal replacement therapy is a combined effort by physicians and surgeons and in most centres it is the physicians who make the initial choice of a patient for a transplant (see Chapter 1). They also assess the patient's fitness for surgery and ensure that he is free from infection and biochemically fit for surgery. When the patient is on haemodialysis and has not dialysed in the 24 hours prior to surgery, pre-operative haemodialysis is likely to be required. When the crossmatch has been reported negative the initial immunosuppression, in most centres cyclosporin A, and steroid is given before the patient is sent to the operating theatre.

Once the patient is anaesthetized by general endotracheal anaesthesia a urinary self-retaining catheter is always introduced under careful antiseptic technique. It is the practice in some units to instil about 150 mL of antiseptic solution such as acroflavine into the bladder and to spigot the catheter. This has an antibacterial action which may help to reduce infection and also has the effect of distending the bladder. The strong yellow colour also facilitates identification of the bladder mucosa during ureteric implantation. The pubic area and the lower abdomen are shaved in theatre and the skin prepared with 0.5% chlorhexidine in 70% spirit or a similar solution. The patient is towelled for operation in either the right or left iliac fossa: a steridrape is useful to fix the towels to the skin around the operative field.

Choice of operative site

The kidney may be implanted in either iliac fossa and the choice is dependent on a number of factors. If the patient has had a previous transplant on one side it is usual to choose the other. When multiple previous transplants have been performed it is usual to chose the side with only one previous operation. The presence of previous surgery for other reasons in either iliac fossa is an indication for choosing the opposite side.

When operating on young people with healthy arteries it is common to use the internal iliac artery for the arterial anastomosis. As the internal iliac artery is medial to the external iliac vein which is almost invariably used for the venous anastomosis, the kidney will fit better anatomically when it is inserted in the side opposite to its origin. Similarly as the external iliac artery is lateral to the external iliac vein the kidney is inserted on the same side when these vessels are used. These are by no means absolute rules but simple guidelines. A kidney can usually be inserted without much difficulty into either iliac fossa using the common iliac, external iliac or internal iliac artery for the arterial anastomosis and the common or external iliac vein for the venous anastomosis.

Incision

An oblique skin incision is used running from the midline anteriorly about 1 cm above the pubic symphysis to a point 2–3 cm superior to the anterior superior spine. The external oblique aponeurosis and muscle is incised in the direction of its fibres; the internal oblique and transversus abdominus are divided by diathermy, care being taken not to enter the peritoneal cavity. This is best done by entering the extraperitoneal space just lateral to the rectus abdominis muscle with scissors and thereafter gently freeing the peritoneum from the transversalis fascia and transversus abdominis with two fingers prior to cutting the muscle with diathermy. Previous operations may have made the peritoneum very adherent and inadvertent entry through the peritoneum occurs frequently. The defects in the peritoneum are usually repaired when the extraperitoneal approach to the iliac vessels is complete. Occasionally the rectus abdominis muscle is very wide and it is appropriate to enter the extraperitoneal space through the linea semilunaris.

The inferior epigastric vessels are ligated and divided as is the round ligament in female patients. The testicular vessels and the vas deferens are usually freed and secured but may be divided particularly in older men when this seems appropriate for the purposes of access. The bladder is identified and gently cleared of surface adipose tissue. It is our practice at this stage to insert two stay sutures in the dome of the bladder on each side of the planned ureteric implantation site prior to preparing the recipient vessels.

Arterial dissection

The peritoneum and its content are retracted upwards and medially using deep retractors. Wound packs soaked in acroflavine solution are used in some units partly as wound towels to protect the skin edges and partly as packs to aid retraction.

The loose areolar tissue in front of the iliac vessels contains an abundance of lymph vessels and it is wise to ligate this tissue prior to dividing it in order to prevent post-operative lymphocoele formation. The external iliac, the internal iliac and the distal part of the common iliac arteries are all freed. The internal iliac is freed down to its division into anterior and posterior divisions, when it is proposed to use these for anastomosis of multiple renal arteries. There are occasional small branches from the back of the common iliac bifurcation which require ligation. Careless dissection may cause troublesome bleeding. When the internal iliac artery and its branches are used for the arterial anastomosis it is advisable to use transfixion 3.0 neurolon or Prolene to secure the distal end of the divided artery.

Venous dissection

The external iliac vein descends in the iliac fossa medial to the external iliac artery. It is easily freed from the lymphatic-rich loose areolar tissue around it. The lymph vessels should be secured by ligature or coagulation before division. Sometimes it is more appropriate to make use of the common iliac vein for the anastomosis particularly in children and small adult patients. On the right side this runs down postero-laterally to the common iliac artery but on the left side it runs down postero-medially. Dividing the internal iliac veins significantly helps mobilization of the common iliac and external iliac vein. This allows a more satisfactory anastomosis and positioning of the kidney particularly when the renal vein is short. The divided internal iliac vein is best secured with a continuous 5-0 Prolene suture rather than simple transfixion ligation.

TRANSPLANTATION OF THE KIDNEY

This part of the transplant operation is the same whether the kidney comes from a living or cadaver donor. When the preparatory dissection is complete in the recipient, the kidney is removed from its cold storage and brought to the operating field in a kidney dish filled with ice-cold saline. The best position for the kidney in the recipient is determined and the renal vessels fashioned accordingly. If a patch of aorta and/or vena cava is to be used for the anastomosis this is now prepared. When a patch is not required the vessels are cut to correct length. The kidney is thereafter wrapped in a gauze swab and is regularly soaked with ice-cold saline to keep it cool during the implantation period.

Most surgeons including ourselves perform the venous anastomosis first[6]. Some surgeons prefer to start with the arterial anastomosis and claim that this is easier[7]. There is also disagreement as to whether systemic heparin is required. We empirically use 5000 units of heparin given intravenously prior to clamping of the vessels in patients with a haemoglobin of more than 9 g per 100 mL.

Venous anastomosis

It is our practice to cross-clamp the iliac vessels with Fogarty clamps with rubber inserts. The venous anastomosis is commonly made to the front of the external iliac vein, but in small patients when we prefer to put the kidney in the right iliac fossa we usually make the anastomosis laterally in the common iliac vein. A narrow ellipse of vein 2–3 cm long is removed. When the kidney has two major renal veins on a caval patch the venotomy may need to be longer. 5-0 Prolene sutures on 16 mm needles are used for the continuous anastomosis. On completion of the anastomosis a clamp such as a Blalock clamp is applied across the renal vein to prevent blood entering the kidney retrogradely when removing the clamps from the iliac veins. Bleeding despite heparinization is usually minimal.

Arterial anastomosis

The preferred anastomosis in a young patient receiving a kidney with one renal artery is an end to end anastomosis between the divided internal iliac artery and the renal artery. The clamped and divided internal iliac artery is carefully distended and the divided end of the artery is trimmed of excess adventitia. When this artery is used in older patients it is common to have to perform a limited endarterectomy up to its origin. Three everting 5-0 Prolene sutures 120° apart are used to approximate the renal artery and the internal iliac (Figure 2.1). These stitches must be carefully placed such as not to twist the artery when the kidney is in position in the iliac fossa. To complete the anastomosis the suture line may be rotated by pulling on the appropriate stay sutures and either interrupted or continuous sutures may be used. In children interrupted sutures should always be used to allow growth in the diameter of the anastomosis with increasing size of the child.

Kidneys are now frequently harvested with an aortic patch whether they have single or multiple arteries. A single artery patch is usually approximately 20 mm long but when the kidney has two or more arteries the patch may be twice this length. Occasionally when the arteries are far apart two patches may be used.

The patch is anastomosed to either the external iliac (Figure 2.2) or the common iliac artery depending on length of the patch, size of the recipient and status of recipient arteries. In children the common iliac or even the aorta may be the most appropriate site for the arterial anastomosis. In older patients with extensive atheroma which is usually maximal at the origin of

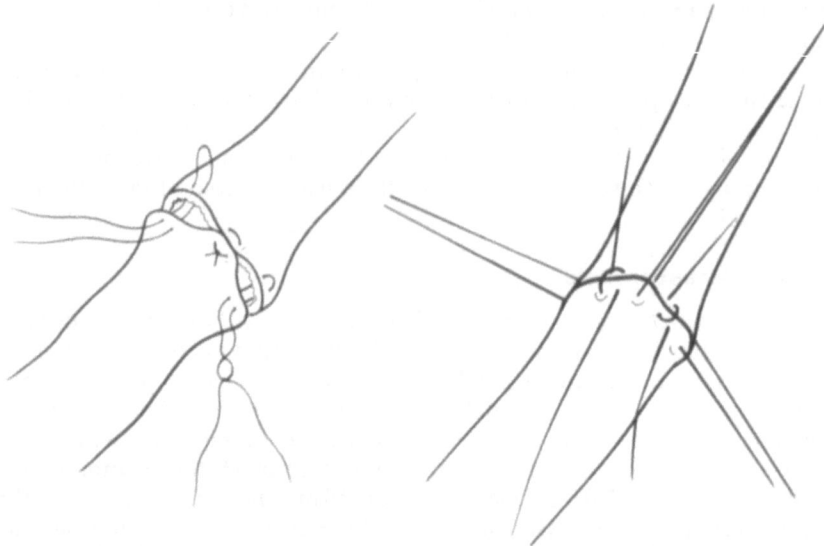

Figure 2.1 Interrupted suture techniques for end to end anastomosis

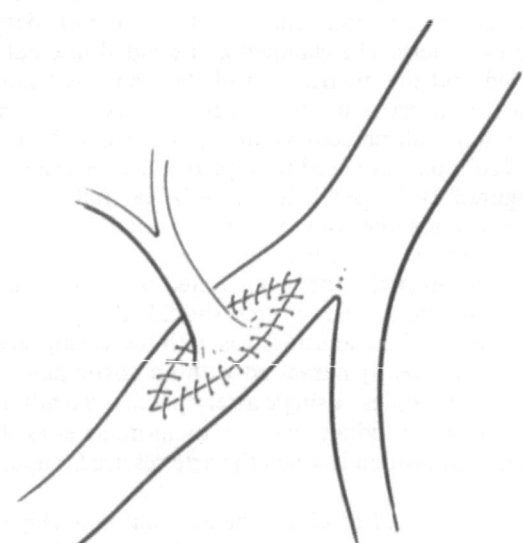

Figure 2.2 Renal artery with aortic patch inserted into the external iliac artery

the external iliac artery it may be best to fashion the patch over the junction of the common and external iliac arteries (Figure 2.3). A narrow ellipse of arterial wall may be removed particularly when the artery is atheromatous and rigid. Continuous 5-0 Prolene suture is used for the anastomosis.

About 25% of kidneys have more than one artery. As long as these are on a patch the arterial anastomosis is dealt with as described above (Figure 2.3). A small upper polar artery is a common finding and this can be dealt with by ligation without danger to the kidney although an upper polar infarct results. A lower polar artery frequently supplies the ureter and should therefore be preserved and revascularized. Figure 2.4 shows a method which we have used in this situation. An infant feeding catheter introduced into the main renal artery is passed through a small side hole into the lower pole artery to act as a stent during the anastomosis which is made with 6-0 interrupted Prolene sutures.

When dealing with two renal arteries of similar size we may join these together as shown in Figure 2.5. These arteries are open longitudinally over a distance of about 10 mm in juxtaposition and anastomosed together to form one common origin which can be joined end to end to the internal iliac artery or end to side to the external. Another possible method when the internal iliac artery is free of atheroma is to divide this artery beyond its

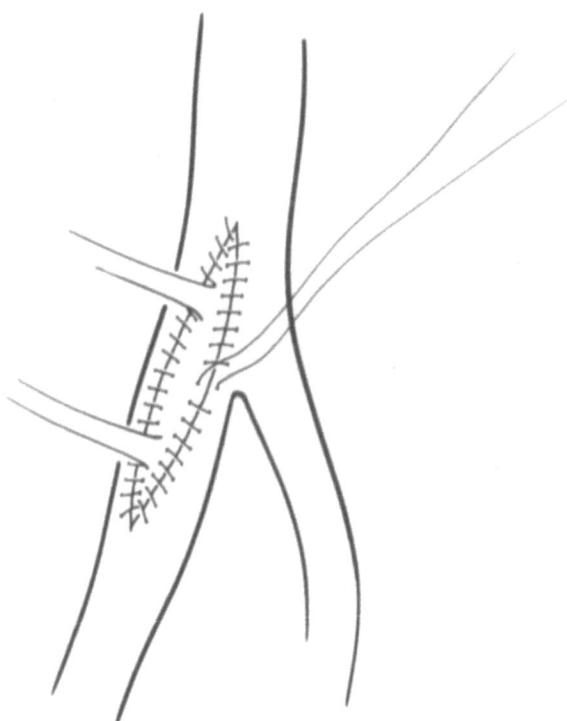

Figure 2.3 Renal arteries on aortic patch implanted into the common iliac/external iliac artery

branching into anterior and posterior divisions and to make use of these for end to end anastomosis to the renal arteries (Figure 2.6). Small visceral branches usually require ligation.

When the arterial anastomosis is complete and tested the clamps on the iliac vessels are removed. When an end to side anastomosis is used the renal arteries are occluded by finger pressure so that any debris or air which might be in the area of the anastomosis goes down the leg rather than into the kidney. The clamp on the renal vein is removed at the same time. Haemostasis is secured in the renal hilum and from the renal capsule.

Ureteric implantation

Following completion of the vascular anastomosis the kidney is positioned in the iliac fossa and attention is focused on the ureteric implantation. Three different methods are commonly used – each with its protagonists. The

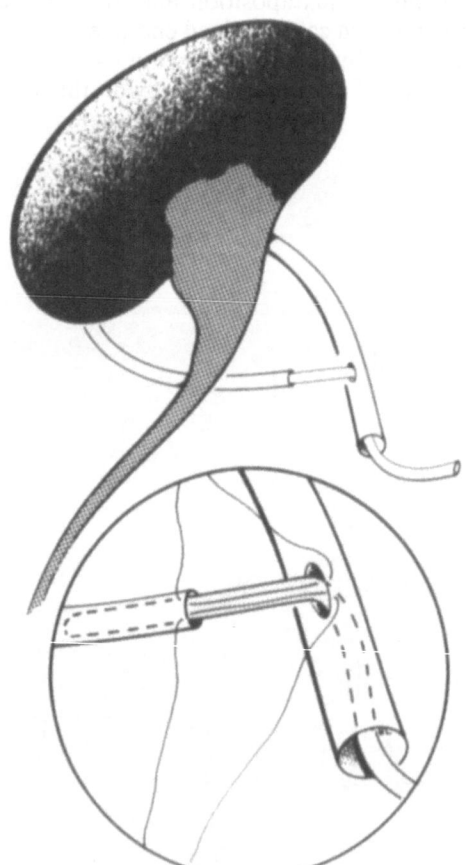

Figure 2.4 Method used to implant small lower pole artery into the main renal artery

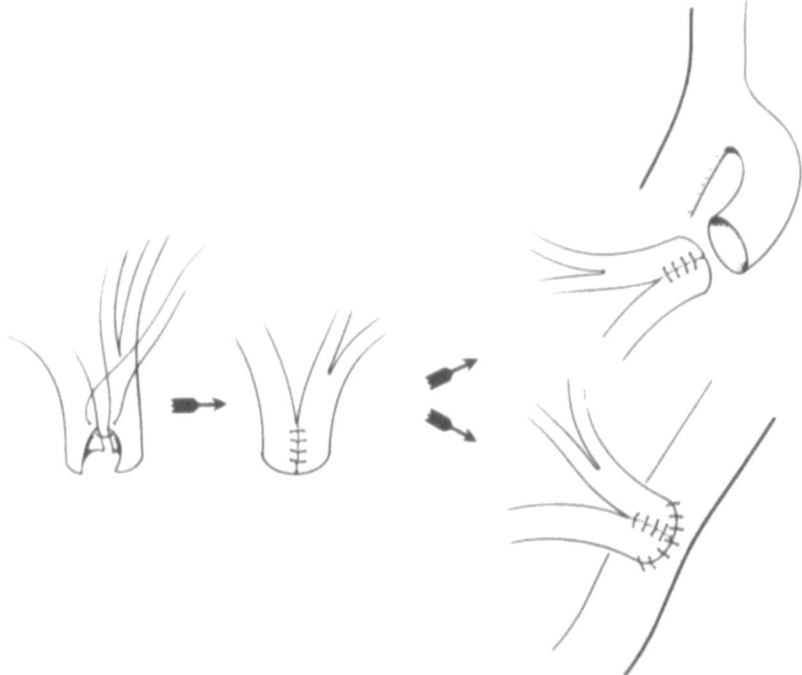

Figure 2.5 Two equal-sized renal arteries joined to form one common renal artery stoma to be anastomosed end to end to the internal or end to side to the external iliac artery

Politano Leadbetter technique[8] or a variant of it is probably the most commonly used method. It involves opening the bladder anteriorly and the mucosa only posterolaterally to the ureteric orifice to create a submucosal tunnel 15–20 mm long. A small hole is then made in the bladder wall at the distal end of the tunnel through which the ureter is pulled. The mucosa of the bladder is sutured to the ureter with chromic catgut sutures at the initial mucosal incision. Others prefer to make use of the recipient's own ureter when this is healthy and to perform a uretero-ureteral anastomosis[9].

We prefer to perform an anterior ureteroneocystostomy in the dome of the bladder. This method, which we have found very satisfactory, will be described in some detail.

A Foley catheter is inserted into the bladder when the patient is anaesthetized. The bladder is distended with approximately 150 mL of acroflavine solution and the catheter spigotted. Others use povidone iodine or neomycin solution instead. This distends and sterilizes the bladder and also colours the mucosa strongly yellow, making its identification easier when the bladder is incised. The two stay sutures inserted in the bladder dome anterosuperiorly are gently used as retractors on the bladder wall. At the same time Langenbeck retractors are used to retract the lower medial edges of the

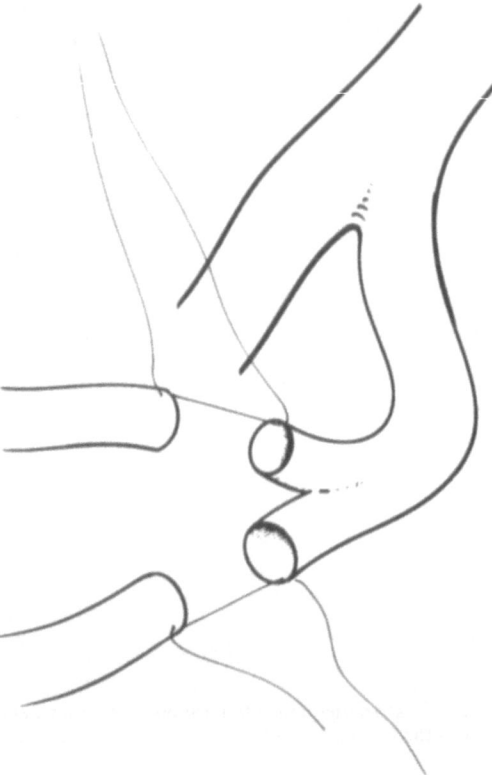

Figure 2.6 End to end anastomoses of two renal arteries to anterior and posterior divisions of the internal iliac artery

wound in order to expose the anterior aspect of the bladder maximally. A 3 cm incision is made in the bladder wall using diathermy, exposing the bladder mucosa which bulges into the bladder wound. The mucosa is incised in the lower part of the wound for a distance of about 1 cm and the bladder emptied of its contents (Figure 2.7).

The ureter is trimmed to the correct length and great care is taken to avoid rotation. The distal 1 cm of the ureter is opened longitudinally on its posterior aspect and joined to the bladder using 4.0 absorbable PDS suture (Figure 2.7). Three interrupted all-coats sutures are placed at the apex of the bladder incision and at the corners of the opened ureter (Figure 2.7). A further all-coats interrupted stitch is used at the other end of the ureteric incision. A few interrupted mucosal stitches are required on each side of the ureter. The bladder wall is closed over the ureter with 3 interrupted PDS sutures making sure that the ureter is not obstructed (Figure 2.7). No splint is required but the bladder catheter is usually retained for one week post-operatively.

Wound closure

Once haemostasis is seen to be adequate and the kidney looks in satisfactory position with good perfusion, the wound is closed in layers with continuous 0 or 1 PDS suture. A small bore closed system suction drain is used for drainage. The skin is closed with interrupted monofilament non-absorbable sutures or continuous subcuticular absorbable sutures such as 4.0 vicryl.

POST-OPERATIVE MANAGEMENT

The post-operative management of kidney transplant patients differs little from that of other surgical patients apart from their drug therapy which is dealt with in Chapter 1. The patients usually tolerate drink and food within 24 hours. Physiotherapy is directed at preventing chest complications. Venous thromboembolism prophylaxis is provided by early mobilization, the wearing of graded compression stockings and, in patients with pre-operative haemo-globins of more than 9 g/dL, by 5000 units of heparin subcutaneously twice daily.

The suction drain can usually be removed on the 2nd to 4th day when the drainage is less than 30 mL per 24 hours. The stitches are left 14 to 21 days depending on the patient's state of health and post-operative course. The bladder catheter is removed on the 7th post-operative day.

POST-OPERATIVE COMPLICATIONS

Complications following kidney transplantation are common. Most of these are immunological or infective and at least partly a consequence of the immunosuppressive medication administered to the patient. These problems are dealt with in other chapters. In this section only the surgical complications

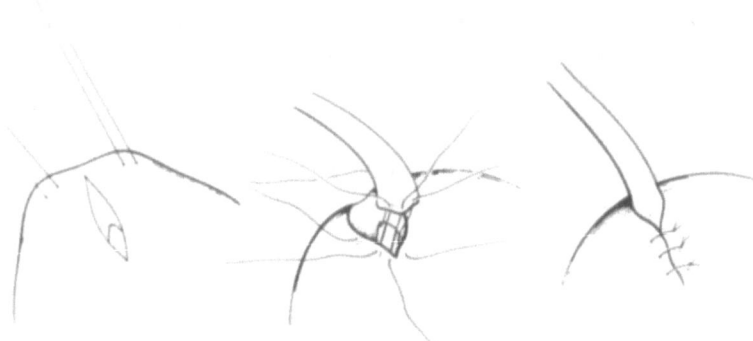

Figure 2.7 Method of anterior ureteroneocystostomy in the dome of the bladder

are considered. These include wound infections, acute early vascular problems such as haemorrhage, arterial and venous thrombosis, late renal arterial stenosis and ureteric necrosis and stenosis.

Wound infections

The infective agents are usually *Staphylococcus aureus* or gram negative organisms. A number of transplant recipients having had frequent hospital contacts prior to their transplants, harbour staphylococci in their skin and airways. Most of the recipients are also oliguric and many have frequent urinary tract infections, commonly with *Escherichia coli* which may indeed be present in their urinary tract mucosa at the time of the operation[10]. As these patients are in addition chronically ill, hypoproteinaemic, anaemic and immunosuppressed, it is clear that meticulous surgical technique is required to avoid wound infections.

Many transplant units routinely instil antiseptic solution into the bladder pre-operatively and use wound towels soaked in antiseptic solution during the operation to protect the wound edges. Haemostasis must always be meticulous and lymph vessels should be ligated to avoid the collection of protein-rich fluid in the wound. For the same reason it is our practice to use a closed system suction drain routinely: other workers never use drains which they suggest may introduce infection[11].

Prophylactic antibiotics are routinely given at the time of surgery in some centres[12] but this is not universal practice. We use appropriate antibiotics in patients with recent positive cultures from sputum or the urinary tract. Cloxacillin or gentamicin as a single pre-operative dose is the usual choice.

The emphasis must, because infection is so serious in these patients, be firmly on prevention. When wound infection does occur it is treated by opening the wound adequately and administering appropriate antibiotics. Healing can be expected to be very slow.

Early vascular complications

Vascular complications are rare but life threatening when they occur. Acute arterial haemorrhage resulting in haemorrhagic shock is sometimes seen associated with early infection and septicaemia and is due to infection in the arterial suture line with dehiscence of the anastomosis. Surgical intervention is obviously required but loss of the kidney graft is probably inevitable. The iliac artery may well have to be ligated and circulation to the leg be provided by an extra anatomic bypass such as a femoro-femoral graft.

Rupture of the transplanted kidney is occasionally seen in association with severe rejection. Such kidneys rarely require removal because of bleeding, but may ultimately do so because of the rejection.

Renal artery thrombosis is a treatable condition if recognized early[13]. Belzer and colleagues recommended that recipients who suddenly become anuric in the first two post-operative days should be immediately returned to the operating theatre for exploration without any diagnostic test. A warm ischaemia time, that is the time the kidney is without circulation at body temperature, of more than 90 minutes leads to death of the kidney. Urgency is therefore mandatory if the kidney is to be salvaged.

Renal vein thrombosis is usually heralded by sudden onset of massive haematuria associated with clinically detectable enlargement of the kidney. This may occur as a separate entity or as part of an iliac venous thrombosis. The incidence of renal vein and deep venous thrombosis in transplant patients is not known but thromboembolism accounts for 6% of all deaths after transplantation[14]. The best treatment is again prevention by the use of subcutaneous heparin, the wearing of graded compression stockings and early mobilization rather than by surgical thrombectomy.

Renal artery stenosis

Hypertension in transplanted patients is a common problem, but it is not known how often stenosis of the transplant renal artery may be responsible. In one series of 100 consecutive patients subjected to arteriography, graft artery stenosis was present in 23 and hypertension in 21 of these[15]. Other workers have reported incidences of renal artery stenosis varying between 1.6% and 16%[16].

The stenosis occurs either at the anastomotic site or in the renal artery between the anastomosis and the branching of the renal artery in the renal hilum. When it is at the suture line it probably represents a technical failure due to the wrong choice of suture material or poor suture technique. On exploration of the second type of renal artery stenosis it is striking how the renal artery is embedded in dense scar tissue and it is probable that this represents a response of the periadventitial tissue to the generalized homograft reaction.

Significant transplant renal artery stenosis is usually associated with hypertension which is difficult to control with drugs. The administration of angiotensin-converting enzyme inhibitors results in a loss of renal function which is usually reversible. Such patients should be subjected to angiography.

Surgical repair of transplant renal artery stenosis is technically difficult and carries a substantial risk of graft loss. Percutaneous transluminal angioplasty of the stenosed artery is now routine treatment in many units for these patients and the experience in our own unit has been excellent with no graft loss. Renal function and hypertension have improved in all patients treated.

Lymphatic complications

A lymphocoele is a collection of lymph in the transplant wound resulting from division without ligation of lymph vessels in the perivascular area of the iliac fossa. Obstruction of the iliac and renal veins and of the ureter may result from the size and tension of the lymphocoele. Occasionally an external lymph fistula may follow.

The diagnosis is usually made by an ultrasonic scan and a cystogram and the lymphocyte should be treated by opening into the peritoneal cavity. An external lymph fistula may take months to heal with conservative management.

Urological complications

The common urological problems after transplantation are ureteric necrosis and obstruction. Both complications are on many occasions caused by surgical error and are therefore preventable. Ureteric necrosis with urine leakage occurs early in the post-operative period. Ureteric obstruction may occur early or late.

Ureteric necrosis

Urinary leakage has been reported to occur in up to 10% of patients following renal transplantation. The cause is usually necrosis of the distal end or of the complete ureter due to interference with the ureteric artery at the time of donor nephrectomy or during the implantation operation. Care should always be taken to safeguard lower pole renal arteries which may supply the ureteric artery. Over-enthusiastic stripping of the adventitial coat of the distal ureter or even careless handling of the distal ureter with forceps are thought to be factors responsible for distal ureteric damage. Some surgeons believe that rejection when it occurs in the kidney may also affect the ureter and cause vascular insufficiency in the ureter.

The clinical presentation is usually that of reduced urine output, impaired renal function, abdominal wound swelling and pain. Urinary leakage through the wound or drain may occur. The diagnosis is confirmed by ultrasonic scanning, isotope renogram, intravenous pyelography or examination of the fluid for urea and creatinine content.

Once the diagnosis is made the patient should be given appropriate antibiotic therapy such as an aminoglycoside or a third generation cephalosporin and the wound should be explored. When the ureter is completely necrotic the best treatment is to free the patient's ipsilateral ureter and anastomose this to the renal pelvis. The proximal ureter can be ligated without the need for a nephrectomy. The necrotic transplanted ureter is excised and a pyelo-ureterostomy performed. We have performed this with one layer of interrupted absorbable sutures such as dexon or vicryl with excellent results, but would now use PDS suture instead. Other workers recommend the use of a double J stent or a nephrostomy to protect the anastomoses, but we have not found this necessary.

When the distal ureter only has shown ischaemic change we have always been able to reimplant the ureter in the dome of the bladder with good result. Clearly the patient's own ureter could be used for a uretero-ureteral anastomosis if insufficient length of ureter remains. We have not lost any kidney or patient after surgical repair of a urinary leak.

Ureteric obstruction

The incidence of ureteric obstruction is uncertain as early obstruction is difficult to diagnose. It is caused by compression of the ureter in its passage through the bladder wall by a blood clot in the tunnel or because the tunnel through the bladder muscular wall is too small or intramuscular rather than submucosal. As this complication occurs in the early post-operative period, ureteric and pelvic dilatation rarely occur and the obstruction is therefore not detected by ultrasonic scanning. Isotope renography and intravenous pyleography may show calyceal concentration of isotope or contrast when there is little or no excretion into the bladder in kidneys with good immediate function. Oliguria is of course common particularly in cadaver transplants and under these circumstances such tests may not help to make the diagnosis.

Late ureteric stenosis months or even years after the transplant does occur and is usually diagnosed by ultrasonic scanning in patients with deteriorating renal function. The cause is usually scar tissue obstruction at the implantation into the bladder and both hydronephrosis and hydroureter are found. Reimplantation of the ureter, pyeloureterostomy using the patient's own ipsilateral ureter or interventional radiological Grunzig balloon dilatation may be used to treat the stenosis. In our practice ureteric stenosis has been a rare complication.

References

1. Health Departments of Great Britain and Northern Ireland (1983). *Cadaveric organs for transplantation. A code of practice including the diagnosis of brain death.* (London: HMSO)
2. A kidney to spare? (1985). Leader. *Lancet*, **2**, 926–7
3. Council of the Transplantation Society. (1985). Commercialisation in transplantation: the problems and some guidelines for practice. *Lancet*, **2**, 715–6
4. Najarian, J. S., Gulyassy, P. P., Stoney, R. J. and Brannstein, P. (1966). Protection of the donor kidney during homotransplantation. *Ann. Surg.*, **164**, 398–417
5. Sear, J. W. (1984). Anaesthesia in renal transplantation. In Morris, P. J. (ed.) *Kidney Transplantation. Principles and Practice.* pp. 219–37. (Grune and Stratton)
6. Starzl, T. E., Marchioro, T. L., Dickinson, T. C., Rifkind, D., Stonington, O. G. and Waddell, W. R. (1964). Technique of renal homotransplantation. Experience with 42 cases. *Arch. Surg.*, **89**, 87–104
7. Hume, D. M. (1966). Progress in clinical homotransplantation. *Adv. Surg.*, **2**, 419–98
8. Politano, V. A. and Leadbetter, W. F. (1958). An operative technique for the correction of vesicoureteric reflux. *J. Urol.*, **82**, 932–41
9. Hamburger, J., Crosnier, J., Dormont, J. and Bach, J. F. (1972). Surgical techniques. In *Renal Transplantation*, pp. 249–78. (Baltimore and London: Williams and Wilkins)
10. Hinman, F. Jr. and Belzer, F. O. (1969). Urinary tract infection and renal homotransplantation. I. Effect of antibacterial irrigators on defences of the defunctionalized bladder. *J. Urol.*, **101**, 477–81
11. Belzer, F. O., Salvatierra, O., Schweizer, R. T. and Kountz, S. L. (1973). Prevention of wound infections by topical antibiotics in high risk patients. *Ann. J. Surg.*, **126**, 180–5
12. Tilney, N. L., Strom, T. B., Vineyard, G. C. and Merill, J. P. (1978). Factors contributing to the declining mortality rate in renal transplantation. *N. Engl. J. Med.*, **299**, 1321–5
13. Belzer, F. O., Schweizer, R. T. and Kountz, S. L. (1972). Management of multiple vessels in renal transplantation. *Transpl. Proc.*, **4**, 639–44
14. Rosansky, S. J. and Sugimoto, T. (1982). An analysis of the United States renal transplant patient population and organ survival characteristics: 1977–1980. *Kidney Int.*, **22**, 685–92
15. Lacombe, M. (1975). Arterial stenosis complicating renal allotransplantation in man: a study of 38 cases. *Ann. Surg.*, **181**, 283–8
16. Faenza, A., Spolaore, R., Poggioli, G., Selleri, S., Roversi, R. and Gozzetti, G. (1983). Renal artery stenosis after renal transplantation. *Kidney Int.*, **14**, (Suppl.), May, 54–9

3
Tissue Typing and Immunological Aspects of Organ Transplantation

G. GALEA AND S. J. URBANIAK

Although transplantation of tissues is biologically artificial, it has provided a therapeutically successful approach to the management of functional failure of a variety of organs or systems. It has long been recognized that successful blood transfusion is dependent on matching the blood groups of donor and recipient red cells. In his Nobel lecture of 1931, Landsteiner suggested that similar 'blood groups' would be involved in the acceptance or rejection of other transplanted tissues[1]. By the end of the 1940s both Simonsen and Dempster had confirmed the early rejection of allograft dog kidneys noted previously by Carrell and Guthrie and had drawn attention to the massive intrarenal infiltration of lymphoid cells which accompanied progressive renal failure[2]. These observations and ideas, developed still further in 1953 by Mitchison and Gowans, led to the realization that although cell-mediated immunity was mainly responsible for acute rejection in the first few days after transplantation, humoral mechanisms and cytotoxic antibodies were also involved in the host response to allografts[2].

In the ensuing years, the surgical specialty of organ transplantation has progressed from a novelty to a mature and scientific technology. Kidneys, although the commonest, are by no means the only transplanted organs. Allografts with a reasonable anticipation of success include heart, liver, pancreas, lung, en-block heart and lung, cornea, skin and bone. In some measure this progress can be attributed to the development of appropriate surgical techniques. Without question, however, most gains have been achieved through the increased understanding and control of the major impediment to organ transplantation—immunological rejection.

NOMENCLATURE AND GENETIC ORGANIZATION OF THE MAJOR HISTOCOMPATIBILITY COMPLEX (MHC)

The nomenclature of the MHC is devised by the World Health Organization. The entire complex occupies a segment of approximately $2\,cM^*$ on the short arm of chromosome 6. The complex occupies approximately $\frac{1}{3} \times 10^{-3}$ of the total genome. Figure 3.1 schematically depicts the current concept of the complex, showing the genetic regions containing the HLA (human leucocyte antigen) and related loci†. There are five officially recognized genetic loci: HLA-A, HLA-B, HLA-C, HLA-D and HLA-DR (D-related). The HLA-D/DR region contains both the D and DR loci, which may be identical[3].

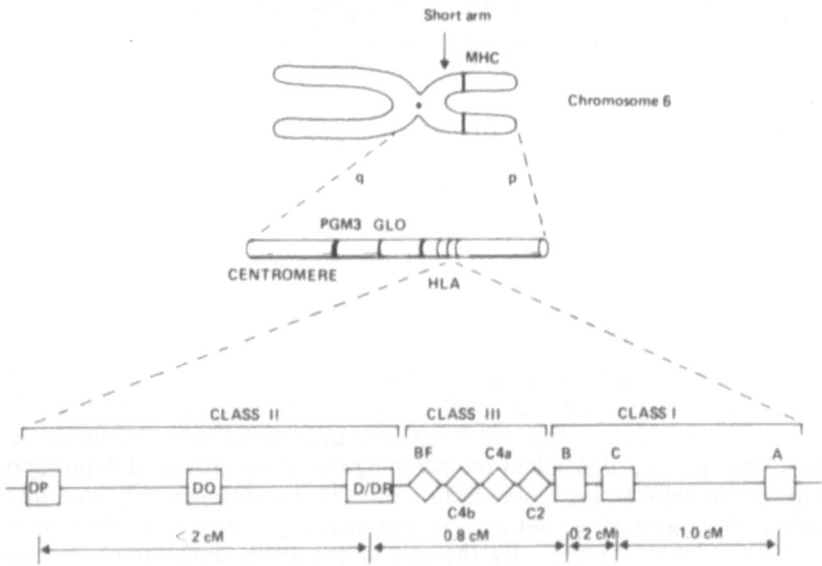

Figure 3.1 The MHC (major histocompatibility complex) on the short arm of chromosome 6. On the upper part of the figure the position of the complex is shown relative to other markers (PGM 3: phosphoglucomutase 3, GLO: glyoxylase) on the short arm of chromosome 6. Approximate distances are given in centimorgans (cM). The lower part of the figure displays an extended version of the HLA complex, showing the relationships of the class I, II and III loci

Several additional genetic regions have been linked to the HLA complex. The complement region, which has been mapped between the HLA-B and D/DR regions, contains genes determining the second and fourth components (C2 and C4) of the classical complement pathway and the properdin factor B (Bf) of the alternate pathway. A series of loci designated HLA-DQ, which determine class II or B cell antigens, are presumed (not proven) to map within or near the HLA-D/DR region. Finally, a locus that determines anti-

*Centimorgan (cM): a unit of physical map distance on a chromosome equivalent to a 1% frequency of recombination between linked genes.

†A locus is the position on the chromosome where a given gene may be found.

gens termed HLA-DP has been mapped between HLA-DR and glyoxylase.

At each locus, one of several alternative forms (alleles) of a gene may be found. Officially recognized alleles at each locus are designated by the locus and a number: thus, HLA-A1 is allele 1 at the HLA-A locus. Alleles that have been tentatively assigned to a given locus but are not yet officially recognized are designated by a w (for workshop) placed before the number, e.g. HLA-DRw1. Official recognition results in the elimination of the w, e.g. HLA-DR1, and occurs when there is international agreement about the 'uniqueness' of the allele.

The HLA system is extremely polymorphic, having multiple alleles at each known locus. For example, there are at least 23 distinct alleles at the HLA-A locus and at least 47 distinct alleles at the HLA-B locus. The entire listing of officially and tentatively recognized HLA antigens is presented in Table 3.1. Each allele determines an immunologically distinct product. The products of the HLA-A, B, C, D, DR, DQ and DP alleles are cell surface molecules that bear the antigenic determinants. Based on their tissue distribution and structure, HLA antigens have been divided into two classes. Class I antigens, also termed the classic histocompatibility antigens, include the HLA-A, B and C antigens. Class II antigens, also termed B cell antigens, include the HLA-D, DR, DQ and DP antigens. Class III antigens include the Bf, C2 and C4 components of complement. With the exception of HLA-D, which is detected by a mixed leucocyte reaction (MLR) and DP which is identified by primed lymphocyte typing (PLT), all of the cell surface antigens are detected serologically, usually by microcytotoxicity. The products of the C2, C4 and Bf loci are soluble serum proteins that can be detected serologically and functionally.

The same term is used to designate the HLA allele and its product, the antigen. HLA antigens found on the molecule determined by a single allele are termed HLA *private antigens*. In contrast, HLA *public antigens* are determinants common to several HLA molecules, each of which bears a distinct HLA private antigen. HLA-Bw4 and Bw6 are the best known examples of HLA public antigens and the distribution of HLA-Bw4 and Bw6 antigens is presented in Table 3.2. This is of practical importance, in that knowledge of the public antigens can on many occasions help identify the specificity of other antigens. If, for example, a person is Bw4 and B16 positive, he will be much more likely to be B38 rather than B39, which is associated with Bw6.

In several instances, an HLA antigen initially thought to be a single private antigen has been subsequently found to be in a group of two or three closely related antigens, each of narrower specificity. These latter antigens are termed 'splits' of the original broad specificity. Conversely, HLA private antigens can be organized into groups based on the apparent serological cross-reactivity between members of the group.

The nomenclature of the HLA antigens is constantly being revised and updated. The DP antigens were previously known as the SB (secondary B cell) antigens and previous specificities known as MT, MB, Te and DC have now been better defined under the DQ system. For example, DQw2 incorporates the previous specificities MB2 and Te24, while DQw3 now incorporates MB2 and MT4[4].

Table 3.1 Complete listing of recognised HLA specificities (WHO 1984)

HLA-A	HLA-B		HLA-C	HLA-D	HLA-DR	HLA-DQ	HLA-DP
A1	B5	Bw4	Cw1	Dw1	DR1	DQw1	DPw1
A2	B7	Bw6	Cw2	Dw2	DR2	DQw2	DPw2
A3	B8		Cw3	Dw3	DR3	DQw3	DPw3
A9	B12		Cw4	Dw4	DR4		DPw4
A10	B13		Cw5	Dw5	DR5		DPw5
A11	B14		Cw6	Dw6	DRw6		DPw6
Aw19	B15		Cw7	Dw7	DR7		
A23 (9)	B16		Cw8	Dw8	DRw8		
A24 (9)	B17			Dw9	DRw9		
A25 (10)	B18			Dw10	DRw10		
A26 (10)	B21			DW11 (w7)	DRw11 (5)		
A28	Bw22			Dw12	DRw12 (5)		
A29 (w19)	B27			Dw13	DRw13 (w6)		
A30 (w19)	B35			Dw14	DRw14 (w6)		
A31 (w19)	B37			Dw15			
A32 (w19)	B38 (16)			Dw16	DRw52		
Aw33 (w19)	B39 (16)			Dw17 (w7)	DRw53		
Aw34 (10)	B40			Dw18 (w6)			
Aw36	Bw41			Dw19 (w6)			
Aw43	Bw42						
Aw66 (10)	B44 (12)						
Aw68 (28)	B45 (12)						
Aw69 (28)	Bw46						
	Bw47						
	Bw48						
	B49 (21)						
	Bw50 (21)						
	B51 (5)						
	Bw52 (5)						
	Bw53						
	Bw54 (w22)						
	Bw55 (w22)						
	Bw56 (w22)						
	Bw57 (17)						
	Bw58 (17)						
	Bw59						
	Bw60 (40)						
	Bw61 (40)						
	Bw62 (15)						
	Bw63 (15)						
	Bw64 (14)						
	Bw65 (14)						
	Bw67						
	Bw70						
	Bw71 (w70)						
	Bw72 (w70)						
	Bw73						

Table 3.2 Distribution of HLA Bw4 and Bw6 on the HLA-B antigens. The listing of broad specificities is indicated in parenthesis after a narrow specificity. Association of 'splits' of a broad antigen (e.g. 12) with either Bw4 or Bw6 aids identification (e.g. B44 (12) with Bw4 and B45 with Bw6)

Public antigen	HLA-B antigens on which it is found
Bw4	B5, B13, B17, B27, B37, B38 (16), B44 (12), Bw47, B49 (21), B51 (5), Bw52 (5), Bw53, Bw57 (17), Bw58 (17), Bw59, Bw63 (15)
Bw6	B7, B8, B14, B18, Bw22, B35, B39 (16), B40, Bw41, Bw42, B45 (12), Bw46, Bw48, Bw50 (21), Bw54 (w22), Bw55 (w22), Bw56 (w22), Bw60 (40), Bw61 (40), Bw62 (15), Bw64 (14), Bw65 (14), Bw67, Bw70, Bw71 (w70), Bw72 (w70), Bw73

Haplotype

Because of their close linkage, the combination of MHC alleles at each locus on a single chromosome is usually inherited as a unit. This unit is referred to as a haplotype. Therefore in first degree relatives, if the donor and recipient are matched for HLA-A and B antigens, there is an excellent chance that other closely linked loci will also be matched. In contrast, with random donors, matching for one or two antigens is a poor marker for other linked loci. This is reflected in better survival figures when the donor and recipient are closely related, as is discussed later in this chapter.

There is a significant degree of crossing-over or translocation between the HLA-A, B and D loci (this happens more frequently with greater distances between loci on the chromosome). Hence there is difficulty in the 'outbred' population of finding HLA-D identity even when there is HLA-A and B identity.

Since one chromosome is inherited from each parent, each individual has two HLA haplotypes. Because all HLA genes are co-dominant, both alleles at a given HLA locus are expressed and two complete sets of HLA antigens can be detected on cells. By simple Mendelian inheritance, there is a 25% chance that two siblings will share both haplotypes, a 50% chance that they will share one haplotype and a 25% chance that they will share no haplotype at all (Figure 3.2).

Linkage disequilibrium

As a result of random matings, the frequency of finding a given allele at one HLA locus in association with a given allele at a second HLA locus should simply be the product of the frequencies of each allele in the population. However, certain combinations of alleles are found with a frequency far exceeding that expected. This phenomenon is termed 'linkage disequilibrium' and is quantitated as the difference between the observed and expected frequencies[5,6]. This is of importance when selecting donors especially with D typing which, as described later, requires an MLR–a laborious and lengthy

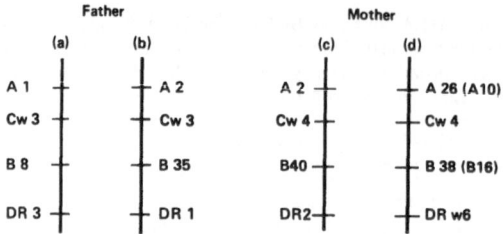

Four combinations of HLA antigens are possible in the offspring of this mating

Chromosome combination		Paternal haplotypes	Maternal haplotypes
1	a c	A 1, B 8, Cw 3, DR 3	A 2, B 40, Cw 4, DR 2
2	a* d	A 1, B 8, Cw 3, DR 1	A 26 (A 10), B 38 (B 16), Cw 4, DR w6
3	b c	A 2, B 35, Cw 3, DR 1	A 2, B 40, Cw 4, DR 2
4.	b d	A 2 B 35, Cw 3, DR 1	A 26 (A 10), B 38 (B 16), Cw 4, DR w6

*S having an example of crossing-over on the 'a' chromosome

Figure 3.2 Inheritance of HLA haplotypes. Haplotype designations in the figure are given as a, b, c, d–offspring of the mating a/b and c/d will inherit one of two possible haplotypes from each parent and so will have haplotypes a/c, a/d, b/c and b/d

procedure. It is known, for example, that HLA-DR3 is closely linked with HLA-B8. Therefore an HLA-B8 random donor would be selected in preference to someone who has a phenotype not closely related to DR3, if one wishes to type for D3, which in turn is closely related if not identical to DR3.

Knowledge of haplotype inheritance and linkage disequilibrium is of great practical importance. It is well established that HLA-DR matching of unrelated individuals gives allostimulation higher than that of HLA identical siblings[7]. This suggests that other unknown loci produce determinants that are sufficient to elicit primary allostimulation, and it is likely that all these loci need to be matched to prevent such stimulation. It follows therefore that the more loci one can identify the better. Investigations in this direction are continuing at present. It is known, for example, that complement proteins have genetic polymorphisms that have been useful in identifying linkage disequilibrium with HLA[8]. These 'complotypes' considered as single genetic units are extraordinarily polymorphic, second only to HLA-B among human genes[7]. They have been studied in some detail and 'extended haplotypes' have been identified. Such extended haplotypes in which the MHC alleles are not randomly associated appear to represent examples of genetic linkage disequilibrium over a large but undefined segment of the short arm of chromosome 6 [8,9].

HLA TYPING

Serological methods

The HLA class I antigens are all defined by serological reactions and typing for these antigens is performed using standard serological techniques. Typing sera are obtained chiefly from multiparous women. These sera tend to have relatively high titres of antibodies directed against a limited number of HLA determinants, since in most cases the women have been repeatedly immunized with the HLA antigens of a single individual. Many attempts have been made to produce monoclonal antibodies with a high titre and sufficient specificity for use as typing reagents: to date the results have been largely disappointing. The most widely used method for HLA typing is the lymphocyte microcytotoxicity assay (Figure 3.3). Multiple antisera against HLA-A, B, C and DR antigens are provided by UKTS (United Kingdom Transplant Service) in Bristol on a UK-wide basis from materials provided by tissue typing laboratories. They are provided in standard plates of defined specificities and these plates are then frozen till needed. In an effort to standardize the techniques for serological typing, quality assurance (QA) exercises are constantly carried out. Standard HLA-A, B, and C typing takes 2 hours to perform.

HLA-DR and DQ antigens are typed by procedures virtually identical to those described above with the exception that the typing is performed on purified populations of B lymphocytes. The typing sera are pre-tested to ensure that they do not detect HLA-A, B or C antigens. The close association and possible identity between HLA-DR and D is of great practical importance. When time is limited, as is most often the case with cadaver donors, it is not possible to perform an MLR (see below) to type for the D locus. Therefore serological typing for the DR antigens is undertaken for selection of recipients. HLA-DR typing takes 4 hours to perform, the longer time being required mostly for the preparation of B lymphocytes.

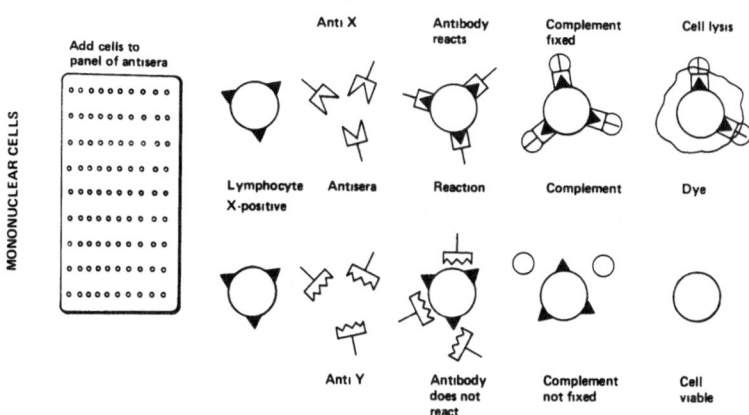

Figure 3.3 Microcytotoxicity test for HLA antigens:

The patient's blood is heparinized, and mononuclear cells are purified. The cells are then added to the wells of a microtitre plate containing anti-HLA antisera. If the antibodies are bound (X positive cell + anti X), they fix complement and cause the cell to lyse. Eosin or other dyes (e.g. trypan blue) enters the cell and the cell appears coloured under phase microscopy. If complement is not fixed, no lysis ensues, and the live cell appears unstained. This assay is used for all class I antigens with some modification to type for DR

Mixed leucocyte reaction

The HLA-D antigens are defined and typed by the mixed leucocyte reaction (MLR). When T lymphocytes from HLA-D non-identical individuals are cultured together *in vitro*, HLA-D antigens on the cells from one individual stimulate blast transformation, DNA synthesis, and proliferation of the second individual's lymphocytes. For HLA-D typing, a panel of HLA-D homozygous typing cells (HTC) which are inhibited from transforming by either irradiation or chemical means (e.g. mitomycin C), and representing all known HLA-D types is used. This is the 'one way' MLR described in Figure 3.4.

In addition to HLA-D typing, the MLR is also useful for matching purposes in the 'two-way' MLR. In bone marrow transplantation, for example, living related donors are first chosen on the basis of class I and DR identity. An MLR is then performed using prospective donor and recipient lymphocytes. On the basis of the MLR result (negative, high or low reactivity) the choice of the donor is then made. The MLR takes 5 days to perform.

The DP antigens are identified and typed by the primed lymphocyte typing (PLT) test. A panel of responding lymphocytes is first primed by stimulator cells matched for HLA-A, B, C, D and DR antigens for approximately ten days in an MLR. Unknown cells are irradiated or treated with mitomycin C and tested for their ability to restimulate the primed responding lymphocytes.

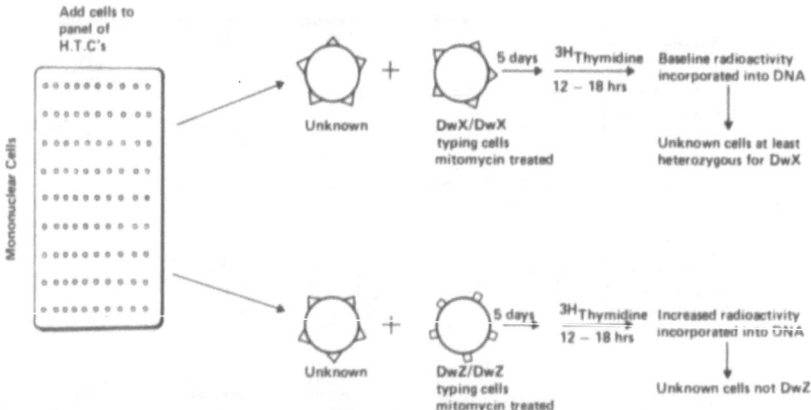

Figure 3.4 HLA-D typing by one-way mixed leukocyte reactions using homozygous typing cells (HTC). Mononuclear cells are added to the wells of a microculture plate containing a panel of mitomycin treated HTCs used as stimulator cells. The cells are incubated for 5 days after which 3H-thymidine is added and incubation continued for an additional 12–18 h. The amount of 3H-thymidine incorporated by the unknown cells into newly synthesized DNA is then determined. The reaction patterns allow the cell to be typed, for example as DwX positive, and DwZ negative

64

Blanks

In general, because individuals possess two haplotypes and because HLA antigen expression is co-dominant, it is possible to type two antigens determined at a particular locus. Occasionally, only one antigen can be determined. The HLA type at that locus is then identified either as being homozygous for the antigen or as having an antigenic specificity that cannot be typed by available reagents. These alternatives can usually be distinguished by family studies. Other explanations which are less likely include the absence of an antigen-producing gene at a particular locus (a true amorph), or the presence of a modifying gene which could act as a suppressor on HLA gene expression.

Possible future methods of HLA typing

It is now possible to apply techniques of molecular biology to the problems of HLA typing. Restriction endonucleases that recognize specific nucleotide sequences are utilized. Genomic DNA clones are used to recognise most or all genes coding for class I and class II proteins[10] and most of the complement components[11]. These new techniques have multiple applications. It is possible that despite drastically reduced expression of HLA antigens on the surface of some patients' cells (they may type as 'blanks') the appropriate gene could still be present. Gene probes will determine whether these people have a defect of antigen expression or a gene deletion. Further studies to elucidate the complex mechanism of gene regulation could ultimately lead to the normal expression of present but malfunctioning genes.

In addition to permitting genotyping in difficult cases (which may be essential, for example, prior to a bone marrow transplantation), these techniques may prove useful tools in prenatal diagnosis of HLA-linked diseases. Fetal DNA may be obtained by biopsy of chorionic villi as early as the 6th to 8th week of gestation. Because HLA probes can detect a high degree of polymorphism, it is likely that they will have considerable clinical value.

TISSUE DISTRIBUTION, STRUCTURE AND FUNCTION

Class I antigens

The HLA-A, B and C antigens are found on virtually every nucleated human cell (Table 3.3). Structurally the class I antigens are found on a two-chain molecule that consists of a polymorphic glycoprotein, determined by genes in the MHC complex, in covalent association with a non-polymorphic protein, a β microglobulin, determined by a gene on chromosome 15 (Figure 3.5).

Much of what is known regarding the function of HLA antigens is based on what has been demonstrated for major histocompatibility antigens in other species. Class I antigens are the principal antigens recognized by the host during tissue graft rejection. In cell-mediated cytolysis, the *in vitro*

65

Table 3.3 Comparison of class I and class II antigens

	Class I	Class II
Antigens included	HLA-A, B, C	HLA-D, DR, DP, DQ
Detection	Serological	HLA-DR, DQ: serological HLA-D: mixed leucocyte reaction HLA-DQ: primed lymphocyte test
Tissue distribution	Wide–on all nucleated cells	Restricted to immunocompetent cells, particularly B lymphocytes, macrophages and activated T cells. (Present in small amounts in resting T cells.)
Functions	Target for cell mediating lympholysis (CML) Recognized during graft rejection Restriction of CML of virus-infected cells	D/DR antigens important for antigen presentation for effective interaction beteween immunocompetent cells

correlate of graft rejection, the class I antigens are the target antigens recognized by the killer T lymphocytes. Both private and public HLA antigens can be recognized independently by these T cells. The true antigens can be recognized independently by these T cells. The true physiological role of class I histocompatibility, however, is probably related to the phenomenon of histocompatibility restriction of cell-mediated lysis (CML) of virus-infected and minor histocompatibility antigen-bearing cells. When T lymphocytes are exposed to a viral antigen, they will recognize it in the context of a class I antigen. This phenomenon is explained in more detail in Chapter 6.

Class II antigens

Class II antigens are found chiefly on the surfaces of immunocompetent cells, including mononuclear phagocytes, endothelial cells, Langerhans cells, activated T cells, and particularly B lymphocytes (Table 3.3). HLA-D antigens are the stimulator antigens of the MLR, and it is this reaction that is used to define and detect these antigens. The ability of anti-HLA-DR antisera to inhibit an MLR by interacting with HLA-DR antigens on the stimulating cell suggests that HLA-DR and D antigens are at least in close proximity on the cell surface[5]. It is unclear whether HLA-D and DR antigens are in fact identical but are recognized by different assay systems, or whether they are discrete. They cannot be isolated serologically and their structure is unknown at present. The remainder of the class II antigens are borne on a two-chain molecule that consists of an α chain and a β chain in non-covalent association (Figure 3.6).

The HLA-D antigens are thought to be the antigens principally responsible for the *in vivo* correlate of the MLR, the graft versus host reaction. Presumably through this role, the HLA-D/DR region antigens have been implicated in

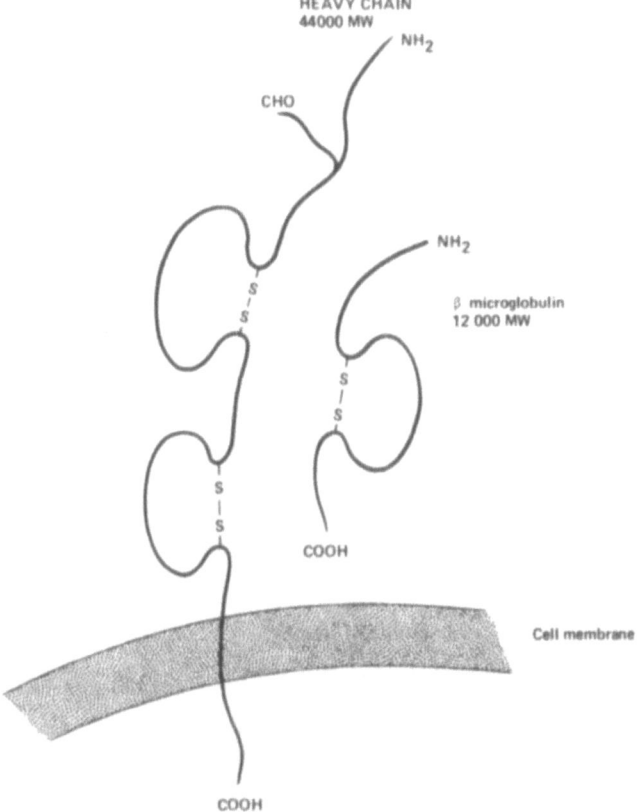

Figure 3.5 A schematic representation of an HLA class I molecule. The molecule consists of 44 000 MW glycoprotein, the heavy chain, which bears the antigenic determinant, in a non-covalent association with a 12 000 MW non-polymorphic $\beta2$ microglobulin. (NH_2 = amino terminal; COOH = carboxyl terminal; CHO = carbohydrate side chain; —S—S— = disulphide bond)

the sensitization phase (i.e. the afferent limb) of cell-mediated cytolysis. This is in contrast to the effector phase where the HLA class I antigens are important as target molecules.

This function relates to the artificial situation in which cells bearing different HLA antigens have been mixed. In the physiological situation where cells bearing identical HLA antigens are required to interact productively, the HLA-D/DR region antigens have been shown to be involved in antigen presentation by macrophages to T lymphocytes, as well as in efficient collaboration between immunocompetent cells. Human suppressor factors that suppress an MLR have been shown to react with anti-HLA-DR alloantisera. In addition, some factors will suppress the MLR response of T cells only if both the factor and the T cell are reactive with the same anti-HLA-DR antiserum.

The DP antigens have been shown to be distinct from all other class II

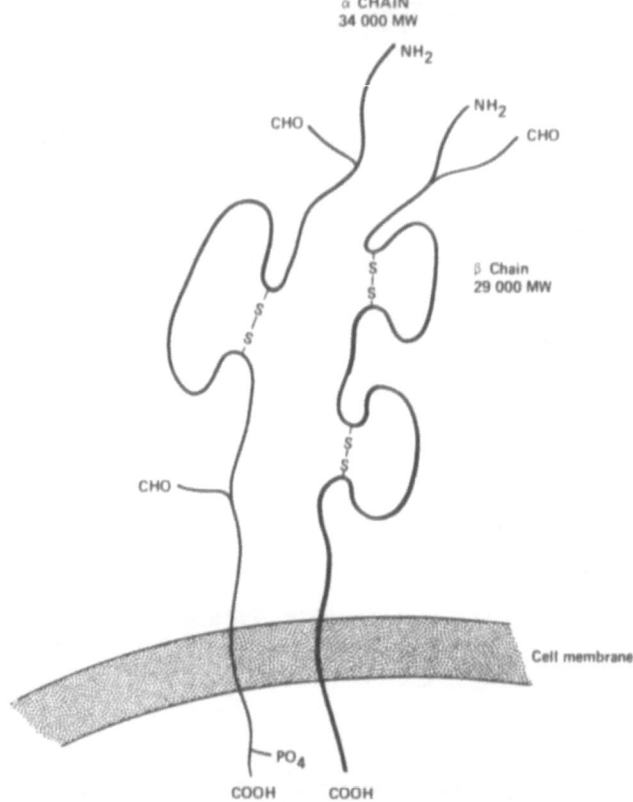

Figure 3.6 Schematic representation of an HLA class II (HLA-DR) molecule. The molecule consists of a 34 000 MW glycoprotein (α chain) on a non-covalent association with a 29 000 MW glycoprotein (β chain). (Abbreviations as for Figure 3.5)

antigens. They can elicit a strong secondary proliferative response and can act as target antigens for cytotoxic T lymphocytes. Their function is presumed (not proved) to be similar to that of the HLA-D/DR antigens.

Immune response genes

Specific immune responses to a variety of antigenic substances are now thought to be regulated by immune response (Ir) genes[12]. In general, Ir gene control is dominant genetically, and the supposition is that individuals who lack that gene are unresponsive. The function of this gene is normally appreciated only when various forms of the gene products exist, such that some individuals respond to a given antigen and some do not. The generally accepted concept is that Ir genes account for the interaction of T lymphocytes with both B lymphocytes and macrophages, which are necessary for T cell activation and expression of T cell function as explained in more detail in Chapter 6.

HISTOCOMPATIBILITY TESTING

Role of the ABO system

Recipient ABO incompatibility to the donor (a mismatched transplant, e.g. a group A organ transplanted into a group B recipient) although not contraindicated in certain clinical situations (e.g. liver transplantation) is avoided whenever possible. However, ABO compatible, non-identical transplants (e.g. a group O donor organ transplanted into a non-group O recipient, or a group A or B organ to an AB recipient) are frequently used[13].

In bone marrow transplantation it has been clearly shown that ABO incompatibility does not significantly affect the outcome[14,15]. The rate of engraftment, incidence and severity of graft versus host disease (GVHD), and patient survival are not related to the ABO group differences or similarities between donor and recipient. These observations, along with *in vitro* experiments, have been interpreted to demonstrate the absence of ABH antigens on the very early pluripotent marrow cells in humans[16,17].

In other organ transplants, e.g. liver or kidney, short-term anti-recipient ABO antibodies occasionally result[13,18]. It appears that immunocompetent 'passenger' B lymphocytes are acquired with the transplanted organ. These cells respond to the recipient ABO antigens in a type of graft versus host reaction. These 'autoantibodies' may cause red cell haemolysis but are usually short-lived (2–4 weeks). It is interesting to note that cyclosporin therapy does not blunt these responses while body irradiation does. It seems that cyclosporin permits this, because it selectively affects T cell function but spares B cell activities[19].

The endothelial-monocyte system

Qualitatively there is mounting evidence that certain cells such as monocytes as well as endothelial cells are important in the graft as sources of antigens which provoke helper T cells to set the cytotoxic cascade in action[20]. This endothelial-monocyte system alone is poorly immunogenic but it can produce an antibody response.

Practical methods of monocyte typing and crossmatching need to be developed to avoid fruitless transplant attempts in patients with donor specific anti-monocyte antibodies. For technical reasons, the standard cytotoxicity assay is difficult to adapt, in part because monocytes are more resistant to the effects of complement than T cells[20]. Moreover, not all monocyte antigens are shared with the endothelium.

Antigens carried on stimulator cells and other lymphoreticular cells of the graft (e.g. 'passenger' leucocytes) constitute a barrier to successful tissue transplantation, and their removal from a graft prior to transplantation has been shown to reduce significantly the immunological strength of the graft[21].

Other antigens

Other antigen systems have shown a reasonably significant association with acceptance of the graft[22,23]. These include the Lewis antigens on the red cells and in the serum, and the H-Y antigens associated with the X and Y chromosomes. Their role is however considered minor.

Other factors

Three non-specific factors are also important[2]:

(1) The site of transplantation,
(2) The form of the allograft, and
(3) Whether or not the graft is on a vascular pedicle.

The effect of the site depends on its proximity to blood vessels and lymphatics. For example, corneal allografts are accepted only if they are grafted into normal avascular corneas: they are rejected if the original pathological condition involves abnormal vascularity. Most experimental work on the form of the allograft suggests that isolated fragments such as pancreatic islets are more vigorously rejected than the solid parent organs. This has never been adequately explained though one possibility might be the ease with which multiple exposed surfaces evoke a response in the recognition phase, together with the susceptibility of small particles to phagocytosis in the effector phase. Finally the effect of primary vascularization is not clear-cut. Simple free skin grafts are as readily rejected as vascularized kidneys and are more difficult to protect with immunosuppressive drugs, though it might be expected that rapid recognition by the host would speed its assault on a renal allograft.

THE VALUE OF HLA MATCHING WITH RELEVANCE TO GRAFT SURVIVAL

Living related donors

From the point of view of clinical transplantation, host-recipient matching is of paramount importance. It is informative to compare the results of transplants from living related donors with those from cadaver donors. Most of the experience gained from living related donors has been from studies on kidney transplantation, although in the UK this approach has been used in the minority of cases. On the other hand, living related donors have been the major source of bone marrow transplantation. In these latter instances, however, the recipients are usually so heavily immunosuppressed, both for their primary haematological condition and in the preconditioning regimes prior to transplantation, that rejection problems are not usually encountered. Amongst first degree relatives, the expected graft success has been shown to be in direct proportion to matching for two, one or no HLA haplotypes as defined by serological typing[20]. Thus 90–95% of HLA-identical grafts, as in identical twins (both haplotypes matched), survive for a year or more. But if the donor is a haplo-identical family member (a parent or sibling who shares one of the recipient's two HLA-A and B haplotypes) one year survival drops to 75% and for HLA incompatible siblings it is 50–60% or little better than the overall average for cadaver transplants. However, it needs to be stressed that a number of poorly matched grafts may in fact do quite well. It is apparent that the usual serological typing for HLA antigens does not necessarily provide a measure of the strength of the immune response in a given case.

Family members who are haplo-identical on HLA-A and B typing may show a wide range of responses (from high to low) on MLR assay. This has been shown in several studies[24,25,26]. Although the MLR assay is relatively imprecise with centre to centre variation, when carefully controlled it may be used to ascertain which HLA haplo-identical donors within a family would provide a graft with the best chance of survival.

It has to be asked why low and high MLR responses occur, and how they relate to matching for the various components of the HLA-D region. Some reports suggest that there is generation of suppressor T lymphocytes which could down-modulate an early vigorous response[20].

Cadaver donors

It has been difficult to assess the role of HLA matching by the usual serological techniques in cadaver-donor grafting. It is accepted that even a 'full house' HLA match of two HLA-A and two HLA-B antigens has a small statistical chance of matching for loci adjacent to the identifiable HLA-A and B loci, in contrast to the situation with first degree relatives in whom HLA-A and B typing is an excellent marker system for other linked loci. Some of these matches will also include compatibility for HLA-D because of the non-random association of linked genes or linkage disequilibrium. The more homogeneous the population, the greater the likelihood that any given marker will be in linkage disequilibrium with another. This may explain in part the cadaver matching results in recent surveys which range from fair in the US (with a very heterogeneous population) to moderate in Europe, where the population is much more homogeneous[20].

The availability of reagents to type for HLA-DR antigens makes indirect approximation of HLA-D compatibility feasible. With DR typing, the results thus far appear to confirm the importance of matching for both alleles, showing 10% or greater improvement in graft survival over one or zero DR matches. Indeed, although some additional benefit may be gained by HLA-A and B matching, the evidence now suggests that HLA-D and DR are the important antigens in typing cadaver transplants[27,28].

Taken together with the MLR results showing that cadaver transplants survive and function better when donor specific reactivity is low, the data make it apparent that a rapid (24 h) MLR assay would be a very useful technical advance. In practice cadaver kidneys cannot at present be D-matched because MLR takes five days, and of course a cadaver kidney cannot be held that long and then transplanted successfully. It has been shown that DNA synthesis is a late result when lymphocytes or other cells are activated. Therefore it ought to be possible to perceive earlier events that will correlate with ultimate DNA synthesis. One such event is the acquisition of insulin receptors on T cells almost immediately after activation. This phenomenon could be assessed within 24 hours. Moreover there is a close correlation between the amount of insulin bound per cell at 18 hours and the amount of DNA synthesis later[20].

A rapid MLR assay takes advantage of the manufacture of new proteins on the surface of activated lymphocytes. However this approach is only practicable with monoclonal antibody techniques, and requires only a small number of cells. Extensive experiments are being evaluated with different monoclonals, studying the relationship of the new proteins thus defined to a proliferative MLR response.

THE ROLE OF PRESENSITIZATION

It is well known that a positive crossmatch of recipient serum with donor T lymphocytes invites immediate vasculitic 'hyperacute rejection'[29,30,31]. The intense arterial and capillary vasculitis is caused by antibodies to class I antigens. This catastrophe is now largely preventable by careful crossmatching. Donor T lymphocytes from peripheral blood are incubated with recipient serum in a cytotoxic assay to detect antidonor antibodies. A positive crossmatch excludes the prospective donor for the recipient in question. However various surveys have shown that patients producing HLA antibodies against a panel of normal lymphocytes, but negative with respect to a specific donor crossmatch, might still be at risk of accelerated rejection[32,33].

An interesting facet emerged when prospective transplant recipients were monitored to define not only the presence or absence of HLA antibodies but also their specificity. Antibody levels and specificity patterns often fluctuated from one month to the next, sometimes but not always in relation to blood transfusions. Thus the fact that an individual lacks an antibody against a specific donor at the time of transplantation is not a sufficient guarantee against a prior sensitization being in the patient's immunological memory. Once priming has occurred, the secondary immune response induced by the transplant would be more intense and more refractory to immunosuppressive therapy. However various centres nowadays use the criterion that if the current crossmatch between a potential recipient and donor is negative, and a match done on a sample taken at least a year before is positive, the recipient is still eligible for that particular donor – the 'peak positive, current negative' crossmatch approach[34,35]. It has been claimed that such grafts have survived as well as those with peak serum negative crossmatches. Most transplant centres however, still use the most recent and the most positive samples for crossmatching purposes at the time of transplantation.

It has become increasingly clear that a positive crossmatch can be due either to antibodies directed against the HLA antigens or to autolymphocytotoxic antibodies[36]. This finding is important because the latter probably have no deleterious effect on graft survival. Therefore a significant number of patients who may appear highly sensitized, i.e. having antibodies against 85–100% of the members of a lymphocyte panel (and therefore practically untransplantable) could in fact be unnecessarily excluded from transplantation. Up to 50% of such highly sensitizied patients may fall into this category. This finding is therefore of considerable clinical and practical significance. These autoantibodies are known to be IgM and are cytotoxic to both T and B cells. They are cold reacting, acting at 5, 15 and 22 °C. They infrequently react with CLL (chronic lymphatic leukaemia) B lymphocytes and could at least in some instances be directed against surface IgM. The stimulus for their production is not known, although there is a suggestion that they may be virus-induced, particularly by CMV. A crossmatch could usefully include an autocontrol and a CLL B cell panel to identify these autoreactive antibodies in highly sensitized individuals.

Other immunological systems

Antibody dependent cell-mediated cytotoxicity (ADCC) may be another sensitive method for the detection of antibodies important in graft rejection[37]. The target cells from the donor are incubated with the serum from the recipient in order to detect donor-specific antibodies. These cells are lysed by a cell population of normal, non-immune lymphocytes called 'K' cells. Several groups of researchers, including Ting and Morris, correlated graft failure with the presence of a positive ADCC crossmatch[38].

Carpenter and Morris found that the presence of lymphocyte-mediated cytotoxicity (cytotoxic T lymphocytes) directed against donor cells had a striking predictive value, especially in association with positive ADCC reactions[39]. Not all these reactions are against the DR antigens[37]. The lack of complete correlation between cytotoxic crossmatches and rejection may be related to the different cell types involved and their susceptibility to immunosuppressive drugs, or may possibly be due to the subtle degrees of interplay between a cellular and humoral factor.

IMMUNOLOGICAL MONITORING IN ALLOGRAFT TRANSPLANTATION

Although the mechanisms by which T cells induce graft destruction are unknown, it is now well established that allograft rejection does not occur in the absence of thymus derived T cells[40]. The ability to predict clinically irreversible allograft rejection has the merit that cessation of energetic immunosuppressive regimes will protect the recipient from the potentially ravaging side-effects of continued therapy and may allow early surgical removal of the rejected organ. Immunological monitoring may be directed along the following lines:

(1) Assay of recipient immune reactivity to donor antigens e.g. ADCC assays, MLR etc. Their accuracy in predicting rejection, once an organ transplant has been accomplished, is questionable, limiting their clinical usefulness[41,42].

(2) Assessment of recipient responsiveness. This may be assessed in several ways e.g. response to mitogens, delayed hypersensitivity skin tests, monitoring circulating levels of T cells, serum complement, or $\beta2$ microglobulin. The assessment of recipient responsiveness has many advantages. The tests are serially reproducible and relatively simple to perform. There is evidence of reasonable accuracy in

73

predicting rejection, providing a clinically useful guide to subsequent action[43].

BLOOD TRANSFUSION IN TRANSPLANTATION MEDICINE

The role of blood transfusions in transplantation medicine has been highly controversial and at times confusing. Most of the experience has been gained from experimental work in renal transplantation. This has mainly been due to the fact that these patients can be kept relatively well on dialysis prior to transplantation. Moreover many of them need transfusion support. Bone marrow transplant recipients on the other hand have, in view of their intrinsic primary pathology, almost invariably been multi-transfused. In these patients no comparisons could therefore be made between those who have been transfused and those who have not.

Hyperacute rejection was first reported in transplant patients by Kissmeyer -Nielson and Terasaki. They demonstrated the presence of lymphocytotoxic antibodies against the donor as shown in a positive crossmatch in the pre-transplant serum of the recipient, and suggested that these antibodies could be induced by blood transfusions[44,45]. However, in 1973 Opelz et al. reported that the outcome of renal allografts in patients never transfused before transplantation was much worse than that of recipients who had been transfused[46]. Initially their claim was greeted with much scepticism, but later studies, both retrospective and prospective, from numerous transplant centres confirmed the beneficial effect of blood transfusions[47].

Various studies have shown that the more transfusions, the greater the transplant benefit[47,48]. In contrast, others have reported that a single transfusion yielded the maximum benefit[49]. Others still have reported that maximum benefit could be achieved with one to five transfusions, and that more than five transfusions afforded no additional benefit[50,51]. It is unclear whether each transfusion should be a standard unit of blood or whether smaller aliquots (30 mL) would be equally effective. The component of blood required to achieve maximum benefit from pre-transplant transfusions has not yet been established, but it would appear that the buffy coat is critical[52]. In primates, platelet transfusions were reported as being as effective as whole blood without inducing cytotoxic antibodies. In man, however, platelet transfusions were shown not to be effective[53].

The available data indicate that it does not matter whether blood transfusions are given several months or just a few days prior to the transplant, but standard practice is to give up to five planned transfusions at monthly intervals before renal transplantation. Today the benefit of transfusions is no longer in doubt and they are given routinely to all patients awaiting a kidney transplant. A more recently developed and extensively applied method of inducing the beneficial effects of blood transfusion is the deliberate giving of donor-specific transfusions, involving the administration of approximately 300 mL of whole blood on three separate occasions at two-weekly intervals. The graft survival and renal function in patients receiving donor-specific transfusions has been comparable to that of recipients who have received kidneys from HLA-identical sibling donors[54,55] (Chapter 4).

Despite the overwhelming evidence indicating a beneficial effect in renal transplantation, little is known about the mechanism which produces such an effect. There appears to be some relationship to the HLA-DR locus. It has been found that patients who are not transfused will do better if they are DR-matched, but with transfusions the DR-match seems to be less important. Recipients of cadaver grafts having HLA-DR-matched kidneys and those receiving multiple blood transfusions have a transplant success rate of about 90% at one year but these results are not additive[56]. Several mechanisms have however been proposed including:

(1) *Selection of non-responders* Approximately 15–20% of patients receiving multiple blood transfusions are strong responders who become hyperimmunized and are thus essentially eliminated as candidates for transplantation by a positive crossmatch. Thus blood transfusions, by inducing such lymphocytotoxic antibodies, lead to the selection of patients who cannot form donor-specific antibody. Results from several studies indicate, however, that although this type of indirect selection may play some role, it cannot account for the entire beneficial effect of transfusions[57].

(2) *Inactivation of alloreactive clones of cells by immunosuppression* Recently Terasaki has advanced the theory that the renal transplant acts as a secondary stimulus to the transfusion and that the high dose immunosuppression, given at the time of transplantation, kills or inactivates clones of alloreactive cells[58]. He hypothesizes that allo-immunization results from blood transfusions and that subsequent immunosuppression is necessary to achieve the beneficial effect of transfusions. However, transfusions have not been shown to result in alloimmunization as determined by changes in cellular and humoral responses. Also approximately 70% of patients do not develop cytotoxic antibodies following blood transfusions[59]. Therefore this explanation cannot account for all the observed effects of transfusion.

(3) *Induction of suppressor cells* There is considerable evidence to suggest that blood transfusions can induce enhancement or active immunological unresponsiveness to donor's alloantigens in man. This reaction could be induced either by suppressor T cells or by antibodies directed against the T cell antigen-specific receptor i.e. anti-idiotypic antibodies. These antibodies inhibiting proliferative responses of the MLR against antigens on the donor kidney were demonstrable in transplant recipients with functioning allografts but not in patients who rejected the graft[60]. Blood transfusions have been shown to induce non-cytotoxic Fc-receptor blocking antigens[61] and anti-immu-noglobulin antibodies[62]. The relationship between such antibodies and the MLR-inhibiting anti-idiotypic antibodies is not clear.

75

ORGAN TRANSPLANTATION

Four types of grafts are recognized according to the genetic relationship between the donor and recipient. An *allograft* is one transplanted between genetically non-identical members of the same species e.g. transplants between humans excepting those between monozygotic twins. A *syngraft* is one transplanted between genetically identical people e.g. monozygotic twins. An *autograft* is tissue transplanted from one part of the body to another in the same individual. A *xenograft* is one transplanted between members of different species e.g. a baboon kidney into a human. Allografts and xenografts differ from autografts and syngrafts in that they are usually made across histocompatibility barriers.

Kidney

The majority of renal transplants performed in the UK are from non-related cadaver donors and a nationwide system is organized by UKTS to provide the best possible service. Regional transplant centres supply centrally, on a regular basis, to UKTS, names and serological details of all the potential kidney recipients in their region. The main purpose of this register is to ensure that, if a kidney cannot be used locally, either for serological or clinical reasons, then the donor with the best possible match is chosen from a computerized nationwide search of this register.

All potential recipients are ABO grouped, and HLA-A, B, C and DR typed. Moreover they are screened for HLA antibodies on a regular basis. When a donor becomes available, the donor is also grouped for ABO, and HLA typed for class I and DR antigens using standard serological techniques. On the basis of these data a short list of potential recipients is drawn up. Depending on the clinical state of the particular patients at the time of the transplant, some of those short listed may be excluded on clinical grounds. After a final selection is made a serological crossmatch between the donor and the potential recipients is performed and on the basis of this a final recipient is chosen for the transplant operation. If nobody is found to be suitable locally, then the kidney is exported to another centre. Data regarding the donor's serological details are notified to UKTS and the kidney is then offered to the patient with the best chance of successfully receiving that particular kidney.

Although an identical match is an ideal state of affairs, in the vast majority of cases this is not possible. However it has been shown that with a negative crossmatch at the time of the transplant, matching for the HLA-B and particularly DR loci is very important. With the advent of cyclosporin, some centres have performed kidney transplants in the face of complete mismatches and claim that such matching is not important[63]. If these findings are confirmed, the practice of renal transplantation will change. If tissue typing is not even necessary at the DR locus then most kidneys will be transplanted in the local centre. However, in view of the side effects, expense and lack of knowledge of the long-term sequelae of cyclosporin one has at present to be cautious about its overuse and close HLA matching should be the aim.

Patients with multispecific HLA antibodies present a major problem because they are very difficult to transplant. As previously described, the activity of these antibodies varies with time. Therefore many centres use the current sample for crossmatching in these patients along with the sample with the highest reactivity over the recent past (one year). It has been claimed that the long- and short-term graft and patient survivals in such peak positive crossmatch patients is equivalent to those with a negative crossmatch on all available sera[34,35].

Bone marrow

ABO identity between bone marrow donor and recipient is not essential for the successful outcome of bone marrow transplantation[14,15]. In fact numerous centres have transplanted bone marrow in the face of major ABO incompatibilities[14].

With the accumulation of the experience obtained in renal transplantation, the importance of the HLA-D related region was appreciated[64,65,66,67]. Patients and their usually related potential donors are matched for the D-region using the MLR, and even if they are incompatible for the HLA-A, B and C loci they may still be grafted with increasing success when appropriate pretreatment is prescribed. The major immunological complication of bone marrow transplantation is graft versus host (GVH) disease. It was realized that GVH could be minimized by depleting the marrow transplant of its mature lymphocyte population, particularly T-cells[68].

Bone marrow transplantation has been almost exclusively undertaken using family members who are fully HLA-matched–thus imposing a considerable restriction on the availability of the technique. Clinical studies will determine whether full HLA matching is a prerequisite for success. Initial results indicate substantial difficulties unless the patient is quite young. Relatively little is known about the use of unrelated HLA-phenotypically matched donors. As panel registries become better established such an approach may be feasible. Both the UKTS and private enterprises (e.g. The Anthony Nolan Foundation) have set up Bone Marrow Voluntary Registries. As a result of an increased number of requests for bone marrow transplantation, there has been a sudden increase in the number of potential donors who need typing. This has caused significant problems in terms of workload and reagent availability, particularly for DR typing. The ideal situation would be to have all potential donors DR typed, but DR typing sera are in short supply. Therefore HLA-A and B typing are done by the 'donor' centres and the DR typing is done by the 'patient' centres after selection of potential donors for a particular recipient on the basis of HLA-A and B identity.

Preliminary data indicate that the ideal unrelated donor would be HLA-DR identical and MLR negative. However, only 10% of HLA-A and B identical donors who are DR typed are identical with the patient, and of these only a quarter are MLR negative. Moreover, preliminary data indicate that there is an increased incidence of GHVD when using unrelated donors for bone marrow transplantation[69].

Liver

Few centres throughout the world have a wide experience in hepatic transplantation, with only a few institutions having performed more than a dozen cases[70]. Recipient ABO incompatibility with the donor is avoided wherever possible[13] but due to problems with organ procurement and the clinical circumstances that prompt a liver transplant this is not always possible. The influence of tissue typing on human liver transplantation is still somewhat unclear. It appears, however, that rigorous HLA crossmatching may increase the survival rate in liver transplants[71], although donors and recipients are not usually immunologically matched[72]. Some information is available on the influence of donor-specific T cell antibodies in the serum of the recipients[73]. Most of this work has been done on patents who require a retransplant. Interestingly, retransplantation did not occur with greater frequency in those with positive crossmatches than in those with negative ones.

The liver allograft is less sensitive to acute rejection than most other organs even in the face of ABO incompatibility and when lymphocytotoxic antibodies are present[74]. Whether the resistance is a consequence of the vascular architecture of the liver or results from an immunological property of the liver has yet to be determined.

Pancreas

Pancreatic transplantation is still in its infancy. Most pancreatic transplants have been performed in diabetic patients with advanced complications. Most have had diabetic nephropathy treated with a renal transplant either before or after the pancreatic transplant. If the pancreatic and renal transplants are obtained from the same donor, the usual selection criteria for renal transplants apply. Pancreatic transplants have, however, been performed in the face of HLA mismatches, from both cadaver and living related donors[75]. Particularly high survival rates are obtained either in HLA-identical siblings, as expected, or with related donors who have previously donated kidneys to the same recipients irrespective of the HLA match. Conversely the graft survival rates for HLA-mismatched grafts are low from either related or cadaver donors in recipients who have not received kidney transplants, or in those who have previously received a kidney transplant from a different donor to the one providing the pancreas. Methods of depleting the transplanted pancreas of DR-carrying passenger leucocytes help to reduce the incidence and severity of the rejection process[76].

Heart and valves

This group of transplantations encompasses allogenic and xenogeneic valve replacements. Xenogeneic valve replacements performed now are either bovine or porcine. Initial reports with unmodified valve allografts showed a reasonably high proportion of cell-mediated and humoral immunity developing to the grafts[77]. Therefore modification of the grafts using chemical or physical means to reduce the antigenicity of these valves has been employed.

Patients receiving xenoallografts of heart valves are not immunosuppressed post-operatively because only very minor graft rejection reactions take place in the modified valves.

The criteria for selecting the donor and recipient combination for cardiac transplantation are essentially those used for cadaveric renal transplantation. Prospective recipients are usually screened using standard microcytotoxicity assays. If the results are negative or if the reactivity is very low (and only with uncommon HLA antigens) a heart transplant can safely be performed with a prospective crossmatch.

Patients with reactivity against the HLA panel should have a prospective crossmatch, especially if the reactivity occurs against common HLA antigens[78]. The desperate clinical circumstances that prompt cardiac transplantation do not lend themselves to a good HLA match. Most grafts are therefore performed despite multiple HLA incompatibilities[79,80].

Cornea

Corneal transplantation has an extremely high success rate because of the ease in obtaining and storing viable corneas. Because of the avascularity of this tissue and its relatively low concentration of class I antigens and essential absence of class II antigens, rejection episodes are uncommon. Avascular corneal grafts exclude lymphocytes and vascularized grafts undergo rejection. Immunosuppression is not provided routinely. It has been shown that in vascularized grafts, the likelihood of graft failure is closely related to the degree of matching for HLA[81].

Lung

Technical, logistical and immunological reasons have made the development of lung transplantation very difficult. Lungs are extremely sensitive to ischaemic damage and preservation techniques have been unsuccessful. Rejection is common and extremely severe because of the large number of passenger leucocytes trapped within the alveoli and blood vessels. The only immunological criterion for selection used in various centres is ABO compatibility[82]. Therefore, because of the massive immunosuppression necessary to maintain engraftment, many recipients have ultimately succumbed to severe infections[83]. Occasionally combined heart and lung transplants have been performed. Technically the procedure is less difficult than single organ transplantation.

Bone

The solid matrix of bone and its lack of significant quantities of immunological material make transplantation a potentially easy procedure with little need for immunosuppression[84].

Skin

The immunology and pathology of rejection has been studied most extensively in animal models of skin-graft rejection. Skin has an extremely high density of class I and class II histocompatibility antigens, thus facilitating sensitization and recognition of antigen differences and resulting in vigorous rejection. The use of skin allografts has been practised in major burn centres, with rather unpredictable survival times. Many factors affect graft survival but prolonged acceptance of such allografts is more likely if the donor and recipient are well matched for HLA[85]. With the development of non-immunogenic skin replacement materials, allografts of skin are needed less today.

CONCLUSION

Over the past several decades, there has been enormous progress in the understanding of the major histocompatibility complex. Although many questions have been resolved, a greater number remain to be answered. It is clear that the MHC plays a major role in transplantation medicine. It is hoped that future studies will result in new ways of manipulating the responses to MHC gene products, allowing clinical improvements in organ transplantation and the treatment of immune disease.

References

1. Roitt, I., Brostoff, J. and Male, D. (1985). *Immunology*. p. 41. (Edinburgh: Churchill Livingstone)
2. Green, C. (1983). *Organ Transplantation*, p. 1–21. (Oxford: Medical Publishing Foundation)
3. Hackel, E. and Fisher, R. (1982). Theoretical Aspects of HLA Genetics and Biology. In Hackel, E. and Mallory, D. (eds.) *Theoretical Aspects of HLA*, pp. 5–8. (California: AABB)
4. Bodmer, J. and Bodmer, W. (1984). Histocompatibility 1984. *Immunol. Today*, **4(7)**, 253–4
5. Schwartz, B. D. (1982). The Major Histocompatibility HLA Complex. In Stites, D. P., Stobo, J. D., Fudenberg, H. H. and Wells, J. V. (eds.) *Basic and Clinical Immunology*, pp. 52–64 (Lange Medical Publications)
6. Bodmer, W. F. and Bodmer, J. G. (1978). Evolution and function of the HLA system. *Br. Med. Bull.*, **34**, 309–16
7. Awdeh, Z. L., Eynon, E., Stein, R., Alper, C. A., Alosco, S. M. and Yunis, E. J. (1985). Unrelated individuals matched for MHC extended haplotypes and HLA identical siblings show comparable responses in mixed leucocyte culture. *Lancet*, **2**, 853–5
8. Awdeh, Z. L., Raum, D., Yunis, E. J. and Alper, C. A. (1983). Extended GLA/complement allele haplotypes: evidence for T/t like complex in man. *Proc. Natl. Acad. Sci. USA.*, **80**, 259–63
9. Pollack, M. S., Chin-Louie, J. and Callaway, M. (1983). Unrelated bone marrow transplantation donors for patients with HLA B/DR haplotypes with significant genetic disequilibrium. *Transplant Proc.*, **15**, 1420–3
10. Marcadet, A., Cohen, D., Dausset, J., Fisher, A., Durandy, A. and Griscelli, C. (1985). Genotyping with DNA probes in combined immunodeficiency syndromes with defective expression of HLA. *N. Engl. J. Med.*, **20**, 1287–92
11. Burger, R. (1986). Complement research – the impact of molecular genetics. *Immunol. Today*, **7(2)**, 27–33
12. Paul, W. E. (1984). Immune response genes. In Paul, W. E. (ed.) *Fundamental Immunology*, p. 15. (New York: Raven Press)
13. Ramsay, G., Nusbacher, J., Starlz, T. and Lindsay, G. D. (1984). Isohaemagglutinins of graft origin after ABO-unmatched liver transplantation. *N. Engl. J. Med.*, **311**, 1167–70
14. Berkman, E. M., Caplan, S. and Kim, C. S. (1978). ABO incompatible bone marrow transplantation: preparation by plasma exchange and *in vivo* antibody absorption. *Transfusion*, **18**, 504–8

15. Buckner, C. D., Clift, R. A., Sanders, J. E., Williams, B., Gray, M., Storb, R. and Thomas, E. D. (1978). ABO incompatible marrow transplants. *Transplantation*, **26**, 233–8
16. Heishko, C., Gale, R. P., How, C. and Fitchen, J. (1980). ABH antigens and bone marrow transplantation. *Br. J. Haematol.*, **44**, 65–73
17. Kachi, K. K., Andersson, L. C., Vuopio, P. and Gahenberg, C. G. (1981). Expression of blood group A antigens in human bone marrow cells. *Blood*, **57**, 147–51
18. Mangal, A. K., Growe, G. H., Sinclair, M., Stillwell, G. F., Reeve, C. E. and Naiman, S. C. (1984). Acquired haemolytic anaemia due to 'auto' anti A or 'auto' anti B induced by group O homograft in renal transplant patients. *Transfusion*, **24(3)**, 201–5
19. Britton, S. and Palacios, R. (1982). Cyclosporin A – Usefulness, risks and mechanism of action. *Immunol. Rev.*, **65**, 5–22
20. Carpenter, C. B. and Strom, T. B. (1982). Transplantation: immunogenetic and clinical aspects – Part 1. *Hosp. Pract.*, **17(12)**, 125–34
21. Lafferty, K. J., Prowse, S. J. and Simeonevic, C. J. (1983). Immunobiology of tissue transplantation: A return to the leucocyte concept. *Ann. Rev. Immunol.*, **1**, 143–73
22. Sholz, D. and Mebel, M. (1983). The significance of sex determined antigens for kidney transplantation prognosis – an analysis of 500 transplantations at a centre. *J. Urol. Nephrol.*, **76**, 209–17
23. Wick, M. R. and Moore, S. B. (1984). The role of the Lewis antigen system in renal transplantation and allograft rejection. *Mayo Clinic Proc.*, **59**, 423–8
24. Cross, D. E., Coxe-Gilliland, R. and Weaver, P. (1979). DR antigen matching and B cell antibody crossmatching: their effect on clinical outcome of renal transplants. *Transplant. Proc.*, **11**, 1908–10
25. Kristensen, T. and Madsen, M. (1983). One way positive cellular reactions between two HLA-A, B, C, D/DR genetically identical brothers following active allogeneic immunization. *Tissue Antigens*, **22**, 359–71
26. Pollack, M. S., Chin-Louie, J. and Callaway, C. (1983). Mixed lymphocyte reactions for individuals with phenotypic identity for specific HLA-B, DR determinants. The role of linkage disequilibrium and of specific DR and other class II determinants. *J. Clin. Immunol.*, **3**, 341–51
27. Kreisler, J. M. (1982). The role of immunological parameters in kidney transplantation. *Proc. EDTA*, **19**, 407–23
28. Muller, G. A., Muller, C. and Wernet, P. (1982). Improved kidney graft survival through HLA-DR matching. *Proc. EDTA*, **19**, 464–8
29. Opelz, G. and Terasaki, P. I. (1976). Significance of a positive crossmatch prior to renal transplantation. *Transplantation*, **21**, 483–7
30. Cicciarelli, J. C. and Terasaki, P. I. (1983). Vasculitis rejection with donor lymphocytotoxic antibodies. *Transplant. Proc.*, **15**, 1208–10
31. Kocandrle, V., Macunova, H., Ivashova, E., Reneltova, I., Sajdlova, H., Kupkova, L. and Jirka, J. (1985). Presensitization of recipients and its significance in kidney transplantation. *Transplant. Proc.*, **17**, 2457–60
32. Bradley, B. A., Klouda, P. T., Ray, T. C. and Gore, S. M. (1985). Negative crossmatch selection of kidneys for highly sensitized patients. *Transplant Proc.*, **17**, 2465–6
33. Klouda, P. T., Ray, T. C., Bowerman, P. and Bradley, B. A. (1985). The prediction of a negative crossmatch in highly sensitized patients. *Transplant. Proc.*, **17**, 2467–8
34. Cardella, C. J., Falk, J. A. and Nicholson, M. J. (1982). Renal transplantation with a positive historical crossmatch. *Lancet*, **2**, 1240–3
35. Goeken, N. E. (1985). Outcome of renal transplantation following a positive crossmatch with historical sera: the second analysis of the ASHI Survey. *Transplant. Proc.*, **17**, 2443–5
36. Ting, A., Williams, K. A. and Morris, P. J. (1978). Transplantation: immunological monitoring. *Br. Med. Bull.*, **34**, 263–70
37. Carpenter, C. B. and Strom, T. B. (1980). Transplantation immunology. In Parker, C. W. (ed.) *Clinical Immunology* p. 376. (Philadelphia: W. B. Saunders)
38. Ting, A. and Morris, P. J. (1980). Matching for B cell antigens of the HLA-DR series in cadaver renal transplantation. *Lancet*, **1**, 575–7
39. Carpenter, C. B. and Morris, P. J. (1978). The detection and measurement of pretransplant sensitization. *Transplant. Proc.*, **10**, 509–13
40. Marks, C. (1983). Immunological determinants in organ transplantation. *Ann. R. Coll. Surg. Engl.*, **65**, 139–44

41. McWinnie, D. L., Curter, N. P., Taylor, H. M., Chapman, J. R. and Wood, R. F. M. (1985). Is the T4/T8 ratio an irrelevance in renal transplantation monitoring? *Transplant. Proc.*, **17**, 2548–9

42. Curtoni, E. S., Amoroso, A., Vercelloni, A., Practico, L., Tacconella, M. and Crepaldi, T. (1985). Antibody monitoring after kidney transplantation. *Transplant. Proc.*, **17**, 81–2

43. Loveland, B. E. and Mckenzie, H. C. (1982). Which T cells cause graft rejection? *Transplantation*, **33**, 217–9

44. Kissmeyer-Nielson, F., Olsen, S., Peterson, V. P. and Fjelborg, O. (1966). Hyperacute rejection of kidney allografts with pre-existing humoral antibodies against donor cells. *Lancet*, **2**, 662–5

45. Terasaki, P. I., Thrasher, D. L. and Hauber, T. H. (1968). Serotyping for homotransplantation. Immediate kidney transplant rejection and associated performed antibodies. In Dausset, J., Hamburger, J. and Mathe, T. (eds.) *Advances in Transplantation*, pp. 225–229. (Copenhagen: Munksgaard)

46. Opelz, G., Singar, D. P. S., Mickey, M. R. and Terasaki, P. I. (1973). Effect of blood transfusion on subsequent kidney transplants. *Transplant. Proc.*, **5**, 253–9

47. Terasaki, P. I. (ed.) (1982). First international symposium on the role of blood transfusion and transplantation. *Transplant. Proc.*, **14**, 247–433

48. Opelz, G. and Terasaki, P. I. (1978). Improvement of kidney-graft survival with increased number of blood transfusions. *N. Engl. J. Med.*, **299**, 799–803

49. Persijn, G. G., Cohen, B., Lamburger, Q. and van Rood, J. J. (1979). Retrospective and prospective studies on the effect of blood transfusions in renal transplantation in the Netherlands. *Transplantation*, **28**, 396–401

50. Vincenti, F., Duca, R., Amend, W. J. C., Perkins, H. A., Cochrum, K., Feduska, N. J. and Salvatierra, O. (1978). Immunologic factors determining survival of cadaver kidney transplants. *N. Engl. J. Med.*, **299**, 793–8

51. Suchia, G., Mercuriali, F., Pizzi, C., SanSecondo, V. E. M. R., Borzini, P. and Ariasi, A. (1982). Blood transfusion and kidney transplantation: effect of small doses of blood on kidney graft function and survival. *Transplant Proc.*, **14**, 263–71

52. Okazaki, H., Takahashi, H., Muira, K., Ishizaki, M., Oguma, S. and Taguhi, Y. (1985). Effect of buffy coat transfusions in living related and cadaveric renal transplantation. *Transplant. Proc.*, **17**, 1034–7

53. Chapman, J. R., Fisher, M., Ting, A. and Morris, P. J. (1985). Platelet transfusions before renal transplantation in humans. *Transplant. Proc.*, **17**, 1038–40

54. Anderson, C. B., Sicard, G. A., Rodney, G. E., Anderman, C. K. and Etheredge, E. E. (1983). Renal allograft recipient pretreatment with donor specific blood and concomitant immunosuppression. *Transplant. Proc.*, **15**, 939–42

55. Mendez, R., Iwaki, Y., Mendez, R., Boggard, T., Self, B. and Terasaki, P. I. (1983). Donor specific blood transfusions: their immunological effect and allograft outcome. *Transplant. Proc.*, **15**, 946–51

56. Strom, T. B., Tilney, N. L. and Merrill, J. P. (1981). Renal transplantation: clinical management of the transplant recipient. In Brenner, B. M. and Rector, F. C. (eds.) *Kidney*. pp. 2618–58. (Philadelphia: W. B. Saunders)

57. Iwaki, Y., Kirukawa, T., Terasaki, P. I., Mickey, M. R. and Ono, Y. (1983). Donor specific transfusions from unrelated dogs and evidence against the selection mechanism. *Transplant. Proc.*, **15**, 979–84

58. Terasaki, P. I. (1984). The beneficial transfusions effect on kidney graft survival attributed to clonal deletion. *Transplantation*, **37**, 119–25

59. Opelz, G., Mickey, M. R. and Terasaki, P. I. (1981). Blood transfusions and kidney transplants: remaining controversies. *Transplant. Proc.*, **13**, 136–41

60. Singal, D. P. and Joseph, S. (1982). Role of blood transfusions on the induction of antibodies against recognition sites on T lymphocytes in transplant patients. *Human Immunol.*, **4**, 93–108

61. MacLeod, A. M., Mason, R. J., Stewart, K. N., Power, D. A., Shewan, W. G., Edward, N. and Catto, G. R. D. (1983). Fc receptor blocking antibodies develop after blood transfusions and correlate with good graft outcome. *Transplant. Proc.*, **15**, 1019–21

62. Chia, D., Horime, T., Terasaki, P. I. and Hermes, M. (1982). Association of anti Fab and anti IgG antibodies with high kidney transplant survival. *Transplant. Proc.*, **14**, 322–4

63. Calne, R. Y. (1985). Organ transplantation from laboratory to clinic. *Br. Med. J.*, **291**, 1751–4
64. Dupon, B. and Hansen, J. A. (1978). Donor selection for bone marrow transplantation: the predictive role of HLA-D typing for MLR compatibility between unrelated individuals. *Transplant. Proc.*, **10**, 53–6
65. Hansen, J. A., Clift, R. A. and Thomas, E. D. (1979). Histocompatibility and marrow transplantation. *Transplant. Proc.*, **11**, 1924–9
66. Hansen, J. A., O'Reilly, R. J. and Good, R. A. (1976). Relevance of major histocompatibility determinants in clinical bone marrow transplantation. *Transplant. Proc.*, **8**, 581–9
67. Neithammer, D., Goldman, S. F. and Haas, R. J. (1978). Bone marrow transplantation for severe combined immunodeficiency with HLA incompatible but MLC identical mother as a donor. *Tansplant. Proc.*, **10**, 43–6
68. DeWitte, T., Raymoker, R. and Plas, A. (1984). Bone marrow repopulation capacity after transplantation of lymphocyte depleted allogeneic bone marrow using counterflow centrifugation. *Transplantation*, **37**, 151–5
69. Hansen, J. A., Clift, R. A., Thomas, E. D., Buckner, C. D., Storb, R. and Giblett, E. R. (1980). Transplantation of marrow from an unrelated donor to a patient with acute leukaemia. *N. Engl. J. Med.*, **303**, 565–7
70. Starlz, T. E. Iwatsuki, B., Shaw, B. W. and Gordon, R. D. (1985). Orthoptic liver transplantation in 1984. *Transplant Proc.*, **17**, 250–8
71. Takacs, L., Szende, B. and Monostori, E. (1983). Expression of HLA-DR antigens on bile duct cells of rejected liver transplant. *Lancet*, **2**, 365–6
72. Starlz, T. E., Iwatsuki, S. and Van Thiel, D. H. (1982). Criteria for hepatic transplantation. *Hepatology*, **2**, 614–8
73. Shaw, B. W., Gordon, R. D., Iwatsuki, S. and Starlz, T. E. (1985). Hepatic transplantation. *Transplant. Proc.*, **17**, 264–71
74. Houssin, D., Gugenheim, J., Bellon, B., Brunaud, M. D., Gıgou, M., Charra, M., Crougneau, S. and Bismuth, H. (1985). Absence of hyperacute rejection of liver allografts in hypersensitized rats. *Transplant. Proc.*, **17**, 293–5
75. Sutherland, D. E. R., Goetz, F. C., Kendall, D. M. and Najarian, J. S. (1985). Effect of donor source, technique, immunosuppression, and presence or absence of end stage diabetic nephropathy on outcome in pancreas transplant recipient. *Transplant. Proc.*, **17**, 325–330
76. Nocera, A., Leprini, A., Fontana, I., Arcini, V., Barocci, S., Damianı, G., Celada, F. and Valente, U. (1985). HLA-DR bearing cells in human pancreas. *Transplant. Proc.*, **17**, 144–6
77. Barbarash, L. S. (1972). Immunobiological aspects of cardiac allo- and xenovalve transplantation. *Kardiologia*, **12(3)**, 150–7
78. Bieber, C. P., Oyer, P. E. and David, L. (1974). Serum antithymocyte globulin (ATG) and anti ATG levels in cardiac recipients. *Surg. Forum*, **25**, 285–7
79. Thomas, F. T., Wolf, J. S. and Thomas, J. M. (1974). Specific immunosuppression in cardiac allografting using anti thymocyte sera and soluble transplantation antigens. *Ann. Thor. Surg.*, **18**, 241–9
80. Bolman, R. M., Anderson, R. W., Elrick, B., Ascher, N. and Simmons, R. L. (1985). Cardiac transplantation without a prospective crossmatch. *Transplant. Proc.*, **17**, 209–10
81. Kissmeyer-Nielson, F., Ehlers, N. and Kristensen, T. (1977). HLA system – new aspects. In Ferrrara, G. B. (ed.) *Proceedings of the International Symposium. Bergamo, Italy*, pp. 69–91. (Amsterdam: Elsevier)
82. Hakim, M. and Wallwork, J. (1980). Heart lung transplantation. *Hosp. Update*, **9**, 653–63
83. Kusijama, K. (1985). Hyperacute pulmonary rejection. *J. Jpn. Ass. Thor. Surg.*, **23**, 1412–20
84. Solinger, A. (1985). Organ transplantation and the immune response gene. *Med. Clin. N. Am.*, **69**, 565–83

4
The Blood Transfusion Effect

J. M. BONE AND A. N. HILLIS

INTRODUCTION

The transfusion effect in clinical transplantation today refers to the beneficial effect on renal allograft survival from blood or blood products given to the patient in the weeks, months or even years prior to his operation. Fifteen years ago, a discussion on the effects of blood transfusions would have emphasized the dangers from the increased risk of accelerated graft loss from hyperacute rejection (see Chapter 1). The reversal of opinion and practice that has taken place in the last 5 years illustrates one of the more interesting paradoxes in modern medicine, and it is one of the purposes of this account to attempt its resolution.

The same period has also seen a major improvement in the results of transplantation. In 1970 the average patient awaiting a cadaveric graft might live in the rather forlorn hope of barely a 50% chance of being alive, well and off dialysis two years after surgery. For a kidney from a poorly matched relative, the results were only slightly better. Today many centres achieve cadaveric graft survival rates of 80%, and poorly matched relatives can undergo a major and painful operation with a 95% expectation that their gift will not have been wasted. While improvements in other directions have made major contributions, there can be few doubts now that planned blood transfusions can make their own very significant impact. It will be argued that the potential benefit of blood transfusions now greatly outweighs the risks.

Future prospects can only be predicted after careful analysis of past experience. For this reason much of the following account is historical, if such an adjective can be applied to only forty years of clinical and experimental endeavour.

BLOOD TRANSFUSION

The history of blood transfusion itself abounds with similar twists and inconsistencies[1]. The ancients believed that the spirit of life circulates in the blood and might thus be transferred to another individual. Advice given to Noah in a personal communication from God* was incorporated into Mosaic and Islamic law and underlies the refusal of Jehovah's Witnesses to accept transfusions of blood or blood products today.

The first experiment to question this advice was performed in Oxford in February 1666 when Dr Richard Lower took blood from two very large mastiffs and gave a much smaller dog what was essentially an exchange transfusion. There must have been some disappointment when the smaller dog did not take on the physical form or the temperament of the larger, more aggressive animal, but no thunderbolt fell.

In the seventeenth century, deeply held convictions were not easily dispelled and further attempts were made to modify behaviour using blood transfusions. The following year in France, Professor Denis and a surgeon, Mr Emmerez, transfused five patients with the blood of a lamb or calf. The last patient, a noted lecher, was given calf's blood in order that 'its mildness and freshness might allay the ebulition of his blood'. He had a bad reaction to his second transfusion, and died after the third. Although his wife was subsequently convicted for his murder by arsenic poisoning and executed, the news halted the progress of transfusion for more than one hundred and fifty years.

In the early 1800s, when Mary Shelley was writing *Frankenstein*, Dr Blundell at Guy's and St Thomas's Hospitals showed that dogs would tolerate blood transfusion from dogs but not from different species. He also safely performed the first transfusions between humans. Nevertheless, so many doctors continued to use lamb's blood, that by the 1890s a not so jocular observation was that three sheep were needed: the donor sheep, the 'sheepish' human recipient, and the even more sheepish physician who had been persuaded against his better judgement.

Identification of the major red cell antigens by Landsteiner in 1901 allowed the safe transfusion of some battle casualties in the First World War. The Second World War gave a further impetus to investigate mechanisms of allograft rejection when skin homografts were used to treat severely burned aircrew.

Origin of the blood transfusion effect

The classical observations made by Medawar during the Second World War[2] indicated that rabbits could be immunized against skin grafting by intradermal injection of leukocytes, but not red cells, from their prospective donor. Signs of accelerated rejection were similar to those seen when skin itself was used for immunization, suggesting that leukocytes and skin share antigens that distinguish 'self' from 'non-self'.

The route of administration was important, however, as the same dose of leukocytes given intravenously had no effect, and only minimal sensitization followed the massive donation (for a rabbit) of 72 mL whole blood. Experience in man had already shown that transfusions were safe after red cell crossmatch–although later studies demonstrated that viable leukocytes could

*But the flesh with the life thereof, which is the blood thereof, ye shall not eat. (Genesis IXv4)

induce antibody formation in patients given multiple transfusions. It was therefore suggested that antigens which could harm a transplant might exist in blood. Indeed, transfused blood might itself be viewed as a 'liquid allograft'. These and other studies demonstrated an *adverse* effect of blood transfusion on subsequent transplantation. At the same time, however, the nature of 'tolerance' by an animal of foreign tissues was also being explored, raising the possibility that prior exposure to donor-specific antigen might be *beneficial*[3].

The earliest clinical blood transfusion effect might even date from these wartime experiences, but was not recognized by the plastic surgeons working with skin homografts. All grafts were ultimately rejected and absorbed but survival ranged widely from days to weeks. While infection, the type of graft used, and difficulties in recognizing rejection contributed to the differences reported, blood transfusions were occasionally given and may have had some influence. An example, and guide to earlier literature is provided by Gibson and Medawar[4].

The transfusion effect in clinical practice might be summarized in terms of the algebraic sum of tolerance and sensitization. Throughout the following account, the balance between these two major but opposite influences will be a recurring theme.

Induction of unresponsiveness (tolerance) by administration of donor antigens

The original observations of tolerance by one animal of the tissues of another arose from one of nature's own transplant experiments in the farmyard[5,6]. A freemartin is the female of a pair of twin calves of unlike sex that shows imperfect development through mixture of cells in a fused placenta. The word appeared in English in the same century as the first experiment in blood transfusion, and its biological significance was equally slow to emerge. Before and after birth, a freemartin and its twin although exposed to foreign tissue antigens on each other's blood cells, yet tolerate their presence with no antibody response. This chimeric state continues until adult life: tolerance of antigens in other tissues was shown when skin grafts between the two animals were not rejected[6]. The next step for scientists was induction of neonatal tolerance in other animals by the introduction of foreign antigen just after birth, before maturation of immunity allowed recognition of non-self from self[3].

In adults, however, it was (and still is) much more difficult to achieve unresponsiveness which allowed successful homografting, and in the laboratory both specific and non-specific measures were required (Table 4.1). The ultimate goal in experimental and clinical transplantation is to develop tolerance to foreign tissues with minimal need for non-specific measures and their attendant risks. Prior administration of donor antigen appeared to offer the best approach. A wide variety of cells and sub-cellular extracts have been given intravenously and intraperitoneally for this purpose[7].

From the outset, the dosage of antigen was recognized as crucial. This was first seen when large amounts of a non-tissue protein, diphtheria toxin,

Table 4.1 Methods of inducing tolerance in adults

Antigen non-specific	Antigen specific
Drugs:	Blood cells:
prednisolone	whole blood, red cells, white cells, platelets
azathioprine	
cyclophosphamide	Cellular suspensions from lympho-reticular tissues:
cyclosporin A	lymph nodes, spleen, bone marrow, thymus, liver, skin
antilymphocyte globulin	Subcellular extracts from lympho-reticular tissues:
Total lymphoid irradiation	cell membrane, soluble antigen
Thoracic duct drainage	

surprisingly failed to produce immunization[8]. As noted already, small doses of leukocytes given intradermally did not induce tolerance but immunized against skin grafting[2]. The response to larger doses of tissue antigens was soon found to have an effect similar to large doses of other foreign proteins[7].

Since cellular mechanisms of immune regulation had not been discovered, unresponsiveness was attributed to the production of 'enhancing' antibodies[9]. Such humoral factors are still thought to have a role. However, once the lymphocyte pool had been sub-divided and the functional characteristics of the different components appreciated, suppressor T cells had also to be considered.

BLOOD TRANSFUSION EFFECT IN CLINICAL TRANSPLANTATION

In clinical practice, the effect of prior administration of blood or blood products has been explored in two different contexts, depending on the source of the kidney.

Living related donor (LRD) transplantation: effect of donor-specific transfusion (DST)

The voluntary donation of a kidney by a living relative (LRD) allows planned transfusion of blood from donor to prospective recipient. Such donor-specific transfusion (DST) provides the closest analogy in man with animal studies. Furthermore, it should be relatively easy in theory to control the conditions under which donor-specific antigen is presented, and to observe changes produced. In practice this has not always proved possible.

Early attempts were successful if somewhat cumbersome. Batchelor and colleagues[10] immunized the father of a uraemic child with serial injections of leukocytes from the mother. Lymphocytotoxic antibodies which developed in the father were extracted and rendered harmless by enzyme digestion followed by separation of immunoglobulin Fc fragments. These 'enhancing antibodies' were given to the child intravenously when the mother's kidney was transplanted, and for the treatment of acute rejecton: only small doses of azathioprine and prednisolone were subsequently required as maintenance anti-rejection therapy.

Newton and Anderson[11] gave lymphocytes from two related (but mismatched) and two unrelated kidney donors by subcutaneous and intravenous injection to prospective recipients immunosuppressed by azathioprine. Transplantation was successful in all four: three patients escaped with no acute rejection, a phenomenon then unique in the authors' experience. Lymphocytotoxic antibodies against donor cells were found in sera from one patient at the outset, but the injections were given safely, and the kidney tolerated. Not surprisingly the benefit was ascribed to enhancing antibody.

Salvatierra and his colleagues[12] were encouraged by this, by animal studies, and by the apparent benefits of third party blood transfusions given pre-operatively to recipients of cadaveric transplants[13]. They determined to try to improve graft survival in 45 patients receiving kidneys from antigenically disparate living relatives by giving donor-specific blood transfusions prior to transplantation. Earlier results with LRD transplants, which were mismatched for one or both HLA haplotypes and which had highly reactive mixed lymphocyte cultures (MLC) were poor: the one-year graft survival in 34 patients was only 56%. From 1978, such patients were given three fortnightly transfusions of 200 mL fresh whole blood from their kidney donor and were transplanted usually 3–6 weeks after the last transfusion. No immunosuppression was given to cover DST. Azathioprine and prednisolone were used after transplantation in a regimen that had been unchanged since 1972, and was used for the 34 haplo-mismatched LRD patients not given DST.

Graft survival in 30 patients transplanted after DST increased to 94% at one year. Episodes of acute rejection occurred earlier (1–4 d after transplantation in 5 out of 10 patients) but less frequently and were more easily reversed. No graft was lost from hyperacute rejection. Many patients, however, had also been given bank blood from unrelated donors (third-party blood) before transplantation.

Experience in 172 patients with 101 planned transplants over 4 years was reported in 1983[14] (Figure 4.1)–the three-year graft survival was 87%. There was benefit, too, from third-party blood alone, in 24 haplo-mismatched patients not given DST, but graft survival fell from 70% at one year to 66% at three years, indicating that protection was not as good.

Unfortunately, the price of DST was sensitization of 30% of recipients to their potential donors. Many also developed antibodies against random panel lymphocytes, but none were broadly sensitized and DST did not adversely affect the chances of a subsequent transplant from a cadaveric donor or indeed from another living relative. Sensitization both to donor and to panel lymphocytes was greater in patients receiving third-party blood in addition to DST.

While induction of donor-specific immunological unresponsiveness might best explain the DST mechanism, DST might merely have selected patients whose immunological systems were naturally more responsive to their donor. These high responders would be more readily sensitized and would develop lymphocytotoxic antibodies preventing transplantation. Excellent results

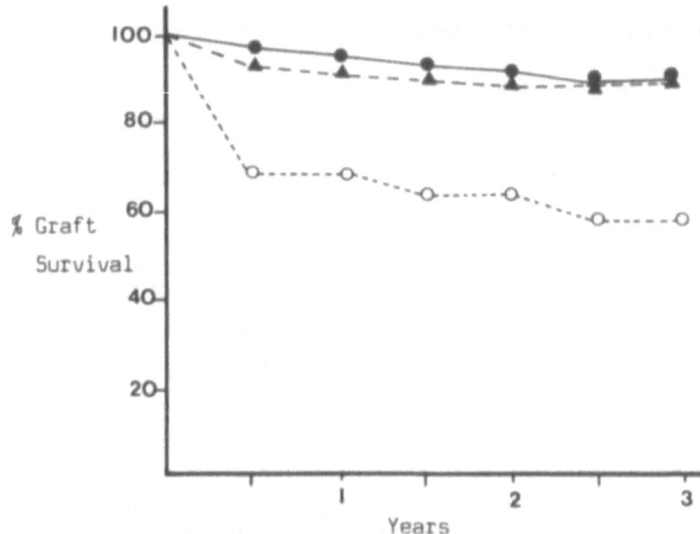

Figure 4.1 Effect of DST on survival of non-identical, MLC-reactive LRD grafts. ● DST; ○ one haplo-mismatch, no DST; ▲ HLA-identical. Redrawn from reference 14

would follow since only weak immunological responders would be grafted. DST could thus be used to identify biologically acceptable donor–recipient pairs, and to prevent unnecessary graft loss in the high responders. It was also difficult to know what contribution third-party blood had made.

Many other centres have confirmed the benefit from DST[15-26]. Generally, results were compared with earlier experience using similar post-transplant immunosuppression, and most patients had been given third-party blood as well as DST. This has made it difficult to assess the effect of DST alone. Three or more third-party transfusions with no DST at all, were even claimed to be as effective[16,18]. Both these studies, however, included patients with low MLC responses to their kidney donor, and included some given only one DST. The excellent results achieved by comparison could have arisen, in part at least, from these other factors. The question could probably best be answered by a randomized controlled trial using the original inclusion criteria of Salvatierra and colleagues[12], to compare three DSTs with three or more transfusions from unrelated donors.

The greatly improved experience with haplo-identical relatives caused Salvatierra et al. (1985)[24] to extend the DST protocol to distantly related and even unrelated donor recipient pairs sharing no HLA antigens, and results were equally good.

In all series a proportion of recipients were sensitized against their donors. Several attempts have been made to overcome this problem.

Sensitization

Pre-sensitization, in both LRD and cadaveric transplantation, refers to immunization of the patient against the prospective donor with formation of antibodies against tissue antigens. Because these antigens are shared by

T and B lymphocytes, monocytes and platelets, patients can be sensitized by transfusions. This might have been predicted from Medawar's original studies: in fact he found that injection of leukocytes intravenously rather than intradermally was a relatively ineffective means of antibody induction[2], although anti-lymphocyte agglutinins were later demonstrated in other patients receiving multiple blood transfusions[1].

Lymphocytotoxic antibodies were so named because of the screening tests that evolved. They are commonly found in untransfused women who have been pregnant, through exposure to haplo-disparate fetal antigens, and in any patient exposed parenterally to foreign tissues, as in non-identical kidney transplantation. Not surprisingly, parous women and patients who have rejected an allograft show re-activation and develop antibodies more readily if blood transfusions are given subsequently.

By contrast 'immunological virgins', like Medawar's rabbits, are less easily sensitized by transfusions of fresh whole blood. Normal heathy male volunteers had to be transfused repeatedly from single donors in order to produce lymphocytotoxic antibodies. The degree of sensitization depended critically on the volume of blood, the number and frequency of transfusions. Lymphocytotoxic antibodies developed in 11 out of 12 subjects given 70–80 mL whole blood weekly for 4–6 weeks, provided that the course was repeated several months later, and further booster transfusions given. By contrast only 3 out of 17 subjects developed antibodies when blood was given in larger volumes of 250–300 mL at longer intervals of 1.5–2 months.

In patients with renal failure, lymphocytotoxic antibodies were soon recognized as causing hyperacute rejection within 24 h of transplantation and accelerated graft loss within the first week (see Chapter 1). Both conditions are analogous to accelerated rejection in laboratory animals, and are extremely refractory to immunosuppressive treatment. This may be prevented by testing serum from the patient against donor lymphocytes in the crossmatch test before transplantation (see Chapter 1). However, the properties and therefore the significance of different classes of antibodies which develop against antigens on the various cell types can differ widely.

In crossmatches carried out before LRD transplantation, recipient serum is incubated with donor peripheral blood lymphocytes, which are predominantly T cells and which exhibit class I (HLA-A and B) antigens. By contrast, spleen or lymph nodes are more commonly used for the final crossmatch before cadaveric transplantation and contain an increased proportion of B lymphocytes which carry class II (HLA-DR) as well as class I antigens. However, if the B and T lymphocytes are separated (see Chapter 1), then crossmatches against the individual cell types can be carried out.

T cell antibodies

Detected by incubation at 37 °C, these are usually of the IgG class of immunoglobulins and are directed to class I antigens. They are associated with hyperacute or accelerated graft rejection, and when present in recipient sera, transplantation is contraindicated.

B cell antibodies

These can be detected after incubation at 4 °C, 22 °C and 37 °C. Cold reactive B cell antibodies are often of the IgM immunoglobulin class, react with the patient's own lymphocytes and are said to be autoreactive. Sera containing such antibodies do not exhibit specificity to class I or class II antigens, react widely in the crossmatch test but are harmless, and are not associated with increased graft loss. Antibodies against antigens shared by monocytes and vascular endothelium can cause a positive B cell crossmatch, and may persist indefinitely. They may also cause hyperacute rejection and should be distinguished from true anti-B cell antibodies. Persisting B-warm antibodies in very low concentration have been ignored safely, but poor results have followed transplantation in patients with stronger sensitization–possibly because of undifferentiated anti-monocyte/vascular endothelial antibodies[21,23,27], or weak anti-class I activity detectable only with flow cytometry[24].

Patterns of sensitization

Three patterns of T and B cell sensitization have been observed following DST, in autocrossmatch-negative patients[12,14–26].

(a) Antibodies reactive against T and B cells on warm incubation develop in approximately 30% of patients treated on the unmodified DST protocol of Salvatierra[13]. These can be detected more than 12 months after the last transfusion, and do not appear to diminish with time.

(b) In a further proportion (perhaps 15%), the T-warm and then the B-warm antibodies disappear over 12–16 weeks. Once this transient sensitization has resolved and crossmatch is negative, transplantation can be safely carried out.

(c) Occasionally a patient will develop cytotoxic antibodies only against B cells on warm and cold incubation. Sensitization is usually transient, and successful transplantation delayed only 8–12 weeks.

Reduction in sensitization

Sensitization has been reduced by several modifications to the original DST protocol, generally with little or no loss of the DST effect: this is, however, often difficult to assess because of the numbers of third-party transfusions also given, and because of differences in inclusion criteria.

(1) Single DST

Sensitization fell to 4% in 24 patients when only one unit of 200 mL donor blood was given[16]. The one-year graft survival was 85%. However, most patients had been transfused previously, and not all had highly reactive MLC. Patients given more than 3 units of third-party blood and transplanted without DST had a 91% graft survival at one year.

A single DST of 400 mL improved graft survival in 21 haplo-identical living relatives, only ten of whom had been given third-party blood[19]. Sensitization was, however, high (24%).

(2)   Storage of donor blood

Most T cells and platelets disappear rapidly from blood stored under standard bank conditions, but B cells persist[17]. Sensitization has been reduced to under 10% by bleeding donors only once, and transfusing three or four stored aliquots at 7–14-day intervals[17,25]. Sensitization was more common in women who had previously been pregnant and in patients transfused with third party blood. Overall results of transplantation following stored DST were good, but a high incidence of acute rejection[17] suggested that storage had abrogated the transfusion effect to some extent, although only one graft failed in a mean nine-month follow-up period.

(3)   Immunosuppression given with DST

Immunosuppressive drugs could reduce sensitization, but could also impair induction of donor-specific unresponsiveness. Unfortunately studies attempting to answer this question have usually included patients given third-party blood, making interpretation difficult.

(a) *Azathioprine*: Azathioprine (2 mg/kg) was given from 2 days before the first DST to 31 patients without prior sensitization[15]. Only one developed a weak anti-T cell antibody which nevertheless led to hyperacute rejection. Two others, who developed weak anti-B cell antibodies, were transplanted successfully. One-year graft survival was 90% but 20 patients had been transfused before DST and 15 received third-party blood transfusions during the protocol, making it difficult to judge whether DST was still effective. Donor–recipient pairs weakly responsive on MLC were also included.

Glass and colleagues[20] used the same protocol and reduced sensitization from 31% to 14%. Two-year graft survival (80%) was, however, somewhat lower than in patients given DST alone (90%), although the difference did not achieve statistical significance. Many patients had already received third-party blood, but the number of transfusions was not indicated.

Both groups used azathioprine and prednisolone for maintenance treatment after transplantation and found that many patients given azathioprine before transplantation developed marrow depression. Salvatierra and colleagues[24] found azathioprine, 1 mg/kg, to be effective in reducing sensitization to 12%, but only in patients who had not been transplanted previously and who showed minimal reactivity (<10%) against random panel lymphocytes

(b) *Cyclosporin*: In a randomized controlled trial, cyclosporin A (10 mg/kg daily) was given from one week before the first DST to 21 prospective recipients exhibiting a reactive MLC with their haplotype-mismatched donors[22,23]. Twenty-six control patients received DST alone. All were given cyclosporin after transplantation.

Four control patients (15%) were persistently sensitized with antibodies against T and B lymphocytes. This relatively low incidence may relate to storage of donor blood for 3 days before transfusion. By contrast, there was no persistent sensitization in patients receiving cyclosporin with DST, although 30% developed transient anti-B cell antibodies which disappeared over 8–12 weeks. There was no morbidity associated with cyclosporin pre-treatment, and graft survival was comparable with control patients (approximately 95% at 1 year). Several recipients had, however, been given third-party blood previously.

Cyclosporin and DST

Donor-specific transfusion is still beneficial in patients given cyclosporin after LRD transplantation. In 118 patients given cyclosporin but no DST, graft survival in one haplotype mismatched donor–recipient pairs was 87% after 200 days, compared with 97% in 65 patients given DST as well as cyclosporin[18].

Mechanisms

Since the DST effect persists in protocols achieving low rates of sensitization, selection of non-responders cannot alone explain the improved results. Both cellular and humoral mechanisms for inducton of donor-specific unresponsiveness have been identified, and will be considered later.

Cadaveric transplantation: effect of third-party blood transfusions (TPT)

Patients on dialysis awaiting transplantation from cadaveric donors are variably exposed to blood given for clinical reasons or as part of a planned programme. There will usually be random variations in HLA mismatching between blood donor and recipient and in storage time. Most patients are given plasma-reduced or packed cells but leukocyte-poor, leukocyte-free and frozen blood have also been used. Occasionally patients will need emergency platelet transfusions from a large number of donors.

The first clear description of a transfusion effect in 1972 was greeted with considerable scepticism[13]. It was not until five years later that unqualified corroboration was provided from more than one other centre. By 1985, however, Tiwari[28] was able to quote over 70 reports showing benefit from one or more units of blood given before or during transplant surgery. Many reports described uncontrolled observations on data collected when skills were evolving, immunosuppression changing and results improving for other reasons.

The size of the effect varied widely. One-year graft survival increased between 9 and 70% in some centres, and between 10 and 35% in most. No difference or even an adverse effect was noted in three. Generally, larger multicentre studies showed a smaller effect, and a larger effect was seen when smaller numbers of patients were studied. Most improvement was seen in units reporting very poor results in untransfused patients. Two centres reporting no effect already had good results with their untransfused patients – possibly because of differences in HLA matching, ethnic factors, more intensive immunosuppression, or perhaps because blood was given to some patients but not recorded. The overall effect of a deliberate blood transfusion policy prior to transplantation was that one-year graft survival rose to 60–70% for patients immunosuppressed with azathioprine and prednisolone.

Type of blood product

The different effects of various blood products emphasize the importance of viable leukocytes. Eight patients who had not previously received blood transfusions, were prospectively transfused with one or three units of blood filtered through cotton wool: this procedure removed 98% of the white cells (leukocyte-free). Graft survival was only 25% at 8 months, compared with 79% in 19 patients transfused with one unit of washed red cells (leukocyte-poor), prepared by a method which removed only 90% of the leukocytes[29].

Opelz and Terasaki[30] found no benefit from giving one unit of blood prepared by freezing and washing, another procedure which removes all but 6–12% of leukocytes. However, graft survival rose if more than one such unit was transfused. They also found that one unit of packed cells was more effective than one of whole blood, but this distinction was also lost if more was transfused. Others found no difference between various red cell products, but did not study patients transfused only one unit.

Buffy coat transfusions given weekly from ten random donors may be slightly more effective than 10 weekly transfusions of whole blood, but numbers of patients studied are small[31].

Platelets exhibit class I but not class II antigens, and might in theory produce less sensitization with greater benefit. Unfortunately in man, platelets have appeared to have an adverse effect[32]. Platelets prepared by cell separation are, to a variable extent, contaminated by leukocytes. When given fortnightly from three random donors sensitization has been high and grafts have been rejected soon after transplantation. Further purification has produced less sensitization but grafts have still been lost early. There may be tissue antigens other than HLA-A, B and DR on platelets and kidney cells but not on lymphocytes.

Number of transfusions

A dose response with leukocyte-free and washed frozen red cells has been noted. A steady rise in graft survival with increasing numbers of transfusions was reported by centres collecting data from hundreds of patients (Figure 4.2). The greatest improvement was found as the number of transfusions rose from one to five, but further benefit resulted if more than ten units were given. After 15–20 units, graft survival fell, a recent observation[37] that echoed experience from the not-so-distant past (see below).

Many other centres reported a transfusion effect but no further improvement in graft survival as the number of transfusions increased. Most studies related to smaller numbers of patients, and the reports of greater benefit

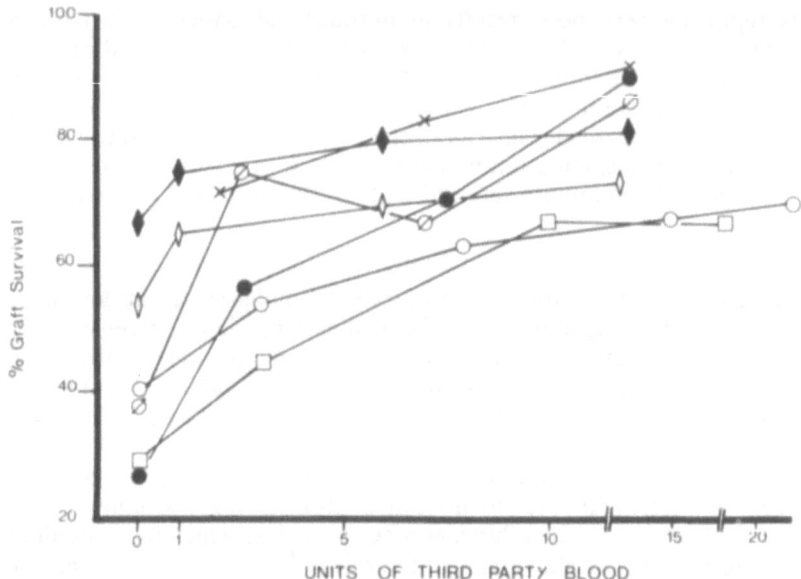

Figure 4.2 Rise in one-year graft survival with increasing numbers of transfusions. ○ Opelz and Terasaki (1980)[30]; □ Spees et al. (1980)[34]; ● Opelz et al. (1980), unsensitized patients[33]; × Bone et al. (1985) with, and ∅ without, cyclosporin A[35]; ◆ Opelz (1986)[36] with, and ◇ without, cyclosporin A

from less blood might have arisen in other ways. For example, an 80% one-year graft survival was reported after patients received only one unit of leukocyte-poor blood[38]. However, out of a total study population of 599, only 40 patients receiving one such transfusion had been transplanted, and only 32 were available for analysis after 200 days. The patients were all Dutch and similar, both racially and in terms of overall clinical management, mismatching was low and DR typing available. These important factors were not always present in other centres reporting poorer graft survival results after only one unit of blood.

Timing

Blood given at the time of transplantation appears to have some effect[39], but only in previously untransfused patients[18]. Single units have an optimal effect if given 30–90 days previously[18]. Some effect may be seen in patients transfused months if not years beforehand[18,33,38].

Unplanned transfusions, however, are not given randomly. Clinical need indicates significant pathology which may affect graft survival or its assessment. Moreover, the most random event for most patients is the date of their transplant operation. Yet blood group, tissue type, matching criteria used by the transplant team, its success in recruiting local donors, and sensitization of the patient will all influence timing of the transplantation and its proximity to the first, last or median unit given. It is not surprising, therefore, that little information is available on the optimal transfusion programme for patients awaiting a cadaveric graft.

Degree of HLA mismatching with transplanted kidney

The degree of mismatching with the cadaveric donor may be significant. The earliest European studies to show a beneficial transfusion effect found improved graft survival only in patients with well-matched donors[40,41]. While receiving some recent support[42], other reports with much larger numbers of patients have found a comparable effect of blood transfusion whether the donor–recipient pairs are fully matched or mismatched at the HLA-A, B and HLA-DR loci[38]. Transfused patients also have a better graft survival if they are given HLA-B and DR matched kidneys. Thus the effects of blood transfusion and HLA matching appear to be additive.

Cyclosporin and third-party transfusion

A transfusion effect in patients given cyclosporin post-operatively was still found by some observers[38,43] (Figure 4.2), but was not seen among smaller numbers of recipients reported from Portsmouth and Scandinavia[44,45]. The increased benefit of blood transfusions given to patients treated with cyclosporin A and reported in the Collaborative Transplant Study[36] was not as striking in 1986 as in 1985[18]. Nevertheless graft survival did rise from less than 70% in untransfused patients treated with cyclosporin A to more than 80% after one year, in similarly immunosuppressed recipients who had received several transfusions. It may become increasingly difficult to demonstrate a transfusion effect, even when present, from analysis of actuarial survival alone, as results improve with better tissue typing and immunosuppression.

Blood transfusion effect on re-transplantation

There is a little information on this clinically important question. Blood transfusions given before the first transplant improved the one-year survival of a second graft from 38% in 29 untransfused patients to 58% in 142 transfused patients[46]. No effect of blood given between the first and second transplants was noted.

In data from over 3000 second and subsequent renal transplants collected by the Los Angeles Registry, the beneficial effect of blood given before the first transplant was confirmed–providing that the graft survived more than six months[47]. No benefit was seen from blood given afterwards, but sensitization increased.

Sensitization following third-party transfusions

Patients with renal failure behave somewhat unpredictably after transfusion. This may arise from variations in antigen disparity between blood donor and recipient, blood storage times, or individual responsiveness. All three may affect sensitization as well as induction of a blood transfusion effect.

97

Fears of sensitization arose from earlier reports that sera from some 52% of transfused pre-transplant patients were cytotoxic to random panel lymphocytes[33]. Unfortunately few comments were made on breadth of sensitization, and the hazards, rather than potential benefits were emphasized[48].

More recent analyses do not confirm these fears. Few patients developed broadly reactive antibodies (Table 4.2). Men especially seemed unresponsive even when the optimal requirements for a transfusion effect were interpreted generously. In two series, ten units sensitized only one in five men: only 1% were sensitized against more than 90% panel lymphocytes. Women were more at risk, but only one in five was broadly sensitized (> 50% panel). However almost one in three who had had more than three pregnancies became broadly sensitized (> 90% panel) after 10 units. The risk of sensitization increased with number of transfusions in both sexes, but the greatest rise was found during administration of the first 5 units[49].

Very few patients remained broadly reactive for long[35,50], and lymphocytotoxic antibodies usually disappeared rapidly even when further transfusions were given. However, the time to cadaveric transplantation was significantly prolonged. Patients sensitized to 3–20% panel lymphocytes waited only 12.2 ± 3.7 weeks, those with 20–80% panel reactivity took 35 ± 7 weeks, and those reacting against over 80% panel were not transplanted for almost two years (90 ± 6 weeks) after planned transfusions[50].

Prevention and suppression of sensitization following third-party transfusion

Few attempts have been made to prevent or suppress sensitization other than by limiting the number of transfusions given or waiting for antibodies to disappear. Azathioprine did not prevent sensitization to three transfusions of buffy coat from the same mismatched unrelated donor[51], in contrast to its effect on DST between haplo-identical relatives[15,20,21], but cyclosporin may have been more effective.

Five broadly sensitized patients whose antibodies persisted were treated successfully by plasma exchange and immunosuppression with cyclophosphamide and high dosage prednisolone, but the protocol was not without risk[52].

Table 4.2 Percentage risk of sensitization against random panel lymphocytes

Source	Patients M/F	Transfusions M/F	Breadth of reactivity against panel			
			<2% M/F	<10% M/F	<50% M/F	>90% M/F
Opelz et al. (1981)[49]	431/306	10*	—	80/67	93/80	1/5
Norman et al. (1985)[50]	40	5**	22.5		77.5	5
Bone et al. (1985)[35]	100/51	12.4/12.0†	—	79/63	96/79	1/4

*Liberal, according to clinical need
**Elective, fortnightly, fresh
†Top-up to 10 'life-time' units, weekly or monthly, then as clinically needed

Significance of lymphocytotoxic antibodies in cadaveric transplantation

Lymphocytotoxic antibodies present at the time of transplantation can profoundly affect graft survival. As with LRD transplants, hyperacute rejection has been largely prevented by standard crossmatching. However, the significance of a positive crossmatch with sera collected months if not years beforehand is less clear. Until recently any sign of presensitization, whether past or present, was thought to increase the risks of rejection. Most laboratories, therefore used historical sera with the broadest response against panel lymphocytes (peak sera) as well as a fresh sample in the pre-transplant crossmatch test. A positive result with either was regarded as a contraindication to surgery.

This policy was questioned when peak sera stored down the years from unlucky transplant candidates ran out and were not available to gainsay later negative results. The 'historical positive–current negative' controversy arose when some centres deliberately ignored positive results from peak sera when more recent samples, including current sera, were negative. Falk *et al.* claimed that graft survival (60% after 2 years) compared favourably with results from unsensitized patients, even when T cell antibodies had been found previously[53].

As with sensitization after DST, cold anti-T and B cell IgM auto-antibodies seem harmless[54]. Weakly reacting B-warm antibodies may also be ignored safely. Hyperacute rejection has, however, followed a stronger response, and may be due to antibodies directed to other antigens present on vascular endothelium. Cells from spleen and lymph nodes which contain an increased proportion of B lymphocytes and which are used for the final crossmatch, may result in a higher detection rate of antibodies to B cells.

Broadly sensitized patients have reduced graft survival rates even when the crossmatch is negative[36,55]. The effect was related to breadth of sensitization ($> 50\%$ panel) immediately before transplantation, rather than that in earlier peak sera. It would seem wise to delay transplantation after planned transfusions until the breadth of sensitization is known, even if a kidney from a potential donor appears compatible on crossmatch.

Mechanisms

Various mechanisms have been proposed to explain the transfusion effect. Few can account for all the phenomena described, but none are mutually exclusive, and all may have some part to play (Table 4.3).

Selection

As noted already, blood transfusions might selectively sensitize naturally responsive patients and identify incompatible donor–recipient pairs. Transplantation would be delayed or prevented, avoiding early graft loss. Improved results would follow in unresponsive patients and from more compatible matches. A dose response would be seen since more transfusions would result in more sensitization and greater selection.

Table 4.3 Mechanisms of the blood transfusion effect

1. Recipient selection
2. Non-specific unresponsiveness
3. Specific unresponsiveness:
   humoral:
      anti-idiotypic antibodies
      Fc-receptor blocking antibodies
   cellular:
      clonal deletion
      clonal inactivation
      suppressor cells

Four observations argue against selection and suggest that biological mechanisms are more important:

(a) In DST protocols, sensitization has been greatly reduced without proportionate loss of the transfusion effect.

(b) In unsensitized patients cadaveric graft survival rises progressively[34] with the number of transfusions (see Figure 4.2).

(c) Graft survival is better in sensitized patients who have been transfused than in untransfused patients who are not sensitized[34].

(d) Graft survival may be even higher in transfused patients showing transient sensitization than in transfused patients with no antibody response[55].

Non-specific unresponsiveness

A single unit of blood depressed cell-mediated immunity in terms of delayed cutaneous hypersensitivity to 'recall' antigens[56]. An effect was detectable after one year but the significance for graft survival is uncertain.

Ferritin can depress lymphocyte function[57] and multiple transfusions might improve graft survival by causing iron overload[58]. This, however, could not account for the benefit from less than 5 units. The overall importance of such non-specific mechanisms in promoting increased allograft survival remains to be assessed.

Specific unresponsiveness

(a) Humoral

(i) *Anti-idiotypic antibodies:* The idiotype on an immunoglobulin molecule is the unique terminal part of the variable region which binds antigen specifically. Anti-idiotypic antibodies develop normally to control the immune response by combining with the idiotype thus blocking its effect. They may be responsible for the eventual fall in lymphocytotoxic activity which often follows sensitization, and allow successful transplantation with a graft to which the recipient has been sensitized[59]. Anti-idiotypic antibodies against donor HLA-DR antigen disparities were found in sera from unsensitized patients following DST who were transplanted successfully. By contrast they were not found in patients with hyperacute or chronic vascular rejection.

Anti-idiotypic antibodies might also control T-cell responses by combining with the idiotype on the T-cell receptor. Sera from transfused mice specifically suppressed MLC responses to donor cells, and the effect lasted longer when the antigen disparity was greater[60]. However, in this species there was difficulty in identifying anti-idiotypic antibodies against specific T-cell receptors[61].

(ii) *Fc-receptor blocking antibodies:* Good graft survival correlated with non-cytotoxic antibodies capable of blocking Fc-receptors on cadaveric donor B lymphocytes[62]. Antibodies developed in a proportion of patients given more than 5 units of blood from unrelated donors, but were detected less frequently if less was transfused. Family studies showed HLA specificity for antibody that was found after only two transfusions from the same donor[63]. In a modified assay[64], Fc-receptor blocking factors were associated with graft survival, but activity found in the high molecular weight fraction on sucrose density gradient centrifugation was thought to represent immune complexes.

(b) Cellular

(i) *Clonal deletion:* Terasaki[65] suggested that blood transfusions might activate clones of lymphocytes against disparate HLA antigens which would be reactivated after transplantation. Immunosuppression would then delete only these activated clones, leaving the individual specifically unresponsive to the graft. However, whole blood DST in one rat strain donor–recipient combination can produce donor-specific unresponsiveness without additional immunosuppression[66]. Moreover, patients given cyclosporin, a non-ablative drug, show a transfusion effect, and many show no clinical signs of significant clonal reactivation in terms of acute rejection. Other arguments for and against clonal deletion as the mechanism underlying neonatal tolerance are linked to the significance and functions of the T suppressor cell[67,68].

(ii) *Clonal inactivation (antigen flooding):* Clonal abortion, exhaustion and functional deletion are terms used to describe failure of T and B lymphocyte activation with different quantities of antigen at different stages of maturation[69]. Clonal inactivation refers to neonatal T cell tolerance recently described in mice that seems unexplained by T suppressor cell activation[70]. While of considerable interest, the significance of these phenomena in adult humans has yet to be explored.

(iii) *Suppressor T lymphocytes:* A number of observations support a role for these cells:

(a) Specific unresponsiveness induced by prior blood transfusion in long surviving renal allograft recipients can be passed from one adult rat to another by transfusing lymphoid cells from the tolerant recipient[66]; this 'adoptive transfer' assays T suppressor cell activity in terms of subsequent allograft survival in the second animal.

(b) Splenic T suppressor cells assayed by this technique are found after a single blood transfusion in rats before transplantation[71].

(c) Splenectomy after DST before transplantation in mice abrogates the transfusion effect[72].

(d) Donor-specific suppressor activity of circulating T cells can be shown in MLC in patients with long-surviving renal allografts[73,74].

(e) Donor-specific unresponsiveness has been shown in MLC and cell-mediated lympholysis assays *in vitro*, following DST in man[75] and in mice[60,76], and has been attributed to T suppressor cells.

Reservations have, however, been expressed over the interpretation of such *in vitro* assays[68,77]. Moreover, other demonstrations *in vitro* of reduced donor-specific cellular unresponsiveness following DST with concomitant immuno-suppression using azathioprine[78] or cyclosporin[22] may have alternative explanations. Most *in vitro* tests have correlated poorly with rejection.

Non-immunological risks of blood transfusion

Two major risks of blood transfusions are serum hepatitis and acquired immune deficiency syndrome (AIDS). Serum hepatitis has been virtually eliminated by screening for HBsAg. If 1 in 1000 donations are from undiagnosed carriers and screening misses 1%, only 1 in 100 000 transfusions will be dangerous. For a centre treating 100 new patients annually the incidence of serum hepatitis will rise by 1 patient in 1000 years for each unit of blood given electively. Similarly, if undiagnosed AIDS affects 600 potential blood donors in the UK, the chances of infection will be 1 in 100 000 per unit of blood. Screening for HTLV III antibody should reduce this risk even further. The risks of viral infection from 5–10 units of blood are thus very much lower than the risks of dying from the transplant operation itself, by a factor of between 100 and 500.

In areas where malaria is endemic, the risk of parasitic infection can be avoided by the use of antimalarial prophylaxis and by excluding donors within three years of clinical infection.

Emergence of the transfusion effect

Residual doubts about the value of planned transfusion programmes of any size may arise from memories of earlier times when fears of sensitization and viral infection were predominant. In addition, recognition of the transfusion effect as a biological phenomenon was greatly delayed, perhaps because of policy changes that these fears themselves produced.

The blood transfusion paradox was recognised in 1968[79]. Since blood transfusion did not affect graft outcome, it was suggested that the adverse effect of presensitization was balanced by a beneficial effect from immuno-logical unresponsiveness. One group, however, showed that graft survival improved as the number of units of transplanted blood increased[80].

Transfusion policies then were extremely liberal to the point of wantonness. Dialysis patients were often given blood at a weekly top-up because they 'felt better'. Dossettor's two groups[80] were given 86 and 40 units, and Morris's[79] averaged 44 (5 to >100) units before grafting. Two factors reduced this river of blood to the merest trickle. Dialysis-associated serum hepatitis claimed lives of both patients and staff in outbreaks between 1966 and 1972. Fears of sensitization arose and perhaps were magnified since more patients survived graft failure and returned to dialysis for more blood to which they were more susceptible. While hepatitis and hyperacute rejection were prevented by screening techniques, it was felt strongly, and correctly, that the best way of avoiding either was to give no blood at all unless life itself was threatened. Centres were affected variably, since risks were perceived differently in each region, and the resulting differences in policies may have influenced both the results of transplantation and the assessment of the transfusion effect.

In 1972 nephrologists were presented with the conflicting data shown in Figures 4.3 and 4.4. The European Dialysis and Transplant Association (EDTA) Registry showed an adverse effect from more than 6, and even worse results from more than 20 units (Figure 4.3)[81]. This was explained only in part by hyperacute rejection. Data presented shortly afterwards to the Transplantation Society (Figure 4.4)[13] clearly showed benefit from 1–10, and even better results from more than 10 transfusions. The most plausible explanation was patient selection, but it was difficult to see why this did not affect Europeans. Alternative reasons were proposed:

(1) The EDTA data in 1972 pooled results from cadaveric and LRD grafts. Patients given LRD kidneys would be better matched and transplanted quickly, thus receiving less blood on dialysis. Better results would apparently follow fewer transfusions. However, EDTA data in 1974 avoided this bias but still showed better one-year cadaveric graft survival in 1899 patients given less than 20 units (52%) than in 314 patients

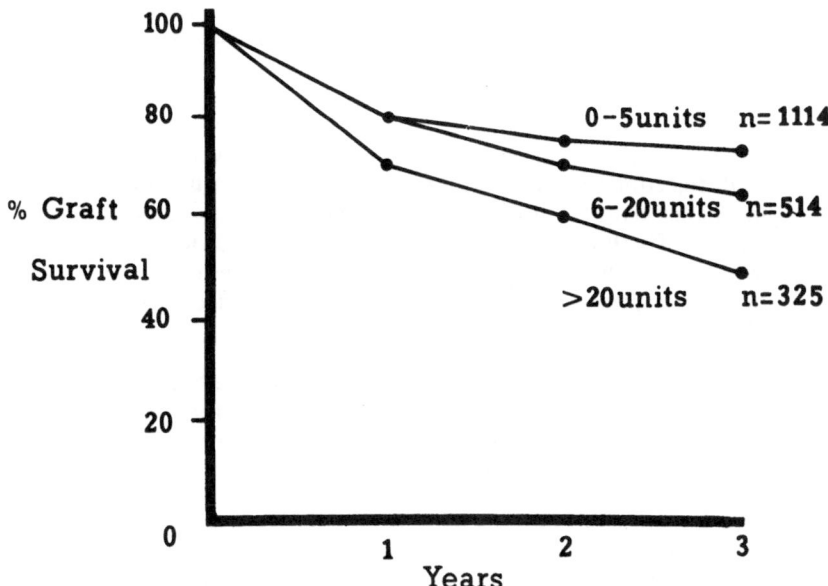

Figure 4.3 Survival of first transplants with increasing numbers of transfusions. Reported by EDTA Registry (1972). Redrawn from reference 81

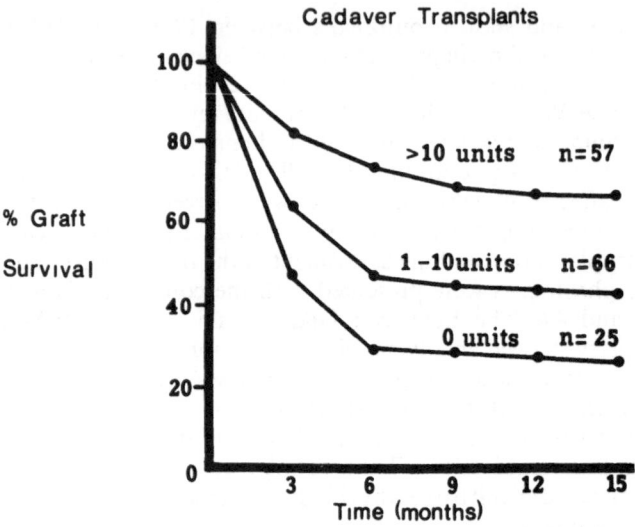

Figure 4.4 Survival of first cadaver transplants with increasing numbers of transfusions. Reported to the Transplantation Society (1972). Redrawn from reference 13

given more (45%). The 684 given no blood fared as well as 612 given 1–5 and 603 given 6–20 units[82].

(2) Opelz and colleagues[13] reported data from only seven closely linked dialysis and transplant centres in the Los Angeles area. Hyperacute rejection was unlikely since they themselves had developed a sensitive microlymphocytotoxicity test for screening pre-transplant sera. By contrast, the EDTA Registry collected data unselectively from many more units of varying size and experience. Larger centres might have better tissue typing and screening, and be transfusing fewer patients. Hyperacute rejection was still being reported, and might occur more frequently in smaller centres with poorer techniques and with an increased proportion of multiply transfused patients who had been longer on dialysis. Whatever the correct explanation, the marked variation in graft survival rates from different transplant units ('the centre effect') is a recognized phenomenon.

(3) Unfit patients are more likely to receive more transfusions while on dialysis and are frequently poor risk candidates for transplantation. This may explain why, in 1976, reduced transplant survival rates were noted in patients given multiple blood transfusions[41].

(4) Many inconsistencies were also found between nurses' notes of transfusions given, patients' memories and blood bank records. Units of blood could be ordered and recorded but not given. Exceptional care was needed to minimize errors: it is easy to appreciate how false information could have been reported to EDTA from many centres.

In 1976, EDTA reported improved graft survival in patients with well-matched grafts given 20 units or more in contrast to the results from patients given no blood: the results from transfused patients with less well-matched grafts were even worse (Figure 4.5)[41]. In keeping with the centre effect (discussed above) reports from London[40] and Leiden[83] showed benefit from transfusions in centres with the best experience in tissue matching and other techniques. Belief in selection and reluctance to risk hepatitis deterred many from planned transfusions until more sensitive tests for HBsAg and effective vaccines for hepatitis B were available, and proof of a biological effect of blood had been conclusively demonstrated. Most were finally convinced in 1981 when Terasaki and Opelz[34] showed a stepwise transfusion effect in unsensitized patients (see Figure 4.2). In the British Transplantation Society centre effect study, elective transfusions began in seven out of eight centres between 1979 and 1982 and blood was the only factor to account for the wide variation in their results[84].

CONCLUSIONS: TOWARDS AN ELECTIVE TRANSFUSION POLICY

It is very likely that the transfusion effect is produced by exposing the prospective recipient to disparate HLA antigens expressed on the subsequent allograft in sufficient dosage to generate specific unresponsiveness. Policies must be devised to achieve this and minimize significant sensitization.

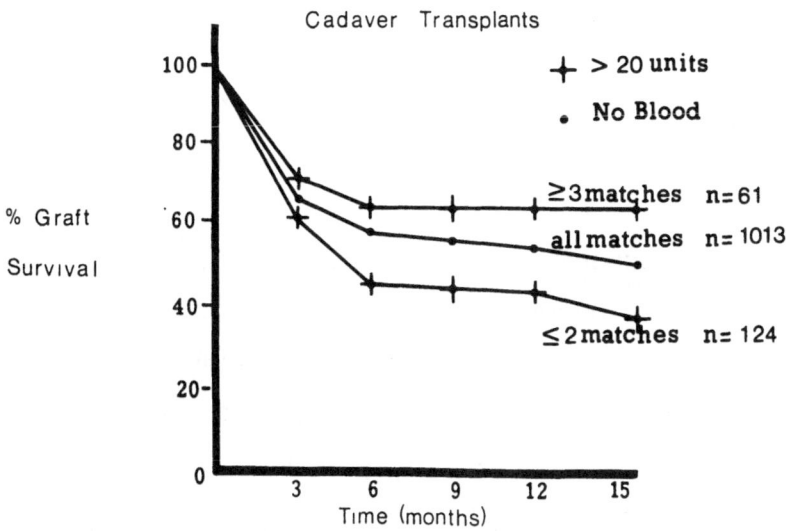

Figure 4.5 Survival of first cadaver transplants in, ◆, transfused (>20 units) patients; and in ●, untransfused patients: influence of matching for HLA-A and B. Reported by EDTA Registry (1975). Redrawn from reference 41

Living donors

Salvatierra's original protocol[12] of three transfusions of 200 mL fresh donor blood given fortnightly still seems best, providing cyclosporin[22] or azathioprine[15] is given to suppress sensitization. Storage of a single donation with transfusion of aliquots is more convenient but sensitization is still seen and some protection lost. Patients given more than three third-party transfusions may be protected already, but there is no way of assessing this before transplantation, and DST still seems the best way to ensure that donor antigens have been presented.

Cadaveric donors

The optimum number of third-party transfusions may lie between 5 and 15 units. In men and non-parous women the requirements should be interpreted generously, unless more transfusions are anticipated for medical reasons. Parous women who may be candidates for transplantation present a special problem. Against the greater risk of broad sensitization must be set the hazards of graft failure. The best policy here may be to transfuse electively before dialysis is needed. Cyclosporin may give protection against sensitization. There appear to be no advantage and many risks in transfusing patients awaiting re-transplantation.

Timing depends on mutual convenience of dialysis centres and their patients. Single units of blood given weekly appear no different from two units given monthly. Since the duration of the effect is not known, no advice can be offered about top-up transfusions. A screening test for specific unresponsiveness would be of considerable help.

ACKNOWLEDGEMENTS

We wish to acknowledge the considerable help of Miss P. Smart in the preparation of this manuscript.

References

1. Mollinson, P. L. (1983). *Blood Transfusion in Clinical Medicine.* 7th edn. (Oxford: Blackwell Scientific Publications)
2. Medawar, P. B. (1946). Immunity to homologous grafted skin. II. The relationship between the antigens of blood and skin. *Br. J. Exp. Pathol.*, **27**, 15–24
3. Billingham, R. E., Brent, L. and Medawar, P. B. (1953). Actively acquired tolerance of foreign cells. *Nature*, **172**, 603–6
4. Gibson, T. and Medawar, P. B. (1943). The fate of skin homografts in man. *J. Anat.*, **77**, 299–310
5. Lillie, F. R. (1916). Theory of the free-martin. *Science*, **43**, 611–3
6. Owen, R. D. (1945). Immunogenetic consequences of vascular anastomoses between bovine twins. *Science*, **102**, 400–1
7. Monaco, A. P. (1972). Immunological tolerance and enhancement in experimental and clinical renal transplantation. *Proceedings of the Fifth International Congress of Nephrology (Mexico).* Vol. I, pp. 92–109. (Basel: S. Karger)
8. Roitt, I., Brostoff, J. and Male, D. (1985). *Immunology.* (Edinburgh: Churchill Livingstone)

9. Flexner, S. and Jobling, J. N. (1907). On the promoting influence of heated tumour emulsions on tumour growth. *Proc. Soc. Exp. Biol. Med.*, **4**, 156–7
10. Batchelor, J. R., French, M. E., Cameron, J. S., Ellis, F., Bewick, M. and Ogg, C. S. (1970). Immunological enhancement of human kidney graft. *Lancet*, **2**, 1007–10
11. Newton, W. T. and Anderson, C. B. (1973). Planned pre-immunisation of renal allograft recipients. *Surgery*, **74**, 430–6
12. Salvatierra, O., Vincenti, F., Amend, W., Potter, D., Iwaki, Y., Opelz, G., Terasaki, P., Duca, R., Cochrum, K., Hanes, D., Storey, R. J. and Feduska, N. J. (1980). Deliberate specific blood transfusions prior to living related transplantation. A new approach. *Ann. Surg.*, **192**, 543–51
13. Opelz, G., Sengar, D. P. S., Mickey, M. R. and Terasaki, P. I. (1973). Effect of blood transfusions on subsequent kidney transplants. *Transplant. Proc.*, **5**, 253–9
14. Salvatierra, O., Vincenti, F., Amend, W., Garovoy, M., Iwaki, Y., Terasaki, P., Potter, D., Duca, R., Hopper, S., Slemmer, T. and Feduska, N. (1983). Four year experience with donor specific transfusions. *Transplant. Proc.*, **15**, 924–31
15. Anderson, C. B., Sicard, G. A., Rodey, G. E., Anderman, C. K. and Etheredge, E. E. (1983). Renal allograft recipient pre-treatment with donor-specific blood and concomitant immunosuppression. *Transplant. Proc.*, **15**, 939–42
16. Squifflet, J. P., Pirson, Y., De Bruyere, J., Littinne, D. and Alexandre, G. P. J. (1984). Preliminary results of one haplotype matched living donor renal transplantation using a single donor-specific transfusion. *Transplant. Proc.*, **16**, 20–3
17. Light, J. A., Metz, S. J. and Oddenino, K. (1983). Donor-specific transfusion with minimal sensitization. *Transplant. Proc.*, **15**, 917–23
18. Opelz, G. (1985). Current relevance of the transfusion effect in renal transplantation. *Transplant. Proc.*, **17**, 1015–22
19. Barry, J. M., Normal, D. J., Bohannon, C. L., Wetzteon, P. and Fischer, S. (1985). Comparison of two donor-specific transfusions protocols. *Transplant. Proc.*, **17**, 1072–4
20. Glass, N. R., Miller, D. T., Sollinger, H. W. and Belzer, F. O. (1985). A four year experience with donor blood transfusion protocols for living donor renal transplantation. *Transplant. Proc.*, **17**, 1023–5
21. Anderson, C. B., Tyler, J. D., Sicard, C. K., Anderman, C. K., Rodey, G. E. and Etheredge, E. E. (1985). Renal allograft recipient pre-treatment with immunosuppression and donor specific blood. *Transplant. Proc.*, **17**, 1047–50
22. Hillis, A. N., Sells, R. A., Bone, J. M., Evans, C. M., Duguid, J., Roberts, F., Evans, P., Kenton, P. and Barnes, R. M. R. (1985). A prospective clinical trial of cyclosporin and donor specific transfusion versus donor specific transfusions alone in living related renal allograft. *Transplant. Proc.*, **17**, 1242–3
23. Hillis, A. N., Bone, J. M. and Sells, R. A. (1986). (Unpublished results)
24. Salvatierra, O., Meltzer, J., Porter, D., Danovoy, M., Vincenti, F., Amend, W., Husing, R., Hopper, S. and Feduska, N. (1985). A seven year experience with donor-specific blood transfusions. *Transplantation*, **40**, 654–9
25. Whelchel, J. D., Curtis, J. J., Kohaut, E. C., Barger, B. O., Luke, R. G. and Diethelm, A. G. (1985). Improved renal allograft survival in patients receiving one-haplotype related transplants and pre-transplant stored, donor specific blood transfusion. *Transplant. Proc.*, **17**, 1077–9
26. Salvatierra, O., Amend, W., Vincenti, F., Potter, D., Iwaki, Y., Opelz, G., Terasaki, P., Duca, R., Hanes, D., Cochrum, K. C., Hopper, S. and Feduska, N. J. (1981). Pre-treatment with donor specific transfusions in related recipients with high MLC. *Transplant. Proc.*, **13**, 142–9
27. Carpenter, C. B. and Milford, E. (1984). Immunological monitoring before transplantation. In Morris, P. J. (ed.) *Kidney Transplantation. Principles and Practice.* 2nd Edn. pp.257–71. (London: Grune and Stratton)
28. Tiwari, J. L. (1985). Review: Kidney transplantation and transfusion in clinical kidney transplants. In Terasaki, P. I. (ed.) *Clinical Kidney Transplants 1985.* (Los Angeles: UCLA Tissue Typing Laboratory)
29. Persijn, G. G., Cohan, B., Landsberger, Q. and Van Rood, J. J. (1980). Retrospective and prospective studies on the effect of blood transfusion in renal transplantation in the Netherlands. *Transplantation*, **28**, 153–8

30. Opelz, G. and Terasaki, P. I. (1980). Dominant effect of transfusion on kidney graft survival. *Transplantation*, 29, 153–8
31. Okazaki, H., Takahashi, H., Miura, K., Ishizaki, M., Oguma, A. and Taguchi, Y. (1985). Effect of buffy coat transfusion in living related and cadaveric renal transplantation. *Transplant. Proc.*, 17, 1034–7
32 Chapman, J. R., Misher, J., Ting, A. and Morris, P. J. (1985). Platelet transfusion before renal transplantation in humans. *Transplant. Proc.*, 17, 1038–40
33. Spees, E. K., Vaughan, W. K., Williams, G. M., Filo, R. S., McDonald, J. C., Mendez-Picon, G. and Niblack, G. (1980). Effects of blood transfusion on cadaver renal transplantation. The Southeastern Organ Procurement Foundation prospective study (1977–1979). *Transplantation*, 30, 455–63
34. Opelz, G., Graver, B. and Terasaki, P. I. (1981). Induction of high kidney graft survival rate by multiple transfusions. *Lancet*, 1, 1223–5
35. Bone, J. M., Hillis, A. N., Taylor, G. T., Barnes, R. M. R. and Sells, R. A. (1985). The benefits of elective transfusion to 10 units whole blood before 1st cadaveric renal transplantation outweigh the risks of sensitization. *Kidney Int.*, 28, 372 (Abstract)
36. Opelz, G. (1986). Immunological factors influencing renal allograft survival. *Proc. EDTA–Eur. Renal Ass.*, 22, 585–602
37. Cecka, M. and Cicciarelli, J. (1985). The transfusion effect. In Terasaki, P. I. (ed.) *Clinical Kidney Transplants 1985*. (Los Angeles: UCLA Tissue Typing Laboratory)
38. Persijn, G. G., Van Leeuwen, A., Parlevliet, J., Cohan, B., Lansbergen, Q., D'Amaro, J. and Van Rood, J. J. (1981). Two major factors influencing kidney graft survival in Eurotransplant: HLA, DR matching and blood transfusion. *Transplant. Proc.*, 13, 150–4
39. Stiller, C. R., Sinclair, N. R., Sheppard, R. R., Lockwood, B. L., Sharpe, J. A. and Hagman, P. (1978). Beneficial effect of operation day blood transfusions on human allograft survival. *Lancet*, 1, 169–70
40. Festenstien, H., Sachs, J. H., Paris, A. M. I., Pegrum, G. D. and Moorhead, J. F. (1976). Influence of HLA matching and blood transfusion on outcome of 502 London Transplant Group renal-graft recipients. *Lancet*, 1, 157–61
41. Brunner, F. P., Giesecke, B., Gurland, H. J., Jacobs, C., Parsons, F. M., Scharer, K., Scyffart, G., Spees, G. and Wing, A. J. (1976). Combined report on regular dialysis and transplantation in Europe, V, 1974. *Dialysis Transplant. Nephrol.*, 12, 3–64
42. Mohanakumar, T., Ellis, T. M., Dayal, H., Du Vall, C., Mendez-Picon, G. and Lee, H. M. (1981). Potentiating effect of HLA matching and blood transfusion on renal allograft survival. *Transplantation*, 32, 244–7
43. Morris, P. J., Thompson, J. F., Ting, A. and Wood, R. F. (1984). Is pre-graft blood transfusion beneficial in cyclosporin treated renal transplant recipients? (Letter) *Lancet*, 1, 98
44. Gardner, B., Harris, K. R., Digard, N. J., Gosling, D. C., Campbell, M. J., Tate, D. G., Sharman, V. L. and Slapak, M. (1985). Do recipients of a cadaveric renal allograft on cyclosporin require prior transfusions? Experience of a single Unit. *Transplant. Proc.*, 17, 1032–3
45. Klintmalm, G., Brynger, H., Flatmark, A., Frodin, B. L., Husberg, B., Thorsby, E. and Groth, C. G. (1985). The blood transfusion, DR matching and mixed lymphocyte culture effects are not seen in cyclosporin-treated renal transplant recipients. *Transplant. Proc.*, 17, 1026–31
46. Persijn, G. G., Lansbergen, Q., D'Amaro, J. and Van Rood, J. J. (1981). Blood transfusion and second kidney allograft survival. *Transplantation*, 32, 392–4
47. Perdue, S. T. (1985). Risk factors for second transplants. In Terasaki, P. I. (ed.) *Clinical Kidney Transplants 1985*. pp. 191–203. (Los Angeles: UCLA Tissue Typing Laboratory)
48. Editorial (1978). Blood transfusions and renal transplantation. *Lancet*, 2, 193–4
49. Opelz, G., Graver, B., Mickey, M. R. and Terasaki, P. I. (1981). Lymphocytotoxic antibody responses to transfusions in potential kidney transplant recipients. *Transplantation*, 32, 177–83
50. Norman, D. J., Barry, J. M. Boehne, C., and Wetzsteon, P. (1985). Natural history of patients who make cytotoxic antibodies following prospective fresh blood transfusions. *Transplant. Proc.*, 17, 1041–43
51. Rafferty, M. J., Lang, C. J., Schwarz, G., O'Shea, J., Varghese, Z., Sweny, P., Fernando, O. and Moorehead, J. F. (1985). Prevention of sensitization resulting from third-party transfusion. *Transplant. Proc.*, 17, 2499–500

52. Taube, D., Williams, D. G., Cameron, J. S., Bewick, M., Ogg, C. S., Rudge, C. J., Welsh, K. I., Kennedy, L. A. and Thick, M. G. (1984). Renal transplantation after removal and prevention of resynthesis of HLA antibodies. *Lancet*, 1, 824–6

53. Falk, J. A., Cardella, C. J., Halloran, P., Robinelk, M., Arbus, G. and Bear, R. (1985). Transplantation can be performed with positive (non-current) crossmatch. *Transplant. Proc.*, 17, 1530–2

54. Ting, A. (1983). The lymphocytotoxic crossmatch test in clinical renal transplantation. *Transplantation*, 35, 403–7

55. Ladowski, J. S., Rosenthal, J. T., Taylor, R. J., Carpenter, B. and Hakala, T. R. (1985). The effect of previous sensitization on allograft survival with cyclosporin immunosuppression. *Transplant. Proc.*, 17, 1218–21

56. Valderabano, F., Anaya, F., Perez-Garcia, R., Olivas, E., Vasconez, F. and Jofre, R. (1983). Transfusion-induced anergy: skin test as an index for pre-transplant transfusions. *Proc. EDTA–Eur. Renal Ass.*, 20, 338–48

57. Matzner, Y., Hershko, C., Polliack, A., Konijn, A. M. and Izak, G. (1979). Suppressive effect of ferritin on *in vitro* lymphocyte function. *Br. J. Haematol.*, 42, 345–53

58. De Souza, M. (1983). Blood transfusions and allograft survival: iron-related immunosuppression? *Lancet*, 2, 681–2

59. Reed, E., Hardy, M., Lattes, C., Brensilver, J., McCabe, R., Reemstma, K. and Suciu-Foca, N. (1985). Anti-idiotypic antibodies and their relevance to transplantation. *Transplant. Proc.*, 17, 735–8

60. Singal, D. P., Joseph, S. and Ludwin, D. (1985). Blood transfusions, suppressor cells, and anti-idiotypic antibodies. *Transplant. Proc.*, 17, 1104–7

61. Sachs, D. H., Bluestone, J. A. and Epstein, S. L. (1985). Anti-idiotype responses in transplantation immunology. *Transplant. Proc.*, 17, 549–52

62. MacLeod, A. M., Power, D. A., Mason, R. J., Stewart, K. N., Shewan, W. G., Edward, N. and Catto, G. R. D. (1982). Possible mechanisms of action of transfusion-effect in renal transplantation. *Lancet*, 2, 468–70

63. MacLeod, A. M., Catto, G. R. D., Mason, R. J., Stewart, K., Power, D. N., Shewan, A. G. and Urbaniak, W. S. (1985). Beneficial antibodies in renal transplantation developing after blood transfusion: evidence for HLA-linkage. *Transplant. Proc.*, 17, 1057–9

64. Forwell, M. A., Cocker, J. E., Peel, M. G., Briggs, J. D., Junor, B. J. R., MacSween, R. N. M. and Sandilands, G. P. (1985). Correlation between high molecular weight Fc-receptor blocking factors and renal allograft survival. *Transplant. Proc.*, 17, 2572–3

65. Terasaki, P. I. (1984). The beneficial transfusion effect on kidney graft survival attributed to clonal deletion. *Transplantation*, 37, 119–25

66. Marquet, R. L., Heystek, G. A. and Tinbergen, W. J. (1971). Specific inhibition of organ allograft rejection by donor blood. *Transplant. Proc.*, 3, 708–10

67. Streilein, J. W. (1985). Suppressor cells are necessary for tolerance. *Transplant. Proc.*, 17, 1558–60

68. Moller, G. (1985). Immunologic tolerance and suppressor cells. *Transplant Proc.*, 17, 1561–5

69. Klein, J. (1985). *Immunology. The Science of Self–Nonself Discrimination.* (New York: John Wiley and Sons)

70. Gammon, G., Dunn, K., Shastri, N., Oki, A., Wilbur, S. and Sercarz, E. E. (1986). Neonatal T-cell tolerance to minimal immunogenic peptides is caused by clonal inactivation. *Nature*, 319, 413–5

71. Marquet, R. L., Heystek, G. A. and Tinberger, W. J. (1971). Specific inhibition of organ allograft rejection by donor blood. *Transplant. Proc.*, 3, 708–10

72. Shelby, J., Wakely, E. and Corry, R. J. (1985). Splenectomy abrogates the improved graft survival achieved by donor specific transfusions. *Transplant. Proc.*, 17, 1083–6

73. Liburd, E. M., Pazderka, V., Kovithavongs, T. and Dossetor, J. B. (1978). Evidence for suppressor cells and reduced CML induction by the donor in transplant patients. *Transplant. Proc.*, 10, 557–61

74. Charpentier, B., Lang, P., Martin, B. and Fries, D. (1981). Evidence for a suppressor cell system in human kidney allograft tolerance. *Transplant. Proc.*, 13, 90–4

75. Klatzmann, D., Gluchmann, J. C., Chapuis, F., Foucault, C., Metivier, F. and Rottemboorg, J. (1985). Independent cell-mediated lympholysis and mixed lymphocyte reaction suppression after blood transfusion in humans. *Transplant. Proc.*, 17, 1051–2

76. Wood, M. L., Gottschalk, R. and Monaco, A. P. (1984). Comparison of immune responsiveness in mice after single or multiple donor-specific transfusions. *J. Immunol.*, **132**, 651–5
77. Bach, F. H. (1985). Immunobiology summary. *Transplant. Proc.*, **17**, 1610–4
78. Tyler, J. D., Anderson, C. B., Sicard, G. A., Murphy, M. K., Anderman, C. K. and Etheredge, E. E. (1985). Decreased mixed lymphocyte reactivity toward donor antigens following donor specific transfusions combined with azathioprine immunosuppression. *Transplant. Proc.*, **17**, 1053–6
79. Morris, P. J., Ting, A. and Stocker, J. (1968). Leucocyte antigens in renal transplantation. I. The paradox of blood transfusion in renal transplantation. *Med. J. Aust.*, **2**, 1088–90
80. Dossetor, J. B., Mackinnon, K. J., Gault, M. H. and Mackean, L. D. (1967). Cadaver kidney transplants. *Transplantation*, **5**, 844–53
81. Brunner, F. P., Gurland, H. J., Harlen, H., Scharen, K. and Parsons, F. M. (1972). Combined report on regular dialysis and transplantation in Europe, II, 1971. *Dialysis Renal Transplant.*, **9**, 3–34
82. Parsons, F. M., Brunner, F. P., Burck, H. C., Graser, W., Gurland, H. J., Harlen, H., Scharer, K. and Spies, G. W. (1975). Statistical report. *Dialysis Transplant. Nephrol.*, **11**, 3–67
83. Van Hooft, J. B., Kalff, M. W., Van Poelgeest, A. E., Persijn, G. G. and Van Rood, J. J. (1976). Blood transfusions and kidney transplantation. *Transplantation*, **22**, 306–8
84. Taylor, R. M. R., Ting, A. and Briggs, J. D. (1985). Renal transplantation in the United Kingdom and Ireland–the centre effect. *Lancet*, **1**, 798–803

5
Experimental Transplantation

I. V. HUTCHINSON

INTRODUCTION

Experimental studies have had considerable influence on the clinical practice of transplantation, including the development of surgical techniques, development of immunosuppressive drugs and therapies, and a better understanding of the rejection process and its regulation.

The aim of this chapter is to review the immunological aspects of experimental transplantation rather than to delve into techniques of grafting or organ preservation. In this chapter, too, we will address the problem of designing meaningful experiments, the limitations on their interpretation and the difficulties encountered when we try to transfer knowledge derived by experiment under carefully controlled conditions to the clinical situation.

THE HISTORY OF TRANSPLANTATION IMMUNOLOGY

Experimental transplantation began in earnest at the turn of the century. Studies of the natural history of cancer in mice led to attempts to propagate tumours by transferring neoplastic cells from one animal to another. Only occasionally was this successful and the conditions required were not known. However, two experimenters happened upon the answer. Jensen (1903) transplanted tumours within a stock of 'Swiss white mice' which were fortuitously inbred and therefore genetically uniform. Loeb (1908) similarly used Japanese waltzing mice inbred for an inner ear defect which caused them to circle and whirl when excited. These observations led to the concept of genetic control of tumour transplantability and the importance of the 'race' of the recipient.

The genetic regulation of tumour graft acceptance was confirmed by Little and Tyzzer (1916)[1], and their work stimulated the development of the inbred strains which are of such importance today. However, the rejection process was assumed to be due to a response to tumour-specific antigens, a notion not in keeping with the overwhelming weight of evidence that immunization against these putative determinants failed to protect.

It was J. B. S. Haldane who suggested in 1933 that the rejection was directed at strain-specific determinants (alloantigens) rather than tumour-specific antigens. These alloantigens, he postulated, were tissue antigens similar to the blood group of other species. A tumour would have the tissue alloantigens of the inbred strain in which it arose and would therefore not be recognized as foreign within an inbred line. By contrast, these tissue antigens would induce an immune reaction in strains of mice which lacked these alloantigens.

The mouse seemed like an ideal experimental animal to test Haldane's hypothesis, with established inbred lines and a range of transplantable tumours. However, nothing was then known about blood group and tissue antigens in mice. The information was provided by the experiments of Sir Peter Gorer[2] who, by absorption studies, using normal human group A serum and rabbit immune serum, defined a series of four antigens, I, II, III and IV, present on red blood cells, on normal tissues and on tumour cells. It was Gorer's antigen II which was associated with tumour histocompatibility[3] (later to become recognized as a complex set of determinants), now known as H-2 in deference to Gorer's original designation and ignoring the fact that antigen II was, in fact, the first histocompatibility (H) gene discovered. Gorer propounded the immunological theory of tissue transplantation and it was not long before others started transplanting normal cells and tissues. Sir Peter Medawar and his colleagues were in the vanguard, using skin allografts in rabbits and later in mice.

George Snell[4] was responsible for an extensive series of studies of the H-2 complex and it was he who coined the terms 'histocompatibility' (H) antigens and genes[5]. Similar studies in humans led to the discovery of the HLA[6,7] system important in clinical transplantation and, more recently, to the recognition that the genes involved in transplant rejection are also pre-eminent in regulation of the immune response in general[8]. The Nobel Prize for Medicine in 1980 was awarded to George Snell, Jean Dausett and Baruf Benacerraf in recognition of their work in this field.

HISTOCOMPATIBILITY BARRIERS

The ferocity of the rejection response is related to the degree of genetic disparity between donor and recipient. *Autografts* from one part of the body to another are not rejected, nor are *isografts* between monozygous twins or genetically identical animals of the same inbred strain. *Allografts* from one non-identical individual to another of the same species (e.g. human to human) are usually acutely rejected in untreated recipients while *xenografts* from one species to another (e.g. monkey to man) are always vigorously destroyed. The mechanisms and tempo of various rejection processes are discussed elsewhere (Chapter 6). Suffice it to say here that *hyperacute* rejection, which occurs in minutes or hours, is due to the fixation of complement by preformed anti-graft antibodies in a sensitized recipient; *acute* rejecton, which takes a few days or weeks, is usually caused by cell-mediated mechanisms; and *chronic* rejection, which evolves over months or years, is a largely undefined process involving both cells and antibodies. Although some studies have been performed with xenografts, their clinical use remains an option of the future since they are so subject to destruction.

Within the allograft category the degree of histocompatibility between donor and recipient is governed by many sets of histocompatibility genes. There are over 25 sets of H genes in mice. One is of paramount importance in skin allograft rejection (the tissue transplanted is important–see below) and is therefore called the *major histocompatibility complex* (MHC). The MHC is known as H-2 in mice, HLA in man, RT1 in rats, DLA in dogs and so forth. The other genes are known as *minor histocompatibility antigens*, although some 'minor' differences, especially multiple minor mismatches, can cause acute skin allograft rejection which is indistinguishable from that observed across 'major' barriers. Matching for the MHC ignores the possible contribution of so-called minor antigens both in terms of acute graft rejection and acceptance (see below).

TRANSPLANTS OF NORMAL TISSUES

The type of transplant itself can have a profound effect on the observed results. Single cell suspensions of bone marrow leukocytes or liver cells may be particularly vulnerable to antibody-mediated damage, antibody-dependent cell-mediated cytotoxicity and natural killer cells. Larger cell aggregates such as pancreatic islets may, too, be susceptible to these malinfluences[9].

The application of microsurgical techniques in rodents has allowed orthotopic or heterotopic transplantation of primarily vascularized kidney[10], heart[11], liver[12,13], pancreas[14], spleen[15,16], lung[17] and small bowel[18]. The rejection of these is usually cell-mediated but the structure of the graft, the differential expression of target antigens (including MHC antigens, minor alloantigens and tissue-specific antigens) on vascular endothelium and parenchyma, the sensitivity of the graft to ischaemia and the possible cotransplantation of passenger leukocytes or lymph nodes can all profoundly influence activation of the rejection response and the progress of graft destruction. Indeed, it is difficult to extrapolate or to compare the results obtained by transplanting one tissue with those obtained with another organ even within a species or, indeed, across the same histocompatibility barrier.

The difficulty of comparison is even worse when using a non-vascularized allograft, especially skin. Because skin grafts are easy to transplant and the progress of rejection is readily monitored by observing epithelial destruction, a great deal of our knowledge was derived from studies conducted with this tissue. It was easy to regard the skin allograft as the benchmark with which to compare normal solid tissues and organs, and to consider as exceptions the results obtained with other tissues due to their immunological properties or some special genetic control of their acceptance or rejection. In fact it turns out that quite the reverse is true. Preventing skin allograft rejection is much more difficult than protecting a primarily vascularized graft. Minor alloantigens can provoke acute rejection of skin while major histocompatibility barriers invariably do: even point mutations in MHC genes leading to single amino acid differences between the donor and recipient MHC antigens can lead to acute rejection. Accordingly, the skin allograft is far more exacting than most other tissues and results obtained with this tissue err towards the pessimistic.

It is pertinent to mention the recent studies of Peugh[19], who has performed a survey of heterotopic cardiac allograft rejection across major and minor barriers in mice. The results are discrepant with skin grafting in the same species. Some hearts are accepted across MHC and minor barriers while, in some other cases, minor differences alone can cause acute graft failure. The differences between skin and heart may be accounted for, to some extent, by route of immunizaton via the local draining lymph node compared with intravenous systemic stimulation, ischaemic necrosis of skin during the revascularization period, non-specific inflammation in the skin graft bed, and the size of the graft. However, other factors such as the greater complexity of skin tissue and consequent expression of a wider array of antigens must play a role such that, if Gorer, Snell, Medawar and others had used cardiac transplants to define the 'major' histocompatibility complex, subsequent progress would have been considerably confused.

SPECIES USED IN EXPERIMENTAL STUDIES

Historically, the mouse was the species of choice particularly as so many inbred lines were available and these were genetically well defined. Several laboratories produced congenic mice such that two inbred strains differed from each other by only one or a few genes. For instance, B10.BR and B10.D2 strains are identical for all their genes (in this case the B10 background genes) except that B10.BR mice have the MHC genes of the H-2^k haplotype and B10.D2 mice are of the H-2^d haplotype. Hence transplants between these strains will be across an MHC barrier only. By choosing the donor–recipient combination one can study grafts across MHC and minor barriers alone or together. The development of congenic lines and the subdivision of the MHC into several loci has made the mouse a favourite subject for immunological studies.

Vascularized allografts in mice are technically very demanding. Rats, being bigger, are most often used for vascularized transplant studies since the requisite skill is readily acquired and an operating rate of 4–5 transplants a day is quite routine. However, rat genetics still lag behind although more congenic rat strains are becoming available.

Rabbits are sometimes used, particularly when the problems of damage caused by antibodies and complement are under consideration. Rats and mice have poor complement systems in so far as hyperacute rejection is not observed without infusion of xenogeneic (e.g. guinea pig or rabbit) serum as a source of exogenous complement components.

Dogs are often used as a preclinical model. The canine MHC, known as DLA, is serologically defined and these animals are more readily obtained than primates. They have been used to study the rejection of islets, and of normal solid tissues and organs, and the immunosuppressive properties of certain agents, notably azathioprine and cyclosporin A. In some areas of the world dogs may have heart worm and are unsuitable for transplantation, especially of the heart.

Pigs have been employed as an alternative to dogs. Recently several lines of inbred miniature pigs have been derived and are being characterized for use in transplant studies.

Primate studies provide the best preclinical data since the anatomy and tissue structure of simians is so similar to that of humans. However, they are expensive to obtain, difficult to handle and may harbour various pathogens. Baboons have been used in South Africa where they are captured from the wild. Elsewhere smaller species such as Rhesus monkeys, macaques and marmosets are imported or purposely bred.

On the whole, with recent advances in microsurgical techniques, rodents can now be used instead of larger animals. The advantages are various, especially the availability of inbred lines. However, there are some important differences between the anatomical, physiological and immunological properties of rodents and humans, in particular differences in the metabolic responses to pharmocological agents. In this case, the use of an animal model more closely resembling humans to assess a new treatment is imperative before clinical application.

EXPERIMENTS IN TISSUE CULTURE

Experiments performed in culture are usually cheaper, quicker and easier than allografting in animals. The amount of information derived from one day's culture work greatly outweighs that obtained even by the quickest and most dedicated surgeon. Why, then, use animals at all?

The data obtained *in vitro* and *in vivo* are of different sorts. For *in vitro* studies, one has to assume that all the relevant cells can survive and function in culture. It used to be thought that a proliferative response of recipient lymphocytes when stimulated with donor leukocytes (the mixed leukocyte response or MLR) reflected recognition of alloantigens by recipient lymphocytes of the T helper subset. However, T suppressor cells may also respond in MLR so that the mere proliferation of cells in culture may not indicate the net function of the reacting cells and their potential for damage *in vivo*.

A better indication of activation of effector cells *in vitro* is to assay the cells stimulated in MLR for cytotoxic activity in a cell-mediated lympholysis (CML) test. In such an experiment, activated 'killer' T cells are mixed with a target cell of donor origin and cell destruction is monitored. This is acceptable if the *in vitro* system is intended to parallel an *in vivo* situation in which the graft is known to be subject to attack by cytotoxic T cells. Unfortunately, this is not always so. In any case, the target cell used in the CML assay (usually a lymphoid blast rather than an organ epithelial or parenchymal cell) may greatly affect the results obtained (see below). Finally, the source of recipient responder cells, whether it be spleen, lymph node, blood or graft infiltrate, may dictate the results obtained *in vitro* since effector cells and suppressor cells may or may not recirculate through the blood-tisssue-lymph node circuit or home to the graft tissue.

In essence, *in vitro* techniques can never substitute for whole animal studies where cells are able to recirculate and reside in their own microenvironment rather than in a flask where lymphoid microarchitecture is completely destroyed. Interpretation of results can be difficult in relation to the *in vivo* model especially where the mechanism of graft destruction is not known. Hence *in vitro* studies can enable us to define certain possible cellular mechanisms but their relevance must always be uncertain. This caveat applies directly to immunological studies in humans which have to be done in culture.

SITE OF TRANSPLANTATION

The site into which an organ or tissue is transplanted may affect the outcome. Orthotopic transplantation is routinely used for the rat kidney where the left kidney is removed and a replacement organ put in its place using end-to-end anastomoses of the artery, vein and ureter. Rat lungs or heart/lung preparations are placed in the thorax. By contrast, hearts are connected across the abdominal aorta and vena cava, onto the renal pedicle or onto the carotid and external jugular vessels, acting heterotopically as an auxilliary organ performing no useful task.

The renal pedicle is useful for anastomosis because the ureter can be used as a drainpipe for exocrine secretions from pancreatic grafts or bile from heterotopic liver grafts. Assay of the 'urine' then becomes one way of determining graft viability and function. However, heterotopic liver grafts are not under a physiological pressure to function in the presence of the recipient's own liver, and suffer terminal rejection episodes in untreated allogeneic recipients. In the same strain combinations, orthotopic liver grafts may survive rejection episodes because physiological pressure causes the organ to be regenerated quickly enough to survive the onslaught.

EXPERIMENTAL DESIGN

How does one go about a series of experiments to answer a simple question? The stages are: (1) ask the question; (2) read all about it; (3) reformulate the question; (4) choose a model and master the requisite techniques; (5) do the experiment; (6) critically interpret the results; (7) pronounce the answer or return to (3). In the following pages we shall consider two illustrative examples of some relevance:

  (a) What is the mechanism of allograft rejection?
  (b) How does the blood transfusion effect work?

(a)   What is the mechanism of allograft rejection?

The world of transplantation awaits the answer to this! However, a review of the literature reveals that the question itself is naive. Firstly, there are several possible mechanisms, humoral or cellular, specific or non-specific, which may play a role at different stages in the rejection process. Secondly, the rejection process in different allografts may be different, depending on the tissue transplanted or the histocompatibility barrier.

Hence one has to be far more specific and ask, for instance, what mechanism (or mechanisms) are most likely to play a role in the acute rejection of kidney grafts transplanted across a major histocompatibility barrier?

A suitable model would be a rat renal allograft system. Inbred rats are available, the microsurgery is straightforward, the model has been extensively reported in the literature, and so on. The choice of strain combination is difficult: DA (RT1^a) to LEW (RT1^l) grafts are vigorously rejected and high doses of immunosuppression are required to prevent graft loss while, in the reverse LEW to DA combination, acute rejection is always observed but this is much easier to reverse either specifically or non-specifically. There is no easy formula to decide which should be used.

The first round of studies would include an assessment of the magnitude and timing of the antibody and cell-mediated immune responses to the graft, and the point of graft failure. Parallel studies might include a histological investigation using haematoxylin–eosin staining to assess pathological changes, immunoperoxidase staining with anti-donor antibodies to examine expression of histocompatibility antigens and with monoclonal antibodies to rat leukocytes to identify infiltrating cells, and recovery of infiltrating leukocytes from the tissue for staining and analysis using fluorescein-labelled antibodies to subsets and activation markers or using DNA/RNA stains to indicate their stage in the cell cycle.

An absolute essential in these (and all other experimental studies) is the inclusion of adequate controls. In this case syngeneic grafts performed under identical conditions are required to account for the effects of surgical trauma on the recipient and ischaemic damage to the graft.

Let us suppose that these studies[10] show an infiltrate of leukocytes on day 3, histological signs of damage beginning on day 5 and termination of graft function between days 7 and 9 coincident with microvascular occlusion and local necrosis. MHC antigen expression is markedly increased by day 5. The infiltrate on day 3 is enriched for lymphocytes with T helper (CD4) markers, by day 5 there is an increase in the T cytotoxic/suppressor (CD8) subset, and by day 7 there are large numbers of macrophages. The recipient animals make a cytotoxic antibody response beginning on day 3 and peaking on day 5 with a second peak between days 10 and 14, their spleens are enlarged and their spleens and lymph nodes contain T cells with cytotoxic activity against donor-derived lymphoblastoid target cells.

The interpretation is complicated. The recipient can and does make antibody and a cell-mediated response to the graft. Both coincide roughly with graft damage, so both could be involved. The sequential appearance of

117

T helper lymphocytes followed by T cytotoxic/suppressor cells in the graft could indicate selective trapping and activation of lymphocyte subsets and the presence of macrophages could be associated either with a delayed-type hypersensitivity reaction or removal of damaged cells. However, the mere presence of an infiltrate may be misleading given that syngeneic grafts too contain trapped leukocytes.

The next step might be to isolate infiltrating cells and demonstrate that they do have cytotoxic activity. When this is done it can be shown that there are potent specific killer T cells and a population of non-specific 'natural killer' cells which lyse sensitive target cells. However, choice of target tissue is difficult and influences the results. Usually lymphoblastoid target cells are used. However, the same cytotoxic cells which kill donor lymphoid cells do not destroy renal parenchymal cells. Perhaps the most relevant target would be donor vascular endothelial cells since these are the likely target during allograft rejection. These are difficult to obtain and may not express the appropriate target antigens until such expression is induced with, say, gamma interferon. Hence it is difficult to state that the cytotoxic cells isolated from the graft are responsible for rejection.

There are two other possible approaches, one indirect and the other direct, namely the use of immunosuppressive treatments to eliminate certain parts of the immune response (e.g. antibody production) to examine the effects of such treatment on rejection, or to isolate each aspect of the response in an inert host and ask if this bit of the reaction can cause rejection. The indirect approach is never clear and interpretation is fraught with difficulties.

The direct approach is most often used. For example, one might lethally irradiate a rat to eliminate the cells of its immune system and then put back into that animal a known population of cells such as pure B cells or cytotoxic T cells. This procedure is termed 'adoptive transfer of immunity'. The reconstituted rat is then given a transplant and the rejection process is observed.

In this way each possible mechanism is examined in isolation. Alas, interpretation even here is difficult because different results can be obtained by transferring normal or immune lymphocytes, by using selected histocompatibility barriers and different tissues and by altering the timing of various manipulations such as adoptive cell transfer relative to grafting.

All we can determine from such studies is whether a particular mechanism is either *necessary* or *sufficient* to cause rejection in that given system. For instance, it can be shown that T lymphocytes are *necessary* to restore acute skin graft rejection in a lethally-irradiated mouse. In addition, by transferring T lymphocytes separated into their various subsets, it can be shown that the subpopulation containing the T cells involved in delayed-type hypersensitivity are *sufficient* to elicit rejection of skin. Uncritical acceptance of this information might lead one to suppose that antibody-mediated mechanisms are insufficient or that cytotoxic cells are unnecessary.

The experimental model in which the observations were made must always be borne in mind. A recent series of experiments in a rat cardiac allograft system have suggested that hearts grafted across class II MHC barriers (equivalent to HLA-D region mismatches) are rejected by delayed-type hypersensitivity reactions[20] while hearts transplanted across class I differences (equivalent to HLA-A, B, C) are despatched by cytotoxic T cells[21]. The different histocompatibility barrier obviously did make a considerable difference to the cells involved in the rejection, but the overall interpretation may be wrong.

One major difficulty lies in the fact that experimental results are *interpreted* in the light of current dogma. Unfortunately, the prevailing view is some-times(!) wrong. For instance, there are two major subclasses of T lymphocyte, defined by possession of either the CD4 (OKT4 or Leu 3 in human, L3T4 in mouse and W3/25 in rat) or CD8 (analogous to OKT8 or Leu 2, Lyt-2 and OX8) antigens. It was erroneously thought that phenotype reflected cell function, and so CD4-positive cells were regarded as the helper/inducer subset and CD8-positive cells as the cytotoxic/suppressor subset. This division is no longer strictly tenable. The CD4/8 markers seem to be associated with cell receptor specificity: CD4-positive T cells recognize class II MHC alloantigens or foreign proteins in association with self-class II while CD8-positive T cells respond to allogeneic class I molecules or foreign antigen plus self-class I.

While there is some preferential division between cell phenotype and function it has now been clearly shown that both the CD4-positive and CD8-positive T cell subpopulations can have helper, cytotoxic or suppressive activity. Hence one might expect that rat hearts transplanted across class I or class II MHC barriers would be attacked by CD8-positive and CD4-positive cells, respectively. The further inference that the transplantation barrier influences the mechanism of rejection is at present unjustified.

Another approach to determining the mechanism of allograft rejection is to look at the transplanted tissue using sequential immunohistological or functional assays to discover what cells are present and what they are capable of doing once isolated. Various caveats apply. Immunohistological evidence is weak: the presence of CD4 or CD8-positive T cells or of macrophages could be associated with either graft damage or local immune suppression. The CD4/8 ratio is unlikely to be informative. Isolated cells can be tested for their function: in a rat kidney allograft model the graft is infiltrated by cytotoxic T cells, natural killer cells and suppressor cells. The main correlation between graft survival and the constituents of the acute infiltrate is a relative dearth of specific cytotoxic cells in organs from treated recipients[10]. There are non-specific, natural killer-like cells in organs from both treated and untreated recipients. Likewise, there are suppressor cells in the transplants of both groups but these may be of distinct lymphocyte subpopulations with suppressive function[22]. Long-term surviving kidneys, too, have infiltrating suppressor T cells, usually seen in sections as a perivascular accumulation of lymphocytes[22].

Testing the function of infiltrating cells poses three problems. The first difficulty is isolation of viable cells and the second problem is cell yield. In experimental animals the whole kidney can be diced, digested and subjected to differential centrifugation to isolate infiltrating leukocytes, an option not open to those studying human material. Here one starts with a Trucut biopsy specimen or a sample obtained by fine needle aspiration cytology. Functional assays on the small numbers of cells recovered in this way are difficult to perform. One approach has been to clone and expand the number of lymphocytes in tissue culture[23]. However, the outgrowth of a clone of, say, cytotoxic cells from the infiltrate indicates only that there was at least one cell in the sample with the potential to be cytotoxic. It should be noted that some cytotoxic lymphocytes can be detected in non-rejecting allografts. Furthermore, the analysis does not mean that the progenitor of the cytotoxic clone was itself cytotoxic *in situ*.

In summary, then, there is not a single major rejection reaction[10]. The possible mechanisms which could contribute to rejection of an allograft have been defined in carefully controlled experimental models but the clinical situation is very different. In the latter case, any or all of the possible rejection reactions could occur depending on the organ transplanted and its physical state (namely whole pancreas or isolated islets), the histocompatibility barrier, or the responder status of the recipient (either genetically determined or affected by drugs or disease).

As a consequence, for the present time at least, clinical immunological monitoring by any of the current methods is unlikely to be useful. The advent of new lymphocyte markers or the better understanding of the association of certain manifestations of the immune response with different histocompatibility barriers or recipient responder status will be required to facilitate prediction and treatment of rejection crises.

(b)   How does the blood transfusion effect work?

This, like question (a), is of great interest to clinicians and there is some frustration that a simple answer is not forthcoming. It must first be recognized that the blood transfusion effect, in other words the improvement of graft survival in pretransfused recipients, may be mediated by very different mechanisms in humans and rodents. Given that, the possible mechanisms are:

(1)   Sensitization and subsequent exclusion of 'high responder' patients,

(2)   Priming of lymphocytes for rapid (secondary) reactivation in the early post-operative period, making these cells more susceptible to immunosuppressive agents, or

(3)   Elicitation of immunoregulatory mechanisms such as suppressor T cells or anti-idiotypic antibodies[24].

Most studies in the rat totally ignore possibilities (1) and (2). Experiments are performed using strain combinations in which prior blood transfusion leads to graft acceptance without immunosuppression. Sensitization is not a problem which has been squarely addressed in rodents: where it occurs it is often an unwelcome complication. Therefore, by selection, these studies are done in low responder recipients. Are the majority of human patients low or high responders? This point surely affects the clinical relevance of the rodent experiments.

A further selection process is usually applied as well. Immunologists are firmly wedded to the concept of specificity, so they choose strain combinations in which specificity of the blood transfusion effect can be demonstrated. It would be wrong, however, to regard the apparent lack of specificity in the clinical effect as an artefact, even if donor-specific transfusion is especially effective. It is only recently that experiments have been directed at the area in which specificity breaks down, although in fact it turns out that lack of specificity itself may have an immunological basis.

Rather than go step by step through the experimental approach as before, suffice it to say that pretreatment with class I, class II or minor histocompatibility antigens on cells can induce graft acceptance in the rat, that timing is usually not crucial (grafting can be done 1–12 weeks after transfusion), that lack of specificity can be attributed to sharing of major and minor alloantigens, and that various aspects of the rejection response (antibody levels and the appearance of cytotoxic cells in the graft may be depressed. As we do not know precisely why grafts reject (see above) we do not know what aspect of the rejection process it is most relevant to study.

Several studies now show that blood transfusion elicits antibodies which block in mixed lymphocyte cultures and so may be anti-idiotypic antibodies[25,26]. In many other studies suppressor T cells have been demonstrated, usually in the post-graft period rather than prior to transplantation[22,27,28].

Suppressor T cells are not a single uniform subset of lymphocytes. There are at least three different suppressor T cells which may form a suppressor pathway[22]. The details will not be discussed here. However, although the T cells in the pathway are immunologically specific the overall effect of the pathway is to arm macrophages for non-specific suppression. We have shown that suppressor T cells specific for donor X will arm macrophages such that when they meet antigen from donor X again they suppress the response to donor Y or Z[22].

This observation may be clinically useful. A potential recipient could be given a blood transfusion from a friend or relative X. When a donor kidney Z becomes available, the recipient would then be retransfused with blood X and should accept kidney Z without being previously exposed to Z antigens. This approach could limit sensitization and elicit an immunologically-activated immunosuppression which probably allows induction of specific mechanisms of unresponsiveness to the graft.

IS EXPERIMENTAL TRANSPLANTATION RELEVANT?

Experimental work has allowed development of surgical techniques, the discovery of new drugs, the improvement of organ preservation procedures, and an understanding of the immunological and immunogenetic bases of rejection and how to treat it. Without these studies clinical transplantation would not be the routine procedure it is today.

Much of clinical practice has been deduced from clinical experience – blood transfusion, the dosage and timing of drug treatment, and so on. This is inevitable: these are experiments performed in the most relevant species – man.

The great and enduring hope of immunologists is to discover enough about the rejection process and its control to manipulate the immune response and engender specific unresponsiveness to donor antigens. The fact that treatments which work well in rats, such as passive transfer of enhancing antibodies or platelet transfusions, are not very efficacious in humans is unfortunate but does not negate the value of experimental studies.

Scientific studies are used to dissect the elements of various phenomena such as the blood transfusion effect, passive enhancement and the process of rejection. Experiments are carried out in defined and selected systems under rigorously controlled conditions. Within such systems it is possible to predict reliably the consequences of any given manipulation. Clearly, clinical practice is bound to be different since there cannot be a systematic change of one variable at a time. For example, if one donor provides kidneys for two recipients these may differ with respect to histocompatibility barrier, transfusion history, prior sensitization, age, sex, immune status, underlying disease and in many other ways. Without defining all of these variables, accurate prediction of the outcome of a particular treatment is not possible. Hence science can predict what could happen but not what will happen!

Laboratory work, then, does not have an immediate bearing on the clinical programme, given that so much selection of experimental conditions is necessary. Furthermore, in isolation, a particular immunological phenomenon might play an overwhelming role in rejection or suppression but this does not guarantee its clinical importance.

It now behoves the experimentalist to lengthen his or her perspective and research the previously ignored questions: the difference between easy and difficult strain combinations and how to convert the latter to the former; the basis of specificity or lack of it especially in outbred populations; and the superior results obtained with haploidentical donors. Current studies on preferential activation of suppression rather than sensitization, and development of new protocols for blood transfusion (see above) based on experimental observations will be of direct clinical relevance too.

CONCLUSIONS

In this chapter we have reviewed some of the background of experimental studies and then tried to explain why experimental observations are difficult to incorporate into clinical practice. Even the best experiments are not watertight and their interpretation, based on the ground of shifting dogma, is not always straightforward. Progress is being made towards solving the rejection problem. However, certain areas remain to be explored.

Clinical practice is based on the concepts derived from experimental studies. The long-term goal of inducing unresponsiveness is, hopefully, going to be achieved in the not-too-distant future.

References

1. Little, C. C. and Tyzzer, E. E. (1916). Further studies on inheritance of susceptibility to a transplantable tumor of Japanese waltzing mice. *J. Med. Res.*, **33**, 393

2. Gorer, P. A. (1936). The detection of antigenic differences in mouse erythrocytes by employment of immune sera. *Br. J. Exp. Pathol.*, **17**, 42
3. Gorer, P. A. (1937). The genetic and antigenic basis of tumour transplantation. *J. Pathol. Bacteriol.*, **44**, 691
4. Snell, G. D., Cherry, M. and Demant, P. (1978). H-2: its structure and similarity to HL-A *Transplant. Rev.*, **15**, 3
5. Snell, G. D. (1948). Methods for the study of histocompatibility genes. *J. Genet.*, **49**, 87
6. Dausett, J. (1958). Iso-leuco-anticorps. *Acta Haematol. (Basel)*, **20**, 156
7. van Rood, J. J. and van Leeuwen, A. (1963). Leucocyte grouping. A method and its application. *J. Clin. Invest.*, **42**, 1382
8. McDevitt, H. O. and Benacerraf, B. (1969). Genetic control of specific immune responses. *Adv. Immunol.*, **11**, 31
9. Mason, D. W. and Morris, P. J. (1986). Effector mechanisms in allograft rejection. *Ann. Rev. Immunol.*, **4**, 119
10. Fabre, J. W., Lim, S. H. and Morris, P. J. (1972). Renal transplantation in the rat – details of a technique. *Aust. NZ J. Surg.*, **41**, 69
11. Ono, K. and Lindsey, E. S. (1969). Improved technique of heart transplantation in rats. *J. Thorac. Cardiovasc. Surg.*, **57**, 225
12. Lee, S., Charters, A. C. and Orloff, M. J. (1975). Simplified technique for orthotopic liver transplantation in the rat. *Am. J. Surg.*, **130**, 38
13. Engemann, R., Ulrichs, K., Thiede, A., Muller-Ruchholtz, W. and Hamelmann, H. (1982). Value of a physiological liver transplant model in rats. *Transplantation*, **33**, 566
14. Schulak, J. A., Franklin, W. A., Stuart, F. P. and Reckard, C. R. (1983). Effect of warm ischaemia on segmental pancreas transplantation in the rat. *Transplantation*, **35**, 7
15. Coburn, R. J. (1969). Spleen transplantation in the rat. *Transplantation*, **8**, 86
16. Lee, S. and Orloff, M. J. (1969). A technique for splenic transplantation in the rat. *Surgery*, **65**, 436
17. Marck, K. W. and Wildevuur, C. R. H. (1982). Lung transplantation in the rat: I: technique and survival. *Ann. Thorac. Surg.*, **34**, 74
18. Monchick, G. J. and Russell, P. S. (1971). Transplantation of small bowel in the rat: technical and immunological considerations. *Surgery*, **70**, 693
19. Peugh, W. N., Superina, R. A., Wood, K. J. and Morris, P. J. (1986). The role of H-2 and non-H-2 antigens and genes in the rejection of murine cardiac allografts. *Immunogenetics*, **23**, 30
20. Forbes, C. R. D., Lowry, R. P., Gomersall, M. and Blackburn, J. (1985). Comparative immunohistologic studies in an adoptive transfer model of acute rat cardiac allograft rejection. *Transplantation*, **40**, 77
21. Lowry, R. P., Forbes, R. D. C., Blackburn, J. and Marghesco, D. (1985). Pivotal role of cytotoxic T cells in rejection of hearts bearing isolated class I disparities. *Transplant. Proc.*, **18**, 227
22. Hutchinson, I. V. (1986). Suppressor T cells in allogeneic models. *Transplantation*, **41**, 547
23. Wee, S.-L., Chen, L.-K. and Bach, F. H. (1983). Cloning of human T lymphocytes in transplantation monitoring. *Transplant. Proc.*, **15**, 17
24. Opelz, G. (1985). Blood transfusions and renal transplantation. In Morris, P. J. (ed.) *Kidney Transplantation: Principles and Practice*, 2nd edn., p. 323 (London and Orlando: Grune and Stratton)
25. Singal, D. P., Fagnilli, L. and Joseph, S. (1983). Blood transfusions induce antiidiotypic antibodies in renal transplant patients. *Transplant. Proc.*, **15**, 1005
26. Suica-Foca, N., Rohowsky, C., Kung, P., Lewison, A., Nicholson, J., Reetstsma, K. and King, D. W. (1983). MHC-specific idiotypes on alloactivated human T cells: *In vitro* and *in vivo* studies. *Transplant. Proc.*, **15**, 784
27. Marquet, R. L. and Heystek, G. A. (1981). Induction of suppressor cells by donor-specific blood transfusions and heart transplantation in the rat. *Transplantation*, **31**, 272
28. Lenhard, V., Maasen, G., Grosse-Wilde, H., Wernet, P. and Opelz, G. (1983). Effect of blood transfusions on immunoregulatory mononuclear cells in prospective transplant recipients. *Transplant. Proc.*, **15**, 1011

6
Rejection, the Immune Response, and the Influence of Cyclosporin A

A. W. THOMSON AND H. F. SEWELL

REJECTION AND THE IMMUNE RESPONSE

Introduction

The major obstacle to successful organ transplantation is the process of immunological rejection. This is particularly and invariably encountered in the situation of allografts (Table 6.1) which involve transplantation of organs or tissues between members of the same species who are not genetically completely identical. The special situation of organ transplantation between identical twins, which is always successful without the need for anti-rejection prophylactic drugs, indicates that it is the genetic differences (expressed as tissue antigens) which play a major part in the rejection process.

The tissue antigens, which define differences between the donor and recipient, are known collectively as histocompatibility antigens. These allo-antigens (i.e. many alternative forms exist amongst members of the species) have an important role in triggering the immune response which mediates rejection. These antigen systems are also the major targets of such a response.

Table 6.1 Types of graft

Type	Example	Outcome of transplantation
Allograft	One human to another (not identical twins)	Varyingly successful, requires immunosuppression
Autologous graft	One part of an individual to another part (similar to situation with identical twins)	Success without immunosuppression
Xenograft	Baboon organ to man	Generally failure

In immunological terms, the histocompatibility antigens stimulate and lead to activation and proliferation of the immune cells, and also function as targets in the resultant effector mechanisms induced by the immune reaction.

The detailed biology of the histocompatibility antigens and the genes encoding them on the short arm of chromosome 6 in man (i.e. the genetic region termed the major histocompatibility complex (MHC)) is expounded in Chapter 3. It should be appreciated that implicit in the term MHC is the acknowledgement that other minor genetic region(s) exist which encode for cell membrane molecules (other than the classical MHC-encoded class I and II histocompatibility antigens) which may play a role in their rejection process. The role of these minor regions, their products and their contribution to transplant rejection in man is not defined. The following discussion will be directed at the MHC and its products expressed at the cell membrane level as the histocompatibility antigens (also termed human leukocyte antigens (HLA)).

The problem of allograft rejection and the immune response will be discussed in general terms, the major information being obtained from extensive studies of renal allografting in man and experimental animals. Some special comments relating to the rejection of certain specific organ allografts will also be highlighted. It is important that the rejection process is seen and understood in the light of our knowledge of the mechanisms involved in the normal immune response[1].

The immune response

For clarity, it should be emphasized that the evolution of an efficient immune response did not occur with the prospect of humans transferring one or other of their body organs amongst themselves. The immune system evolved to combat, contain and/or eliminate 'non-self' substances (foreign antigens) which could disturb the internal milieu. Thus, correctly, allografts which express foreign histocompatibility antigens are attacked and rejected by the host immune system. Before examining in detail the processes involved in rejection, it is appropriate to summarize the major elements of the immune response.

A foreign substance X, entering the body via natural portals of entry, or as the result of medical or surgical intervention, is seen by the recipient's immune cells. The foreign material, termed an immunogen (i.e. it has the capacity to trigger the immune response), is presented to cells of the immune system by the appropriate antigen presenting cells (APC). APC are found at strategic sites and closely juxtaposed to the cells (i.e. lymphocytes) with specificity for the foreign substance X. Familiar APC are tissue macrophages, histiocytes, blood monocytes, Langerhans cells of skin and related cells, follicular dendritic cells in the lymph node follicle areas, interdigitating reticulum cells in lymph node paracortex and other mononuclear phagocytes and dendritic cells found throughout the body. The immunogen X (the term antigen is often used synonymously and will be used henceforth in this chapter), appropriately displayed by the APC, encounters lymphocytes and is recognized specifically via membrane antigen receptors on their surfaces (the lymphocytes being definable as T and B lymphocytes, with respect to their ontogeny, their expression of different differentiation membrane molecules, their function and differing forms of antigen-specific cell membrane receptors).

The receptor for antigen X on the surface of B lymphocytes is immunoglobulin in nature. It is the prototype of antibody which will be secreted by terminally differentiating B cells, recognized as immunoblasts and plasma cells. The receptor on T lymphocytes, which also recognizes antigen X, is not immunoglobulin (though similar in its molecular arrangement) and has very recently been defined. The T cell receptor sees the antigen X in a unique way. It recognizes X in conjunction with the host's own histocompatibility antigen system. Thus in the individual, the T cell sees antigen X (presented on APC) with MHC-encoded histocompatibility antigens, which are an integral part of the membrane of the same APC. This 'dual recognition' (Figure 6.1) of foreignness (antigen X) with self-MHC antigen is the central and pivotal event in triggering of the normal immune response. This also tells us that T lymphocytes are most important in such responses. It is also important to note that the MHC molecules of the host, which are essential in the normal immune response, are the same molecules which, when

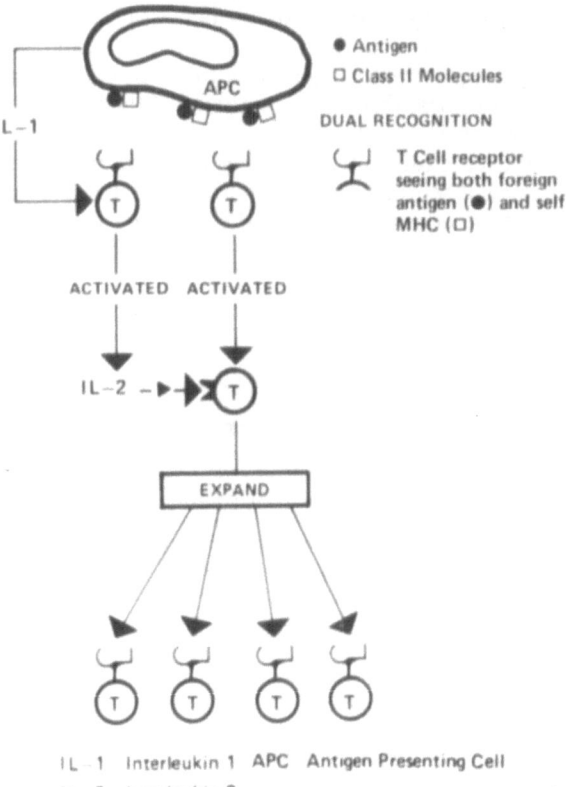

IL 1   Interleukin 1   APC   Antigen Presenting Cell
IL-2   Interleukin 2

Figure 6.1 Activation of T cells by antigen: the process of dual recognition

127

presented as 'donor' tissue to the immune system of a recipient, now function predominantly as the antigen. The recipient sees these in conjunction with his/her own MHC in dual recognition to initiate the rejection processes. They also function as targets in some responses.

Consequences of triggering of an immune response

B cells develop into antibody secreting cells, whilst T cells have a central role as regulatory cells and effector cells in the immune response (Table 6.2). These immunocompetent (i.e. with the ability to respond to antigen) lymphocytes are found within the secondary lymphoid compartments in strategically placed lymph nodes throughout the body (Figure 6.2) and in defined lymphoid aggregates scattered throughout important potential portals of entry, i.e. the intestinal tract, respiratory tract, skin and urogenital tract. Within these compartments the lymphocytes are found in reasonably well-defined but not exclusive locations. In lymph nodes, T cells are mainly in the paracortex, whilst B cells and their progeny are found in primary and secondary follicles, germinal centres, and the medullary region. The lymphocytes in these locations are heterogeneous in their physiology: some cells are migratory; others are predominantly sessile.

The other major lymphocyte compartment is peripheral blood, in which there is a recirculating pool of both T (the major population) and B cells. These recirculating lymphocytes, together with their counterparts in the tissues, have the ability to pass through most tissues of the body (by exploiting cell-to-cell and cell membrane receptor interactions). Such a versatile system, together with the intricate afferent lymphatics draining most tissue spaces, allows for a most efficient sentinel system (Figure 6.2). Thus antigens entering the body are likely to encounter, through the dynamic wanderings and/or strategic location of lymphocytes, cells with the appropriate antigen receptor. Provided the antigen is seen in the context of the appropriate microenvironment, with the appropriate interacting cells, a positive immune response can be elicited.

Table 6.2 Phenotypic and functional heterogeneity among human peripheral T cells

Function	T_4+ Helper/Inducer	T_8+ Cytotoxic/Suppressor
Effectors:		
effector cells for DTH	+	−
effector cells for cytotoxicity	−	+
Regulators:		
help for antibody production	+	−
help for cytotoxicity	+	−
suppressor for antibody synthesis and DTH	−	+
inducer of suppressor	+	−

T_4+: a molecule recognized by monoclonal antibody on T cells of helper/inducer subset. T_8+: different molecule recognized by a different monoclonal antibody on T cells of cytotoxic/suppressor subset. DTH: delayed type hypersensitivity

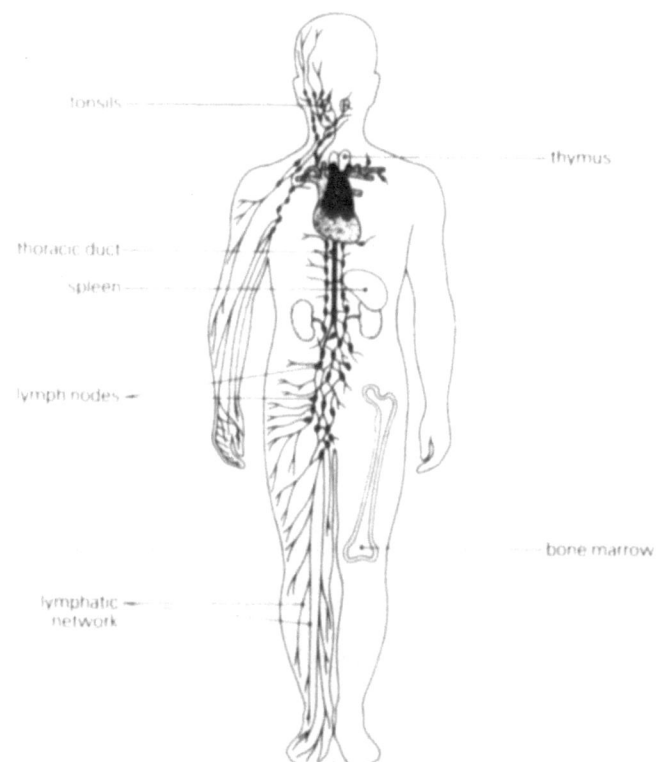

tonsils

thymus

thoracic duct

spleen

lymph nodes

bone marrow

lymphatic
network

Figure 6.2 The human lymphoid system

Modern technology has allowed functional and phenotypic (i.e. marking structurally defined, usually differentiation-associated molecules on the cell membrane) definition of T lymphocytes into subsets, or subgroupings, these divisions correlating to some extent with function. Thus, in mice, rats and humans, by using monoclonal antibody, subsets of T lymphocytes have been defined which correlate with function (Table 6.2). The regulatory T cells of the 'helper/inducer' (H/I) grouping are cells which see antigen in a dual recognition fashion, i.e. they see foreign antigen in association with self MHC class II histocompatibility molecules of APC. T cell reactivity is assisted by soluble factors from APC; particularly well-defined is the molecule called interleukin 1 (IL-1) which is secreted by APC (see Figure 6.1).

The helper/inducer cells, on interacting with the antigen–self complex, undergo biochemical changes. One result of such reactivity (or 'activation') is the elaboration by the $T_{H/I}$ cells of interleukin 2 (IL-2) – one of many soluble factors secreted (the total secreted soluble substances are generically termed 'lymphokines') (Table 6.3). It should be appreciated that for the secreted lymphokines to act upon the appropriate cells and tissues such cells must be receptive to them. Such is the case, and appropriate cell surface receptors for the defined soluble factors can be demonstrated (see Figure

Table 6.3 Lymphokines – synthesized and secreted by T cells

Lymphokine	Action
Migration inhibition factor (MIF)	Inhibits random migration of macrophages
Macrophage activation factor (MAF)	Enhances cytolytic activity of macrophages
Gamma interferon	Same activity as MAF
Macrophage procoagulant inducing factor (PIF)	Induces procoagulant activity in macrophages
Chemotactic factor	Attracts macrophages
Interleukin 2 (IL-2)	Stimulates growth of activated T cells
Interleukin 3 (IL-3)	Colony-stimulating factor activity
B cell growth factor	Stimulates growth and differentiation of a 'subset' of B cells
Colony-stimulating factor	Supports growth and differentiation of monocytes

Other lymphokines have been described

6.1). The reason for such an elaboration of soluble substances by the immune cells is to recruit more cells and more factors into the responding state of activation and proliferation. The aim is to produce a culmination of reactions (the end point being commonly seen as inflammatory reactions) which will eliminate or at least contain the foreign substance, with respect to the host. Thus the reaction generated by the specific immune response of T cells can result in some of the following:

(a) Help for B cells – so that they can, via specific receptor interactions with other determinants on the same antigen X, efficiently produce high affinity, high titre antibodies of various classes. Notably, B cells can produce antibody (although usually of less quality and quantity) against antigen without T cell help.

(b) T helper/inducers also help other defined subsets of T cells, e.g. T 'cytotoxic/suppressor' cells (see Table 6.2 and Figure 6.3), T cells associated with delayed type hypersensitivity (DTH) – a clinically defined entity with histomorphological and immunophenotypic correlates. DTH is represented by prototype reaction states such as contact hypersensitivity, immune reactivity to many intracellular pathogens, and experimental transplantation, and is pathologically defined by the type IV hypersensitivity reaction of Gell and Coombs.

Ultimately, the specific reactions of T cells and of antibodies from B cells destroy antigen, partly by their direct effects, but more consistently by secondarily recruited molecules, cells and their molecular products. The resultant manifestations of these effector mechanisms are the signs which we have recognized historically as inflammation, both acute and chronic. Thus the agents of inflammation (polymorphonuclear leukocytes, lymphocytes, platelets in aggregation, monocytes, factors of the coagulation system, etc.) which also are induced by many physical and chemical methods, are the same agents recruited to varying degrees by the specific immune response. Thus, for example, in T cell killing of target cells (e.g. virally-infected cells),

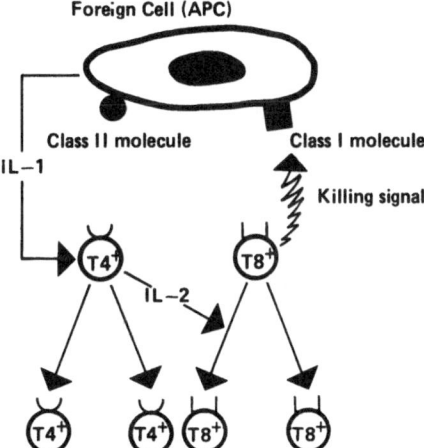

Figure 6.3 Activation of T cells by alloantigen: T_4+ are helper/inducers; T_8+ are cytotoxic/suppressors

the cytotoxic T cells see the foreign viral antigens associated with self MHC class I antigens. Contrastingly, in the efferent limb of allograft rejection (Figure 6.3), the donor MHC class I antigens are targets for the recipient's cytotoxic T cells. These effector cytotoxic T cells kill directly and also recruit other T cells, monocytes and soluble mediators to give efficient killing of the targets.

To highlight the role of histocompatibility antigens in the immune response associated with rejection, it should be remembered (see Chapter 3) that the class II MHC antigens are found on a restricted number of cells (e.g. APC, endothelial cells, B cells, activated T cells). The class I antigens are much more ubiquitous, being found on all nucleated cells of the body. These MHC antigens (coded for by the genes found at differing loci on the short arm of chromosome 6) are expressed as defined molecules on the surfaces of cells (Figure 6.4).

In the situation of organ allograft rejection, some of the major antigens seen on the donor tissue by the recipient's immune cells are the *donor* MHC molecules. Thus the recipient's recognition of the grafted organ's foreignness is of the associated complex of the host's own MHC molecules with soluble MHC molecules of the donor, or the foreign MHC alone. The donor MHC is of course now the foreign antigen.

Processes and forms of rejection

The rejection phenomenon associated with organ allografts can be detailed with respect to clinical histopathological and immunological criteria and their manifestations. These are markedly intertwined, and analysis by any individual aspect is by itself wholly inadequate and somewhat misleading when endeavouring to unravel the mechanisms of the different forms of rejection. Histopathological evaluation of transplant biopsies is invaluable

131

Genetic Loci and their encoded products at the cell membrane

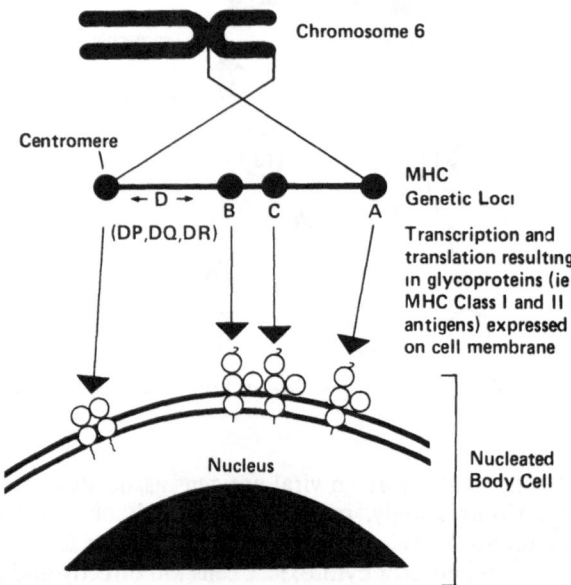

1. Genetic loci designated A, B, C — encode for Class I MHC (HLA) antigens

2. Genetic region designated D—contains at least three sub-loci DR,DQ,DP encoding for the Class II MHC (HLA) antigens

Figure 6.4 The human major histocompatibility complex

in monitoring and diagnosing rejections; but obviously what is seen in the tissue is the sum total of possibly recent specific immune responses and many secondary effector mechanisms, involving inflammatory cells, coagulation systems etc.

In contrast, many extensive animal experiments using well-defined genetic, immune and laboratory-manipulated rodents can give fairly concise insights into the role of specific elements required for rejection, but they still do not approximate to the complexity of far less well-defined interactions in humans, which manifest as rejection.

In the following commentary, we will endeavour to define the forms of rejection, with respect to clinical, histopathological and immunological effects, highlighting where possible the reasonably well-defined and accepted roles of the specific immune response.

Mechanistically, *rejection* like any other immune response, can be defined as having an afferent limb i.e. from the graft antigen(s) interaction with the recipient immune system (dual recognition), followed by the activation and the expansion of the immune response; and an efferent limb, i.e. the recipient's immune system generating reactions within and without the graft, leading to its rejection.

In the afferent limb, data exist which indicate several ways in which the appreciation/presentation of the foreign antigenic determinants of the graft to the recipient's immune cells occur[2,3]. These include:

(a) Histocompatibility antigens (MHC-encoded class II and I), together with other less well-defined antigens, which can be shed from the surface of the graft into intercellular spaces and other body fluids and can thus be transported to sites of strategically aggregated cells of the immune system (e.g. lymph nodes via afferent lymphatics, spleen via blood etc.) In these microenvironments with the appropriate APC, interactions between the antigens and T and B lymphocytes result in the specific immune response being triggered.

(b) There is also overwhelming evidence of triggering of the specific anti-graft immune response within the graft itself. Thus the recirculating T and B lymphocytes of the recipient can, on their movements through the graft, see the foreign antigens. MHC class II antigens on the graft blood vessel endothelium, the MHC class I antigens on similar cells and other graft nucleated cells, and systems such as foreign graft antigens outwith MHC molecules which are expressed on graft tissue[4] can trigger *in situ* the afferent limb response of the appropriate T and B cells.

(c) There is also evidence that donor 'passenger' leukocytes within the graft, which have many MHC-encoded antigens on their surfaces, can trigger the specific immune response of the recipient within and outwith the graft.

Following one or a combination of these afferent limb reactions, there occurs increased activation and amplification of the immune response against the graft antigen, through recruitment of other cell types by the various lymphokines (see Table 6.3). The intense activation/amplification can be seen in regional lymphoid tissues distant to the graft. For instance, many enlarged, activated lymphocytes can be demonstrated by immunological, radioisotopic and histological analyses. These reacting cells are given many names e.g. 'blasts', 'immunoblasts', 'lymphoblasts', 'large pyroninophilic cells', 'activated lymphoblasts' etc. These varying descriptions are a statement of expansion and recruitment of cells generated by the specific afferent limb response. Similar features can also be seen at varying times in the graft itself.

The final effector reactions which lead to graft destruction and rejection are commonly described in terms of cellular (immune effector T cells) and humoral (antibody) components. These simplistic terms fail to indicate the difficulty of defining which reactions are of major consequence in some forms of rejection. This point may be of considerable importance clinically, when endeavouring to treat or prevent such episodes.

Classically, rejection of organ allografts can be divided into at least three categories (these being in patients who may or may not be immunosuppressed by their disease or by desired clinical–pharmacological intervention). The

133

categories of rejection are *hyperacute, acute,* and *chronic*–these designations relating to the rate of destruction of the graft, rate of deterioration of graft function and the nature of the lesions.

Renal allografts provide the most studied and best defined examples of these forms of rejection in humans. Also, the use of animal models to study kidney rejection, plus the availability of methods and reagents such as monoclonal antibodies which define functional subsets of lymphocytes, result in reasonably, broadly accepted statements concerning mechanisms of graft rejection.

Hyperacute rejection

In man and experimental animals, hyperacute rejection is seen as being antibody-mediated, the target antigens being predominantly those on the graft vascular endothelium. The antibody/antigen reaction in such a situation activates complement (this series of protein enzymes, on activation, can generate components which interact with and recruit many agents of the inflammatory process and of the coagulation system, as well as being able to destroy some cells directly). There is evidence of platelet activation and aggregation and thrombosis. These reactions occur a few minutes to hours following revascularization of the graft. In most instances, it is due to 'preformed', circulating, cytotoxic antibody which binds to MHC class I and other antigen systems in the donor organ. The rapidity of the reaction clearly indicates, in this situation, that the afferent limb of the rejection response occurs *before* the recipient received the graft. Thus natural antibodies associated with ABO-incompatible donor–recipient pairs of antibodies generated by previous transfusions of recipients (the transfused blood contains leukocytes with foreign MHC antigens[5], which act as stimulating antigens for the immune system of the potential recipient of a graft) have been shown to be involved in hyperacute rejection. Similarly, multiparous women may be sensitized i.e. have their immune cells triggered by paternally-derived MHC antigens: such women have preformed cytotoxic antibodies to MHC antigens.

Hyperacute rejection processes rapidly result in the obstruction of blood vessels and ischaemia. Clinically, this manifests itself initially as acute inflammation in the patient, who is pyrexial, with a marked leukocytosis. Renal function rapidly declines and the patient becomes oliguric or anuric. The graft itself, in the more immediate forms of hyperacute rejection, becomes dramatically enlarged and cyanotic. Histologically, the effects of polymorph influx, their released enzymes, the lysis of endothelial cells and the aggregation of platelets to exposed vascular basement membrane leading to thrombosis, is characterized as fibrinoid necrosis. Immunological analyses reveal deposition of antibody (usually IgG class) and complement in glomerular and peritubular capillaries.

There is no successful treatment for hyperacute rejection – the organ must be removed. Prevention is the answer. Thus, with improved tissue typing techniques (see Chapter 3), especially cytotoxic crossmatching, hyperacute rejection has become uncommon. Nevertheless, occasionally cases do occur, and sometimes indicate rarer non-MHC antibody–antigen system involvement.

Some authorities describe a form of rejection called 'accelerated rejection' occuring 2–5 days after transplantation. This appears to be a more protracted antibody-mediated episode, but in terms of mechanisms it is essentially as described for hyperacute rejection.

Acute rejection

Classically, acute rejection occurs a few weeks to a few months after transplantation, but clear-cut episodes of acute rejection can develop many months or even years after grafting, possibly due to the modifying influence of the post-transplantation immunosuppressive regimes. The mechanisms involved in this form of rejection have been studied for many years. Detailed examination (histopathological and immunopathological) of post-transplant biopsies at various times, together with detailed examination of elements of the patients' immune responses, have indicated a bewildering number of phenomena relating to cell types, mediators and cellular interactions in the acute rejection situation. Using such acquired knowledge, plus imaginative experimental animal models (e.g. dogs, monkeys, rats and mice), the information now emerging indicates that acute graft rejection is initially and predominantly mediated by T lymphocytes of the helper/inducer phenotype. Other cells and mechanisms such as natural killer cells (NK) and antibody-dependent cell-mediated cytotoxicity (ADCC), though useful *in vitro* models of allograft rejection, are not now seen as playing a major *in vivo* role.

The most recent analyses, using adult thymectomized, irradiated and bone marrow restored animals, together with monoclonal antibody-defined reconstitution with various lymphocyte subsets in such grafted animals, again clearly demonstrate cells of the T helper/inducer phenotype to be the main agents of acute rejection. Much more limited phenotypic analyses of blood cells and cells infiltrating rejecting grafts in humans support the role of T cells as the main population mediating acute rejection.

The fine dissecting out of the main T cells involved is still imprecise: we are now aware that the designation 'T helper/inducer cells' contains several subpopulations of T cells, some being regulatory cells, and others being effector cells. Within the effector group are the cells mediating DTH (see Table 6.2). Some authorities suggest that these are the cells responsible for the effector limb of the acute rejection episode (as postulated more than a quarter of a century ago by Medawar and colleagues). Nevertheless, the answer is not yet complete as regards the true nature of the T cells responsible for acute rejection.

Clinically, early diagnosis is important because prompt treatment of acute rejection episodes may reverse the damage to the allograft. Diagnosis may prove difficult. The renal transplant patient who, after weeks or months develops fever, graft tenderness and deteriorating renal function (proteinuria/ oliguria, with a fall in creatinine clearance), may be experiencing an acute rejection episode, but the same symptoms and signs may be due to an infection or drugs etc. Biopsy of the allograft may help to confirm the diagnosis. As described above, current evidence indicates T cells as the main mediators of acute rejection, but it must be appreciated that once damage ensues, the effects of tissue destruction also bring into operation many other secondary reactions and associated phenomena observable in the graft. Thus in a biopsy, various forms of cellular infiltration are noted, together with secondary features such as vascular occlusion, thrombosis and tissue necrosis. Histopathologically, various changes are described in rejecting tissues, in relation to different components within the tissue, e.g. blood vessels, interstitium etc.

The picture is further complicated by the fact that acute rejection episodes can occur against a background of chronic damage, with all the features associated with chronic changes. Furthermore, identifying the microscopic features noted in the biopsy from a patient undergoing chronic immunosuppressive therapy (some drugs such as cyclosporin A can induce changes in some allografts having many features in common with the microscopic appearances of acute rejection) can prove difficult, hence again differential diagnosis is troublesome. Clearly, it is most important that the study and reporting of biopsies, histologically, immunologically and ultrastructurally, must be done only in conjunction with all the available clinical information and other laboratory tests. The analysis of biopsies, apart from establishing a diagnosis of acute rejection, can also help in patient management and be of prognostic value. Thus, varying features indicating the severity of the rejection episode can be correlated with the likelihood of response to anti-rejection therapy. Thus a predominant cellular infiltration of an allograft with mononuclear cells, with little evidence of fibrinoid necrosis, generally indicates a rejection episode which will respond to anti-rejection therapy.

Chronic rejection

Chronic rejection is seen months to years after successful allograft transplantation with slow and progressive deterioration of function. Thus with a renal allograft undergoing chronic rejection, there are signs of progressive renal failure and possibly secondary hypertension.

The immune mechanisms responsible for chronic rejection are *unclear*. There is no adequate animal model to help unravel the plethora of biopsy findings as obtained in humans. In humans, the transition between the appearances of acute and chronic rejection is indistinct, but the emphasis, histologically, is on the balance shifting from a predominance of cellular infiltration and fibrinoid vasculitis lesions, to a predominance of proliferative and stenosing vascular lesions.

Thus, in chronically rejecting renal allografts, there is thickening of the glomerular basement membrane, interstitial fibrosis and proliferation of endothelial cells. Some authorities suggest that such changes may be due to low grade deposition of antibody and antigen (donor MHC class I–II antigen) complexes in the allografts, together with lower grade T cell-mediated responses qualitatively similar to those found in acute rejection. It is suggested that depressed effects of the T cell reaction are due to the standard therapeutic immunosuppressive regimens (steroids, cytotoxic drugs, cyclosporin A etc.)

on which all allografted patients are maintained. It is also suggested that there may be development within the recipient of some forms of specific tolerance to the graft. Ill-defined mechanisms invoking ideas of anti-idiotypic antibodies, anti-class I MHC suppressive antibodies, contrasuppressor cells etc., presently represent mere speculation.

Patients with chronic rejection do not appear to benefit from current antirejection therapy. As in the case of acute rejection, differential diagnosis of chronic rejection versus drug toxicity can at times be difficult. This is again the situation with possible cyclosporin A toxicity versus microscopic features of chronic rejection in a renal allograft biopsy (see below).

Rejection related to various organ allograft systems

Most of the foregoing relates particularly to renal allografts – we will now indicate a few points of significance to other organ graft systems.

Heart transplantation

Acute rejection

Transvenous endomyocardial biopsy reveals interstitial mononuclear infiltrates with or without myocyte (heart muscle cell) necrosis. Attempts are being made to immunophenotype with monoclonal antibodies the nature of the cellular infiltrate, as is being done with percutaneous needle biopsy analysis of renal allografts.

Chronic rejection

The cardiac lesion resembles coronary arteriosclerosis. Among the factors defined as important in chronic cardiac rejection are some particular forms of MHC class I, A locus incompatibilities.

Liver transplantation

The principles and mechanisms of liver transplant rejection are essentially those outlined above. Importantly, the incidence and severity of the rejection processes (hyperacute, acute and chronic) seems, in the few large series published to date, to be significantly less for liver allografts. The reasons for the somewhat privileged place of liver allografts, with respect to the rejection process, are not clear. Several studies have indicated that MHC class I and II antigens are poorly expressed on liver hepatocytes, hence such cells are less likely to be stimulators and targets in the afferent and efferent limbs of the rejection process. Contrastingly, the bile duct epithelium and sinusoidal cells of the liver do express MHC encoded class II antigens to high levels, which could function as stimulators for acute rejection episodes. These are the sites where cellular infiltrates are pronounced in episodes of acute rejection. Interestingly, the work of Portmann et al.[6] has documented that liver grafts acquire post-transplantation, sinusoidal lining cells of host origin. One would not expect such 'self' cells (being of recipient origin) to be under attack from the recipient's own immune system. These observations go some way to explaining the privileged position of liver allografts, with respect to the rejection process, *but* the explanations are as yet incomplete.

The symptoms and signs of liver allograft rejection are non-specific, i.e. hyperbilirubinaemia, increased liver enzymes, fever and radioisotopic abnormalities. Thus diagnosis again relies heavily on percutaneous biopsies.

Pancreas transplantation

Many medical and surgical aspects of pancreatic allografts have yet to receive consensus opinion of how best to proceed. The techniques to be applied, e.g. islet cells injected into the portal vein, segmental pancreatic transplants, whole pancreas grafts, etc., need to be agreed. It is apparent that, depending on the chosen method, the problem of rejection may vary considerably with respect to antigens displayed in the graft. In fact, ideas of enclosing islet cells in implantable chambers which will allow release of insulin but prevent ingress of immune cells appear most attractive, and one would expect rejection to be a minor problem. There are immense problems in obtaining adequate numbers of viable, hormone-producing islets: these problems must first be overcome before this pancreatic transplant procedure and a discussion of possible rejection problems can be seriously entertained.

Skin transplantation

Skin autografts for covering and replacing areas destroyed by trauma, burns or operation are commonplace, and as discussed above the genetics of such self-to-self situations present no problems of rejection. Contrastingly, skin allografts used in the treatment of severe burns are susceptible to vigorous rejection. This is in part associated with local anatomy and the establishment of a necessary and delicate microvascular circulation which is susceptible to the ravages of inflammation and infection. Skin allografts also possess APC (Langerhans cells and related cell types) which express abundant amounts of MHC class II alloantigens, which in turn are major stimulators of the recipient's immune system (afferent limb). Moreover, APC and keratinocytes in skin allografts possess a lot of MHC class I antigens (good targets for the effector limb of the rejection process).

Prevention and control of the rejection process

From the foregoing discussion of the role of the immune response in mechanisms of rejection, a theoretical working sequence of methods for preventing and controlling rejection can be devised as shown in Figure 6.5. Anti-rejection prophylaxis/treatments are theoretically directed against defined points in the spectrum of the immune response. The ideal situation would be specific immunosuppression directed against the immune cells with the specific receptors for the donor antigens. We are far from reaching such an ideal. The goal of specific tolerance is, of course, realized during pregnancy ('nature's transplant' – a semi-allogeneic graft). Many of the concepts illustrated for specific immunosuppression (Figure 6.5), even in animal

138

IMMUNOSUPRESSION OF THE REJECTION REPONSE

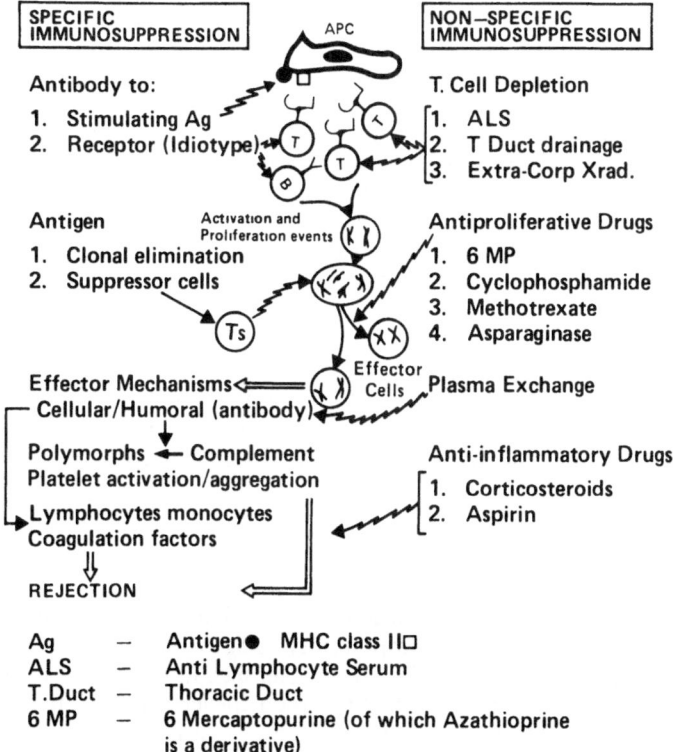

SPECIFIC IMMUNOSUPPRESSION	NON–SPECIFIC IMMUNOSUPPRESSION

APC

Antibody to:
1. Stimulating Ag
2. Receptor (Idiotype)

T. Cell Depletion
1. ALS
2. T Duct drainage
3. Extra-Corp Xrad.

Activation and Proliferation events

Antigen
1. Clonal elimination
2. Suppressor cells

Antiproliferative Drugs
1. 6 MP
2. Cyclophosphamide
3. Methotrexate
4. Asparaginase

Ts

Effector Cells

Effector Mechanisms
Cellular/Humoral (antibody)

Plasma Exchange

Polymorphs ← Complement
Platelet activation/aggregation

Anti-inflammatory Drugs
1. Corticosteroids
2. Aspirin

Lymphocytes monocytes
Coagulation factors

REJECTION

Ag	–	Antigen● MHC class II☐
ALS	–	Anti Lymphocyte Serum
T.Duct	–	Thoracic Duct
6 MP	–	6 Mercaptopurine (of which Azathioprine is a derivative)

Figure 6.5 Methods for preventing and controlling rejection

models, cannot be consistently defined and utilized. Thus the mainstay practical methods of prevention and control of rejection rely on non-specific immunosuppression and other manoeuvres which may be listed as follows:

(1) Minimizing antigenic differences between donor tissue and recipient by good tissue typing – matching procedures (see Chapter 3);

(2) Clinically avoiding procedures which may prime the potential recipient's immune system to non-self MHC antigens, e.g. certain forms of blood transfusion;

(3) Immunosuppressive therapy to prevent and control rejection – relying on agents that destroy immunocompetent cells, or inhibit their differentiation, activation and proliferation, in response to the non-self MHC antigen. Extensive animal experiments have revealed that it is more difficult to inhibit the immune response after it is already underway. Immunosuppression is therefore best commenced before or at the time of transplantation. Nevertheless, some control and success is obtained

with attempts at treating episodes of acute rejection in the already immunosuppressed patient.

All currently practised forms of immunosuppressive therapy have drawbacks. Thus they weaken the recipient's immune system not only against the graft as desired, but also against infections caused by bacteria, fungi and viruses. Prolonged usage of cytotoxics is also associated with an increased incidence of malignancies in recipients of allografts, particularly skin cancers and non-Hodgkins lymphomas. Prolonged usage of steroids also has many well-documented, undesirable side effects.

The mainstays of immunosuppressive agents have, for more than twenty-five years, been azathioprine, corticosteroids and, to lesser extents, antilymphocyte and antithymocyte globulin. All these reagents have proved useful, but suffer from combinations of undesirable effects. Methylprednisolone is still currently the best form of therapy for treating episodes of acute rejection in transplant patients. The drug cyclosporin A has proved to be an effective immunosuppressant for prevention of rejection and in many transplantation centres it now occupies the primary place, superceding azathioprine and prednisolone as the backbone of prophylactic anti-rejection therapy.

CYCLOSPORIN A

The ultimate aim in transplantation is to inhibit selectively the immune response towards donor histocompatibility antigens in the manner achieved with neonatally-induced transplantation tolerance in the mouse thirty years ago[7]. Although no therapeutic agent has yet achieved this goal, the serendipitous discovery of cyclosporin A (CsA) represents a major advance towards the selective impairment of T cell activation, with sparing of non-specific host resistance. Although a great deal has been learnt over the past ten years about the immunological properties of CsA, we still do not fully understand which step in the lymphocyte activation process is blocked by the drug. CsA is effective during the induction phase of the immune response and has been shown to be at least as effective as the most potent immunosuppressant known for each particular graft in the prolongation of allograft survival in both laboratory animals and man (Table 6.4).

Unfortunately, CsA is not without side effects, the most important of which is renal dysfunction, some degree of which occurs in virtually all patients receiving the drug. This problem offers the greatest challenge in the area of renal transplantation, where it may confound the diagnosis of allograft rejection. Much information has been acquired regarding the pharmacokinetics of the drug leading to improved treatment strategies. Moreover, it is possible that particular structural analogues may yet emerge which exhibit less deleterious effects. It is our purpose to discuss the immunological properties and mode of action of CsA, to review clinical results with the drug, the complications which may arise and the strategies which have been devised to avoid or at least minimize the impact of CsA-induced nephrotoxicity.

Table 6.4 Prolongation of allograft survival by CsA in various species

Species	Graft	CsA dose range (mg/kg)
Mouse	Skin, bone marrow, muscle	25–300
Rat	Skin, bone marrow, liver, islets of Langerhans, pancreas, nerve and Schwann cells, kidney, heart (allo- and xenograft), lung, small intestine, limb	10–50
Rabbit	Skin, cornea, kidney (allo- and xenograft), ovary	15–25
Dog	Skin, bone marrow, pancreas, kidney, heart, lung, small intestine	9–50
Pig	Heart, liver	15–25
Monkey	Kidney, heart, heart/lung	10–50
Chicken	Skin	25–50
Man	Kidney, liver, heart, heart/lung, pancreas, bone marrow	6–17

Chemistry of CsA

CsA was isolated by workers at Sandoz Ltd, Basle, Switzerland, from metabolite mixtures obtained from two new strains of fungi imperfecti, *Cylindrocarpon lucidum* Booth and *Tolypocladium inflatum* Gams. It was purified in 1973 and its structure fully elucidated in 1975 using both chemical degradation and X-ray crystallographic techniques. It is a cyclic peptide (Figure 6.6), composed of 11 amino acids (M.W. 1202.6 kD) and displays several distinctive features including (i) a nine-carbon (C9) novel amino acid at position 1 and (ii) a hydrophobic nature (10 aliphatic amino acids; high degree of *N*-methylation). Due to its complex structure, CsA cannot be synthesized in sufficient quantity to meet demand. It is produced by a fermentation process, then refined chromatographically. CsA is not inactivated by gut pH or enzymes: it is insoluble in water but dissolves in lipids and organic solvents. For clinical use it is administered orally or by intravenous injection.

Immunosuppressive properties

In 1976, J. F. Borel and his colleagues first reported the potent immunosuppressive properties of CsA in laboratory animals[8]. They showed that whilst the drug suppressed both antibody production and cell-mediated immunity, it exhibited a selective inhibitory effect on T cell dependent (type IV hypersensitivity) responses. Thus, in normal and congenitally athymic animals, CsA failed to suppress humoral responses to the T cell-independent antigen, lipopolysaccharide.

Additional important observations were that CsA depressed chronic but not acute inflammatory reactions, that the drug was neither lympho- nor myelotoxic and that it had no influence on the viability or activity of mature cytotoxic T cells or antibody-producing B cells. From this information, it

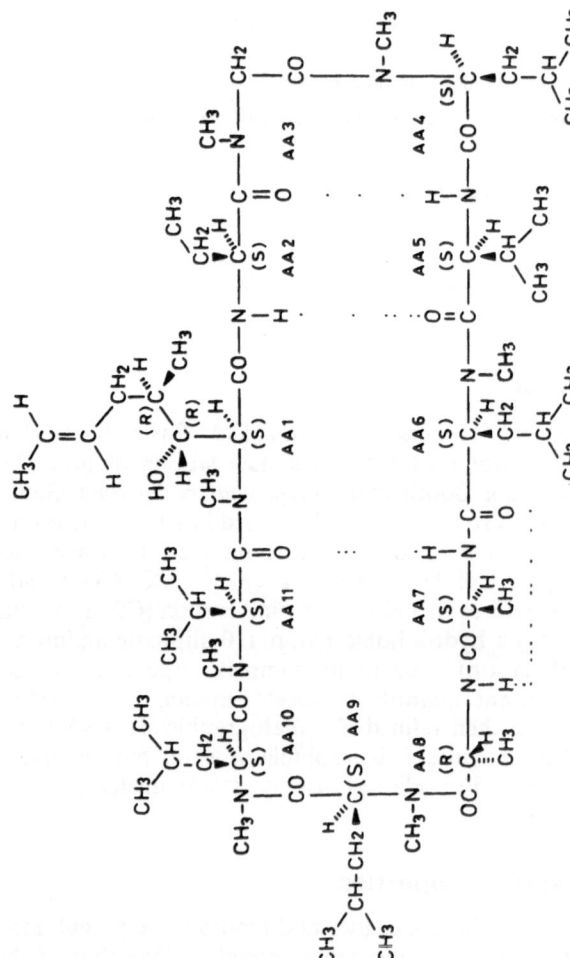

Figure 6.6 The structure of CsA. The novel amino acid is designated AA1. Note also the high degree of *N*-methylation of the molecule

was clear that CsA exhibited unique properties as an immunosuppressant: all other immunosuppressive drugs such as azathioprine lack such a discriminating mode of action and exert varying degrees of toxicity towards haematopoietic stem cells. Subsequent studies have, however, cast some doubt on the absolute selectivity of CsA for T cells: in mice, for example, antibody responses to certain T-independent antigens may be totally inhibited by CsA. Secondary antibody responses appear less susceptible to CsA than primary responses and indeed there is evidence that the helper function of *primed* $T_{H/I}$ cells is resistant to CsA, although that of virgin or primary $T_{H/I}$ cells is highly susceptible. In animals given CsA at doses which prolong allograft survival, there is a marked reduction in the cellularity of the thymic medulla, splenic marginal zone and splenic periarterial sheath – areas believed to contain cells of the T_H lineage.

A considerable amount of phenomenology has now been accumulated regarding the effects of CsA on immune reactions in laboratory species[9-11]. These reports include the inhibition of antibody production in response to a variety of antigens including histocompatibility antigens, impairment of classical delayed-type hypersensitivity to, for example, tuberculin and dinitrochlorobenzene, and the suppression of graft-versus-host reactions induced by bone marrow grafting. Although it induces graft to host tolerance after histoincompatible bone marrow transplantation in rodents, it is not uniformly effective in preventing graft-versus-host disease (GVHD) in dogs or rabbits.

Prolongation of allograft survival in animals

Of particular significance, with respect to this chapter, is the important finding that for many (e.g. kidney, heart) but not all organs, limited courses of CsA commencing at the time of grafting (e.g. on days 0–14), can lead to very prolonged allograft survival[12]. Thus, CsA-induced indefinite, donor-specific transplantation tolerance, with respect to renal allografts in rabbits and both renal and cardiac allografts in rats, is now well recognized. The effect is dependent on administration of the drug at the time of engraftment, is reversed by presensitization of the recipient to donor alloantigens and may prevail despite mononuclear cell infiltration of the graft. As discussed below, such cells may play an important protective role in allograft survival.

In the rat cardiac allograft model, Nagao et al.[13] studied host (PVG) responses to donor (DA) and third-party (WAG) skin grafts in animals given a 14-day course of CsA. They were thus able to examine both the degree and specificity of the unresponsive state induced by the drug. They found that stable, donor-specific immune suppression was only achieved after eight post-transplant weeks. During the 14-day period following engraftment, when the drug was administered, both DA and WAG skin grafts were protected from rejection (this state was however dependent on the presence of the DA heart graft). Between two and six weeks (following drug withdrawal) the capacity to reject DA and third-party skin grafts was restored. Rejection of DA skin grafts was invariably followed by heart graft rejection. After eight weeks, however, specific unresponsiveness to heart donor (DA) skin grafts was observed, whilst the third-party (WAG) skin grafts were once again rejected. The same group of workers have also established that the tolerant state induced by CsA in this cardiac allograft model is dependent on the presence of donor antigen. Thus removal of the primary heart graft following the 14-day course of CsA was found to prevent development of unresponsiveness to subsequent heart transplants from the same donor strain.

On the basis of the evidence obtained using the above and similar rat allograft models, it seems likely that the development of a specific, stable state of CsA-induced unresponsiveness is due to the gradual proliferation of suppressor $T(T_S)$ cells. It also appears that such T_s, derived from the thymic cortex and accumulating within the graft, may ensure its acceptance. Thus thymectomy of prospective CsA-treated allograft recipients prior to transplantation results in rejection, whereas thymectomy post transplant and CsA treatment do not affect induction of the tolerant state. Evidence accumulated by Kupiec-Weglinski and his colleagues[14] suggests that in the rat, CsA allows the development of an active mechanism of suppression mediated by cells (T_S) which are sensitive to cyclophosphamide (an agent reputed to destroy the rapid-turnover precursors of T_S) and that these cells may (i) elaborate soluble mediators responsible for graft survival and (ii) strongly inhibit host effector mechanisms against organ allografts. In addition to these suggested mechanisms, it has been proposed that during the development of the specific non-responsive phase (stage 3) in the CsA-treated allografted rat, there is a sequestration from the circulation of antigen-specific T-cells. A mechanism such as that suggested by Hutchinson and Zola[15], whereby complexes of antigen–antibody and alloreactive cells are phagocytosed by Kupffer cells could be operative in CsA-induced unresponsiveness.

In contrast to renal and cardiac allograft survival in rats, prolongation of skin allograft survival in rats, mice, rabbits and dogs is dependent on continued CsA administration. Maintenance of the drug is also required for indefinite, cardiac allograft survival in monkeys. Other organs and tissues which have been successfully allografted in CsA-treated animals are shown in Table 6.4. These include pancreatic allografts, which are difficult to transplant with conventional drugs.

The minimum effective dosage required to prolong survival of isolated pancreatic islets in histoincompatible rats is considerably in excess of that needed to produce indefinite renal allograft survival in the same species. Isolated pancreatic islets implanted under the renal capsule have also been transplanted to CsA-treated allogeneic diabetic hosts with indefinite survival of the islets. More spectacular has been the marked prolongation of dog lung allograft survival achieved with CsA alone or in combination with other immunosuppressants. Additional evidence suggests that dog lung allograft recipients are specifically unresponsive to their grafts and that this unresponsiveness persists (as in the rat renal/cardiac allograft model) after cessation of CsA treatment. Equally remarkable is the survival of grafts of small intestine in both rats and dogs, whilst corneal allograft rejection in the rabbit has been abrogated by CsA. Clearly though, variability in the effectiveness of CsA is encountered with respect to different tissues and species. Of particular importance is its continued requirement for indefinite allograft survival in primates.

Mode of action

Inhibition of T cell activation and interleukin production

The initial reports of Borel and his colleagues suggested that the inhibitory effects of CsA were restricted to T lymphocytes. Thus the proliferative responses of these cells from various species to phytohaemaglutinin or concanavalin A *in vitro* were suppressed by CsA. Included amongst the *in vitro* T cell responses inhibited by CsA are both primary and secondary mixed lymphocyte reactions. These responses are models of *in vivo* anti-allograft reactions and are manifested by the $T_{H/I}$ cell functions of lymphoproliferation and cell-mediated lympholysis. In contrast, the generation of T_S is unaffected. The sensitivity of these responses to CsA is related to both drug concentration (in addition, antigen-driven responses are more sensitive than those induced by polyclonal mitogen) and to the timing of addition of the drug. Antigen-stimulated T cells become insensitive to CsA within 8 h of stimulation.

The inhibitory effect of CsA on T_H cell activation is believed to be exerted at two levels:

(1) The production of IL-1 by APC, and

(2) The generation of IL-2 (T cell growth factor), which causes proliferation of T cells bearing the appropriate receptors (see Figure 6.1).

Although CsA inhibits the production of IL-2, it does not affect the responsiveness of IL-2 receptor-bearing cytotoxic suppressor T cells ($T_{C/S}$) to proliferation in the presence of exogenous (preformed) IL-2.

Inhibition of IL-1 release, is not due to an effect on the macrophage (whose properties generally are resistant to CsA), but to an inhibitory action of CsA on T cells which stimulate IL-1 production in APC. The inhibitory effect of CsA on IL-2 generation cannot be overcome by addition of exogenous IL-1. An hypothesis that CsA blocks class II (HLA-DR) antigen receptors on T cells has not been confirmed. There is also no evidence that T_H cells have a special affinity for CsA as opposed to T_S or B cells.

The production of lymphokines other than IL-2 is also inhibited by CsA. These include macrophage migration inhibition factor (MIF), macrophage activating factor (MAF), macrophage procoagulant-inducing factor (PIF) and lymphocyte-derived chemotactic factor (essential for delayed-type hypersensitivity reactions)[16]; B cell growth factor (causes polyclonal antibody production); gamma (immune) interferon; colony stimulating factor (causes growth of granulocyte colonies in bone marrow) and IL-3 (induces synthesis of 20α-hydroxysteroid dehydrogenase in certain T cells). With respect to IL-3, it is noteworthy that this lymphokine has been implicated as a T_S cell growth factor in the maintenance of allograft unresponsiveness following short courses of CsA in allografted rats (see above)[17].

145

Earliest reports on the mode of action of CsA indicated that the drug did not impair the responses of B cells, e.g. murine B lymphocytes to LPS, or pig lymphocytes to anti-immunoglobulin (Ig). Also, no effect was observed on human T-independent Ig production induced by the Epstein-Barr virus. Since these early observations, however, much more detailed *in vitro* analyses of murine and human B cell responses to various stimuli in the presence of CsA have been conducted. It now appears that there are both CsA-sensitive and CsA-resistant components of the B cell activation process. Further details of these effects of CsA may be found in the recent review by Shevach[11].

Subcellular action of CsA

As depicted in Figure 6.7, activation of T_H cells and production of IL-2 takes place in several stages. The exact manner in which CsA disrupts this process is unknown, but it is likely that the drug acts either at the membrane level (steps 1-4) or by preventing generation of the cytoplasmic derepressor of lymphokine genes (steps 5, 6). It is clear that CsA does not influence events distal to gene transcription, i.e. mRNA translation and the synthesis and release of lymphokines. Established cell lines producing IL-2 are not affected by CsA.

The lipophilic nature of CsA and its likely incorporation within the plasma membrane may well be important factors in disturbing critical events (e.g. receptor aggregation) in the initial activation process. The specificity of CsA for T_H might be explained by unique, drug-sensitive events during activation

1. Binding of antigen	6. Derepression of IL-2 gene
2. Receptor aggregation	7. Transcription of m-RNA
3. Membrane transduction	8. Synthesis of IL-2
4. Transmembrane signal	9. Transport to cell surface
5. Cytoplasmic signal	10. Release of IL-2

Figure 6.7 The various stages in T_H cell activation and IL-2 production. The sequence of events to the left of the bar is CsA-sensitive. Modified after Kahan[18]

of this cell subset. It has recently been suggested that a cytoplasmic receptor for CsA 'cyclophilin' might exist. Such an interaction could be a key event in prevention of lymphokine gene derepression. It has also been proposed that CsA binds to calmodulin, a calcium-dependent protein essential to normal cell function and intimately involved in early events of cell activation. Inactivation of calmodulin, despite the normal calcium flux into the cell associated with activation, could prevent the signal to activate cyclic nucleotides, protein kinases and phospholipase A_2, messengers necessary to initiate synthesis of nucleic acids, protein and prostaglandins.

Clinical transplantation

There is now abundant evidence that CsA is a potent immunosuppressive agent in man. Most experience has been gained in cadaveric organ transplantation, where advantages over the use of conventional immunosuppressive agents in terms of graft survival and patient management have been demonstrated in numerous centres world-wide.

Renal transplantation

The first clinical trial of CsA in renal transplantation was conducted in Cambridge by Calne and his colleagues and reported in 1978[19]. In addition to demonstrating the capacity of CsA to prevent allograft rejection, they found that combination of CsA with other imunosuppressive agents could lead (due to excessive impairment of the host's immune system) to the danger of life-threatening infections and increased risk of malignant disease (lymphoma). Moreover, they found that CsA was nephrotoxic in man. Subsequent to these important early observations, a number of different treatment strategies have been adopted by different centres with the aims of:

(1) Minimizing the nephrotoxic effects of CsA;

(2) Reducing the risks of insufficient or excessive immune suppression; and

(3) Avoiding the possible unknown untoward effects of long-term CsA administration.

In the European eight-centre trial in which CsA has been compared with conventional immune suppressants (azathiorprine and steroids), prospective cadaveric renal graft recipients were selected on the basis of post-operative graft function (a diuresis of $> 50\,mL/h$ during the first 6 h) in order to reduce CsA nephrotoxicity. The patients were randomly allocated to one of the two treatment groups. Patients in the CsA group received no other immunosuppressive agent, except for short courses of intravenous methylprednisolone for the treatment of rejection episodes.

One year analysis of the results of this trial revealed an increase in graft survival of 20% in patients within the CsA group (72%), compared with those in the conventionally-treated group (52%). At three years, the advantage of CsA treatment has been maintained, with graft survival rates of 66% and 42% for the above groups, respectively (Figure 6.8)[20]. A significant proportion of the patients originally allocated to the CsA group (37%) did, however,

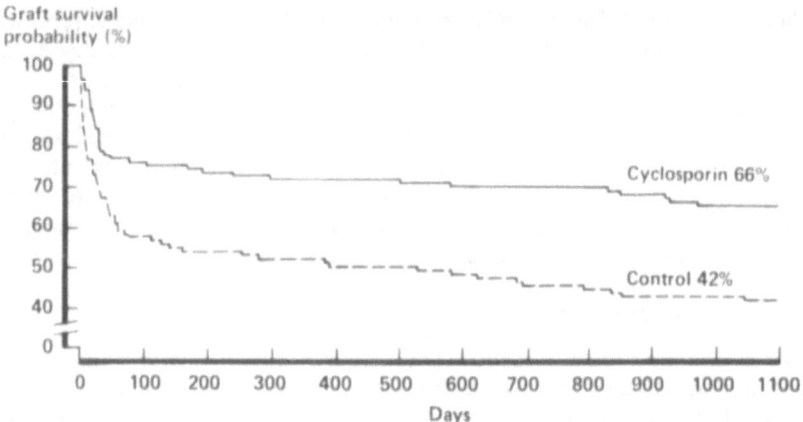

Figure 6.8 Kidney graft survival curves for CsA and conventionally-treated (azathioprine and steroid) patients. Results of European multicentre trial. Reproduced with permission of *The Lancet*[20]

require to have their treatment changed to azathioprine and steroids, principally because of nephrotoxicity. Moreover, renal function was significantly poorer in the CsA group than in the conventionally immunosuppressed patients. The incidence of malignant tumours was similar to that with azathioprine and steroids (no lymphomas were observed).

Although large randomized trials conducted in other centres (e.g. the Canadian multicentre trial) have confirmed the significant improvement in graft survival with CsA, opinions differ as to the best treatment strategy. In particular, the addition of maintenance 'low-dose' steroids has been adopted (e.g. by Starzl *et al.*[21]) to allow non-diuresing patients to be treated and to reduce the possibility of rejection episodes. The disadvantages of this approach are, of course, the well-known side effects of protracted steroid therapy and the increased risk of infection and lymphoma. An alternative approach, initiated in Oxford[22], is to convert from CsA to conventional immunosuppression six months post transplant. This trial has shown improved graft survival with the CsA protocol and demonstrated the reversibility of some of the features of CsA nephrotoxicity. This strategy avoids doubts about chronic CsA nephrotoxicity and the expense incurrred with long-term CsA administration. Indeed, nephrotoxicity and cost would currently be regarded as the long-term disadvantages of CsA.

The severity of CsA-induced nephrotoxicity has, however, been alleviated by the use of lower dosage schedules with relatively aggressive tapering (from 14 mg/kg orally or less to 6–8 mg/kg by 60 days post transplant) and by the introduction of therapeutic drug monitoring by radioimmunoassay. It is also now well recognized that co-administration of drugs which alter hepatic CsA metabolism (e.g. ketoconazole, erythromicin) or induce synergistic nephrotoxicity (e.g. gentamicin, sulpha drugs, non-steroidal anti-inflammatory agents) is an important but avoidable complication. Although it has also been advocated, the avoidance of CsA during the first few days post transplant (when the renal allograft may be most vulnerable to drug-induced injury) and its replacement with azathioprine and antilymphocyte serum has the disadvantage of losing the influence of the drug during the critical phase of $T_{H/I}$ cell priming.

Differentiation between renal allograft rejection and CsA nephrotoxicity

The full potential of CsA in clinical medicine is limited by its nephrotoxicity and use of the drug in renal transplantation is especially difficult since impaired allograft function may be due to either rejection or drug toxicity. Despite studies of clinical parameters, allograft biopsies, intrarenal hydrostatic pressures and CsA levels, no simple guidelines have emerged which facilitate the differential diagnosis of CsA nephrotoxicity and allograft rejection. An important limitation imposed in this context is the non-availability of biopsy material from CsA-treated patients with normal or stable renal function.

Differential diagnosis between nephrotoxicity and allograft rejection is particularly difficult between one week and three months post transplant: thereafter rejection becomes much less likely. Following exclusion of a primary renal disorder, several factors (Table 6.5) need to be taken into account[23]:

(1) Clinical history;

(2) Physical signs of rejection;

(3) The overall renal picture – biochemistry, radionuclide perfusion, urinary lymphocyte count; and

(4) Trough serum CsA levels (> 250 mg/kg is more likely to be associated with nephrotoxicity).

It is however recognized that a proportion of patients, perhaps as many as 20%, simultaneously exhibit nephrotoxicity and rejection. It appears, in addition, that rejection episodes may reveal or exacerbate subclinical, CsA-nephrotoxicity. The use of steroids to treat rejection episodes may, as previously mentioned, interfere with CsA metabolism leading to elevated blood (and intra-renal) levels.

The question of whether morphological changes in kidney transplant are associated with CsA treatment has received much attention. It now appears that there are histological patterns which occur more frequently in CsA-treated patients (Table 6.6), but that these are not specific to CsA. Based on their histopathological findings, Mihatsch et al.[24] have brought forth a new concept for CsA treatment of the renal allograft recipient. They suggest very low trough CsA levels immediately post transplant, with a requirement for additional, conventional immunosuppression. This would be followed, at 1–2 weeks, by a slow increase in CsA trough levels to within the therapeutic range, with concomitant, stepwise reductions in all other immunosuppressants until the patient is maintained on CsA alone.

Table 6.5 Considerations for the differential diagnosis between CsA-induced nephrotoxicity and allograft rejection

Parameter	Percentage likelihood of incidence of:	
	Nephrotoxicity	Rejection
Adverse donor conditions	50–75	10–25
Second transplants	10–25†	50–75
Time post-transplant:		
<40 d	25–50	>75
>40 d	50–75	10–25
Physical signs of rejection	0–10	50–75
Decreased urine output:		
<25%	50–75	10–25
25–50%	25–50	25–50
>50%	10–25	50–75
Rate serum creatinine rise:		
fast	25–50	50–75
slow	50–75	25–50
Extent of serum creatinine rise:		
<25%	>75	25–50
25%–50%	25–50	25–50
>50%	25–50	50–75
Urea/Creatinine ratio of 20/1	50–75	10–25
Decreased perfusion by radionuclide	10–25	50–75
Urinary lymphocytes >20%	10–25	50–75
CsA levels‡		
>250	>75	10–25
<100	10–25	50–75

†Except in instances when CsA was used for the first transplant and the patient was a high drug absorber
‡Plasma trough level by radioimmunoassay, measured in ng/mL. Reproduced with permission from Reference 23

Table 6.6 Morphological patterns in kidneys of CSA-treated transplant patients

Lesions unrelated to CsA	Lesions possibly related to CsA
Classical rejection	Diffuse interstitial fibrosis
Other lesions, e.g. ATN, infarction, *de novo*	Toxic tubulopathy
and recurrent glomerulonephritis	Peritubular capillary congestion
	CsA-associated arteriolopathy
	Interstitial fibrosis, striped form, with tubular
	atrophy

Modified after Mihatsch *et al.*[24]

Heart transplantation

Immunosuppression with CsA has resulted in a distinct improvement in the survival rates of cardiac allograft recipients. It has also allowed substantial reductions in steroid levels ('steroid-sparing') and their side effects compared to historical control patients treated with azathioprine. There have also been marked improvements in the patient's quality of life. There has been a remarkable reduction, at Stanford University and elsewhere, in the death rate due to infectious complications and although rejection episodes continue to occur, two-year actuarial survival rates of 75% have been reported.

There are several difficulties in the use of CsA for cardiac transplantation. Most patients exhibit mild, persistent (but not progressive) impairment of renal function. In addition, however, there may be myocardial fibrosis (possibly drug-induced) and the majority of patients develop systemic hypertension (far exceeding the incidence in azathioprine-treated controls). The latter is usually controlled by diuretic therapy. A further problem is the occurrence of accelerated allograft coronary atherosclerosis. It is presumed that this is due to incomplete control of the immune response, resulting in chronic coronary endothelial damage and triggering of endothelial hyperplasia, leading to obstructive atherosclerosis lesions.

Liver transplantation

Imunosuppression with CsA has contributed significantly to the improved outcome of human liver transplantation. Recent reports indicate that the one-year patient survival rate can exceed 60%[25]. A particular problem in hepatic allograft recipients is the difficulty in maintaining adequate serum CsA levels, due to problems in enteric drug absorption. These may arise due to lack of bile secretion or to impaired hepatic extraction and biotransformation of CsA. Generally, differentiation of rejection from (hepato-)toxicity is easier than with renal transplantation.

Pancreas transplantation

Although the number of transplants performed has increased dramatically in recent years, the success rate of human pancreas transplantation remains low and allograft survival has been only slightly improved with the introduction of CsA. A recent study conducted in the University of Minnesota, which has the greatest experience of pancreatic transplantation (almost exclusively segmental pancreas grafts) shows 24% allograft survival with CsA immunosuppression, compared with 15% in azathioprine-treated controls[26]. These relatively poor results can, however, be ascribed to technical difficulties and the complications of end-stage diabetes which do not allow the influence of CsA on rejection to be evaluated. Ultimately of course, pancreas transplantation should be performed in diabetic patients before the appearance of serious complications. Such a manoeuvre will require immunosuppressive regimens with high therapeutic ratios.

Bone marrow transplantation

CsA has improved patient survival and the severity (but not the incidence) of GVHD in bone marrow transplantation. In a four-year prospective study of CsA compared with methotrexate in allogeneic bone marrow transplantation for leukaemia and severa aplastic anaemia, Speck et al.[27] reported 55% patient survival with rapid and sustained engraftment and a low incidence of infections. The repeated occurrence of GVHD in CsA-treated bone marrow transplant recipients raises interesting questions about the possible resistance of GVHD-inducing cells to CsA in man.

Adverse effects of CsA (other than nephrotoxicity)

The most significant complications encountered in CsA-treated patients, in addition to nephrotoxicity, are tremor, gastrointestinal intolerance and hirsutism (between 20% and 40% of transplant recipients). Other adverse effects (some secondary to renal impairment) seen in a smaller proportion of patients include hepatotoxicity, hyperaesthesia, facial oedema, fits, gum hypertrophy, hyperkalaemia and hypertension. In comparison with conventional, immunosuppressive therapy, there is a reduced incidence of bacterial and fungal infections. There is also evidence that the frequency of severe cytomegalovirus infections is low with CsA therapy.

It is now clear that the incidence of malignant disease with CsA is at least no higher than with other immunosuppressive agents. The selectivity of CsA for T cells may impair resistance to Epstein-Barr virus-induced B cell proliferation. The comparatively high incidence of lymphomas observed in the initial clinical experience with CsA, in which the drug was combined with other immunosuppressants, can be ascribed to excessive immunosuppression.

Prospects

The goal of safely achieving donor-specific unresponsiveness in the transplant patient is still far from being realized. It is clear that for some time to come, clinicians will remain dependent on pharmacological agents to control rejection. The advent of CsA fulfils certain criteria towards the goal, but the full potential of the drug cannot be realized because of nephrotoxicity. Perhaps a cyclosporin analogue will go some way towards reducing this unfortunate side effect. Some interest has been expressed in the properties of cyclosporin G, a naturally occurring, immunosuppressive analogue[28], which differs from CsA in one amino acid. There is recent evidence, however, that cyclosporin G may also exhibit nephrotoxicity in animals[29]. Evaluation of the true potential of any such analogue will be dependent on adequate clinical trials.

An alternative approach, currently being explored at the experimental level, is the use of pharmaceutical agents both to help elucidate the pathogenesis of nephrotoxicity and to alleviate this effect. Thus inducers of hepatic drug metabolism such as phenobarbitone, ameliorate CsA toxicity in rats[30,31]. Nephrotoxicity is also alleviated in experimental animals by prostaglandin E_2, an effect attributed to reversal of the reduced renal blood flow caused by CsA[32]. Both these manoeuvres, however, lead to reductions in the bioavailability of the immune suppressant. More significant perhaps, has been the observation that in animals, the angiotensin converting enzyme inhibitor, enalapril, or the aldosterone antagonist, spironolactone, reduces the extent of CsA nephrotoxicity without a fall in circulating CsA levels[33]. Not only does this finding implicate the renin-angiotensin-aldosterone system in the pathogenesis of CsA nephrotoxicity, but it also suggests that these agents may prove useful in the clinical management of CsA nephrotoxicity.

The recent definition, isolation and cloning of the genes for the human T cell receptor, together with the ability to grow individual T cell clones in culture, now offers the opportunity of investigating both T cells and their receptors specifically in the context of the rejection process. The exciting prospect also arises of modifying these structures prior to transplantation of the graft as a means of preventing induction of anti-allograft responses. Indeed, recently, in adult mice, tolerance to certain protein antigens has been achieved by administration of these together with monoclonal antibody directed against the L3T4 molecule on T_H[34]. Such antibodies may have a future in the induction of specific tolerance for transplantation purposes.

ACKNOWLEDGEMENTS

We thank the Department of Medical Illustration, University of Aberdeen for the line drawings (Mr K. Mutch) and photographic assistance. The manuscript was typed by Mrs I. Watson.

References

1. McConnell, I., Munro, A. and Waldmann, H. (1981). *The Immune System*. 2nd Edn. (Oxford: Blackwell Scientific Publications)
2. Najarian, J. S., May, J., Cochrum, K., Baronberg, N. and Way, L. W. (1966). Mechanisms of antigen release from canine kidney homograft transplants. *Ann. NY Acad. Sci.*, **129**, 76–87
3. Strober, S. and Gowans, J. L. (1965). The role of lymphocytes in the sensitization of rats to renal homografts. *J. Exp. Med.*, **122**, 347–60
4. Paul, L. C. and Carpenter, C. B. (1980). Antibodies against renal endothelial alloantigens. *Transplant. Proc.*, **12**, 43–8
5. Kissmeyer-Nielsen, F., Olsen, S., Petersen, V. and Fjeldborg, O. (1966). Hyperacute rejection of kidney allografts associated with pre-existing humoral antibodies against donor cells. *Lancet*, **2**, 662–5
6. Portmann, B., Schindler, A. M., Murray-Lyon, I. M. and Williams, R. (1976). Histological sexing of a reticulum-cell sarcoma arising after liver transplantation. *Gastroenterology*, **70**, 82–4
7. Billingham, R. E., Brent, L. and Medawar, P. B. (1953). Actively acquired tolerance of foreign cells. *Nature*, **172**, 603
8. Borel, J. F., Feurer, C., Gubler, H. U. and Stähelin, H. (1976). Biological effects of cyclosporin A: a new antilymphocytic agent. *Agents Actions*, **6**, 468–75
9. Thomson, A. W. (1983). Immunobiology of cyclosporin A – a review. *Aust. J. Exp. Biol. Med. Sci.*, **61**, 147–72
10. Kahan, B. D. (ed.) (1984). *Cyclosporin. Biological Activity and Clinical Applications*. (New York: Grune and Stratton)
11. Shevach, E. M. (1985). The effects of cyclosporin A on the immune system. *Ann. Rev. Immunol.*, **3**, 397–423
12. Green, C. J. and Allison, A. C. (1978). Extensive prolongation of rabbit kidney allograft survival after short-term cyclosporin A treatment. *Lancet*, **1**, 1182–3
13. Nagao, T., White, D. J. G. and Calne, R. Y. (1982). Kinetics of unresponsiveness induced by a short course of cyclosporin A. *Transplantation*, **33**, 31–5
14. Kupiec-Weglinski, J. W., Filho, M. A., Strom, T. B. and Tilney, N. L. (1984). Sparing of suppressor cells: a critical action of cyclosporin. *Transplantation*, **38**, 97–101
15. Hutchinson, I. V. and Zola, H. (1977). Antigen-reactive cell opsonization (ARCO). A mechanism of immunological enhancement. *Transplantation*, **23**, 464–9
16. Thomson, A. W., Moon, D. K., Geczy, C. L. and Nelson, D. S. (1983). Cyclosporin A inhibits lymphokine production but not the responses of macrophages to lymphokines. *Immunology*, **48**, 291–9
17. Abbud-Filho, M., Kupiec-Weglinski, J. W., Araujo, J. L., Heidecke, C. D., Tilney, N. L. and Strom, T. B. (1984). Cyclosporine therapy of rat heart allograft recipients and release

of interleukins (IL-1, IL-2, IL-3): a role for IL-3 in graft tolerance? *J. Immunol.*, **133**, 2582–6

18. Kahan, B. D. (1985). Cyclosporine: the agent and its actions. *Transplant. Proc.*, **17**, 4 (Suppl.), 1, 5–18
19. Calne, R. Y., White, D. J. G., Thiru, S., Evans, D. B., McMaster, P., Dunn, D. C., Craddock, G. N., Pentlow, B. D. and Rolles, K. (1978). Cyclosporin A in patients with renal allografts from cadaver donors. *Lancet*, **2**, 1323–7
20. Calne, R. Y. and Wood, A. J. (1985). Cyclosporin in cadaveric renal transplantation: 3-year follow-up of a European multicentre trial. *Lancet*, **2**, 549
21. Starzl, T. E., Hakala, T. R., Iwatsuki, S., Rosenthal, T. J., Shaw, B. W. Jr., Klintmalm, G. B. G. and Porter, K. A. (1982). Cyclosporin A and steroid treatment in 104 cadaveric renal transplantations. In White, D. J. G. (ed.) *Cyclosporin A*, pp. 365–77 (Amsterdam: Elsevier Biomedical)
22. Wood, R. F. M., Thompson, J. F., Allen, N. H., Ting, A. and Morris, P. J. (1984). The consequences of conversion from cyclosporine to azathioprine and prednisolone in renal allograft recipients. In Kahan, B. D. (ed.). *Cyclosporine. Biological Activity and Clinical Applications.* pp. 646–52. (New York: Grune and Stratton)
23. Kahan, B. D. (1985). An algorithm for the management of patients with cyclosporin-induced renal dysfunction. *Transplant. Proc.*, **17**, 4 (Suppl.) 1, 303–8
24. Mihatsch, M. J., Thiel, G., Basler, V., Ryffel, B., Landmann, J., von Overbeck, J. and Zollinger, H. U. (1985). Morphological patterns in cyclosporine-treated renal transplant recipients. *Transplant. Proc.*, **17**, 4 (Suppl.), 1, 101–16
25. Starzl, T. E., Iwatsuki, S., Van Thiel, D. H., Gartner, J. C., Zitelli, B. J., Malatack, J. J., Schade, R. R., Shaw, B. W. Jr., Hakala, T. R. and Rosenthal, J. T. (1984). Report of Colorado–Pittsburg liver transplantation studies. In Kahan, B. D. (ed.) *Cyclosporine. Biological Activity and Clinical Applications*, pp. 366–9 (New York: Grune & Stratton)
26. Sutherland, D. E. R. (1983). Pancreas transplantation: overview and current status of cases reported to the registry through 1982. *Transplant. Proc.*, **15**, (Suppl.), 1, 2606–10
27. Speck, B., Gratwohl, B., Osterwalder, E., Signer, E., Nissen, C., Corneo, M. and Jeannet, M. (1983). Allogeneic bone marrow transplantation: the Basel trial with cyclosporine. *Transplant. Proc.*, **15**, (Suppl.), 1, 2617–9
28. Hiestand, P. C., Gunn, H. C., Gale, J.. M., Ryffel, B. and Borel, J. F. (1985). Comparison of the pharmacological profiles of cyclosporine. (Nva²)-cyclosporine and (Val²) dihydro-cyclosporine. *Immunology*, **55**, 249–55
29. Duncan, J. I., Thomson, A. W., Simpson, J. G., Davidson, R. J. L. and Whiting, P. H. (1986). A comparative toxicological study of cyclosporine and Nva²-cyclosporine in Sprague-Dawley rats. *Transplantation* (In press)
30. Cunningham, C., Burke, M. D., Wheatley, D. N., Thomson, A. W., Simpson, J. G. and Whiting, P. H. (1985). Amelioration of cyclosporin-induced nephrotoxicity in rats by induction of hepatic drug metabolism. *Biochem. Pharmac.*, **34**, 573–8
31. Duncan, J. I., Whiting, P. H., Simpson, J. G. and Thomson, A. W. (1986). Alleviation of cyclosporin A-mediated nephrotoxicity by phenobarbitone, during the suppression of graft-versus-host reactivity. *Transplant. Proc.*, **18**, 645–9
32. Ryffel, B., Donatsch, P., Hiestand, P. and Mihatsch, M. J. (1986). PGE₂ reduces nephrotoxicity and immunosuppression of cyclosporine in rats. *Clin. Nephrol.*, **25**, (Suppl.), 1, 595–9
33. McAuley, F. T., Whiting, P. H., Thomson, A. W. and Simpson, J. G. (1986). The influence of enalapril or spironolactone in acute cyclosporin nephrotoxicity. *Biochem. Pharmac.* (In press)
34. Benjamin, R. J. and Waldmann, H. (1986). Induction of tolerance by monoclonal antibody therapy. *Nature*, **320**, 449–51

7
Kidney Preservation

R. W. G. JOHNSON

INTRODUCTION

For most people successful renal transplantation equals a life free from dialysis. This definition allows a wide range of acceptable renal function from a creatinine clearance of perhaps 10 mL/min to one of 120 mL/min. This range does exist and there are two main reasons for it:

(1) Ischaemic injury during procurement, and

(2) Immunological injury resulting from rejection.

The relative contributions of these two processes are rarely quantified but it is reasonable to assume that the former can be avoided or at least minimized, thus leaving the kidney with more in reserve to meet the latter. Since the introduction of cyclosporin the role of non-immunological injury has assumed a much higher profile – indeed it has become increasingly important to ensure good quality immediate function after renal transplantation just so that recipients can receive the benefit of cyclosporin.

Historically, transplant units have been rather complacent about lack of immediate function, regarding it as a common complication, accepting post-operative dialysis rates of up to 50%, and even suggesting that periods of post-transplant uraemia may be beneficial! It is the very availability of dialysis that has removed the impetus to improve methods of kidney procurement and preservation: in those areas of transplantation where lack of immediate function means death (heart and liver) the wits have remained sharp and tremendous efforts have always been made to ensure donor resuscitation, eliminate warm injury and minimize cold storage time.

Immediate renal function after kidney transplantation brings many advantages. It improves the morale of both the recipient and the staff. The need for heparin and dialysis are eliminated together with the obvious complications they may cause. Diagnosis of rejection is facilitated, as is the management of immunosuppressive therapy. Hospital stay is shortened and cost reduced, but most important of all, non-immunological injury is

155

minimized. In order to produce immediate function after transplantation it is essential to understand the injury processes that can occur as the kidney passes from one host to another.

MECHANISM OF INJURY

The kidney's susceptibility to ischaemic injury is well recognized as is its remarkable ability to recover. The essential difficulty lies in its apparently variable response to injury – seemingly trivial ischaemic intervals occasionally result in irreversible damage whilst prolonged periods of ischaemia often pass without problem.

Kidneys from cadaver donors are at risk during two separate intervals before preservation can even commence:

(1) Immediately before death (the agonal period), and

(2) Immediately after circulatory arrest (the warm ischaemic interval).

Distinguishing between these two intervals may seem academic, since they run into each other and since to some extent the injury processes are common to both. The separation of the two intervals, however, may explain why some kidneys removed rapidly after death are already irreversibly injured. Post-traumatic renal shutdown was first described by Bywaters and Beall in 1941[1]. Diminished glomerular filtration rate and renal plasma flow were subsequently demonstrated in peripheral circulatory failure[2] and found to correlate roughly with the severity of the shock. Renal blood flow was decreased further than could be predicted from the systemic blood pressure. The assumption that vasoconstriction had occurred was strengthened by the fact that renal blood flow did not reach normal levels until 12–72 h after the blood pressure, blood volume and cardiac output had been corrected.

It was confirmed[3] that shock caused renal ischaemia in patterns that correlated roughly with the severity of the injury. A mild state of shock caused patchy ischaemia in the subcapsular area, whilst a severe state of shock caused ischaemia of the entire cortex and corticomedullary area. Renal vasoconstriction produced by shock persists after nephrectomy, and with isolated perfusion and persistence of vasoconstriction, is the most common cause of post-transplantation renal failure.

Various vasoactive substances liberated during shock, notably the catechol-amines, have been shown to produce vasoconstriction, and the degree of vasoconstriction is equal in kidneys removed at either 5 or 25 min after cardiac arrest[4]. This substantiates the belief that vasospasm occurs during the agonal period and not after cardiac arrest. Pretreatment of donors with phenoxybenzamine significantly improves the perfusion characteristics and reduces the number of recipients requiring post-transplantation dialysis.

Once vasoconstriction has occurred most vasodilators are unable to reverse it. The resulting underperfusion of the kidney produces significant changes in intracellular water and electrolytes as a result of anoxia and metabolic acidosis. In addition red cells and debris are trapped in the renal microcirculation. When the kidney is reperfused with blood after ischaemic injury there is maldistribution of blood in the microcirculation resulting in a patchy mottled appearance, and there is an increase in vascular resistance which is more pronounced in the deeper parts of the cortex and in the renal medulla. This medullary vascular congestion gives rise to a dark dis-colouration at the cortico-medullary junction which has been described as 'the blue line'[5].

Failure to re-establish flow after ischaemic injury is the single most critical factor in determining whether or not the kidney will survive the ischaemic insult. There appear to be three main elements in this 'no reflow' phenomenon: vasospasm, cellular swelling and red cell sludging. Clearly, if the problem is to be avoided, renal protection must commence in the donor prior to the agonal period.

DONOR SELECTION AND PREPARATION

Ideally all potential donors should be managed in an intensive therapy unit where adequate monitoring facilities exist. Stable donors present few problems but many donors are unstable, having suffered multiple injuries and perhaps having had at least one cardiac arrest.

In situ protection is aimed at resuscitation of the donor during the agonal phase and preparing the kidney by pharmacological means for the anticipated anoxic insult. The aims are (1) to prevent prerenal failure, (2) to conserve the kidney's intrinsic energy stores, and (3) to delay autolysis.

Ventilation of donors prior to nephrectomy has been shown to influence the early onset of renal function favourably. However, ventilation alone does not ensure early onset of renal function[6]. Good results are most likely to be achieved if the period of *antemortem* hypotension does not exceed 6 h[7]. Hypotension and prerenal oliguria are commonly seen in potential kidney donors: they are most often caused by dehydration related to the management of the head injury and are easily treated by fluid replacement with blood, saline, dextrose or an albumin solution. Large volumes are often required. Infusion of Dextran 40 is particularly useful.

It is important to distinguish between the effects of dehydration and decline in cardiac function. Failure in cardiac output can be supported pharmacologically with a number of agents but dopamine is the treatment of choice, since it raises blood pressure by improving myocardial function and cardiac output, whilst specifically increasing renal blood flow. Resuscitation of severely hypotensive oliguric donors with dopamine for up to 12 h leads to a high rate of immediate function after transplantation[8].

Once the central venous pressure has been raised a diuresis usually follows: promoting the diuresis with mannitol or frusemide provides further protec-tion as renal plasma flow increases. At the same time vasodilatation with phenoxybenzamine 150 mg I.V. or chlorpromazine 250 mg I.V. ensures that cooling will be rapid through a widely dilated renal circulation.

Warm ischaemia

Warm ischaemia, that is the interval between cardiac arrest and cooling, can be avoided by removing kidneys with the heart still beating. However, as this is not always possible, it is important to know how much warm ischaemia the kidney can tolerate. Immediately after circulatory arrest cells begin to die. The progress towards death may be divided into three phases:

(1) *Reversible deterioration* in which the cell is injured, but the damage is not so extensive that recovery is impossible

(2) *Dying* in which the cell sustains injury to pass 'the point of no return' and cannot be revived, and

(3) *Death* in which cellular organization is disrupted and integrated cellular functions cease altogether.

The speed with which different cells pass through these stages and the extent to which they are able to recover depends upon their innate characteristics, as well as on the stresses to which they are subjected.

The cause of cell death after circulatory arrest is loss of energy which is essential for maintenance of cell membrane potential, cell volume and the synthesis of proteins and other macromolecules. The maintenance of cell volume in particular is a continuous energy-consuming process which is dependent on the active extrusion of sodium at the cell membrane.

The lack of energy resulting from hypoxia causes the sodium pump to fail and as a consequence sodium and water accumulate in the cell which then begins to swell. This correlates with the microscopic swelling which occurs in isolated ischaemic tissues and which is reversible in its early stages and also with the increase in weight found in hypoxic tissues *in vitro*.

Cellular swelling following hypoxia may be the cause of breaks sometimes seen in cell membranes, resulting in leakage of cytoplasm from the injured cells. Hypoxia also results in a switch to anaerobic metabolism, causing cellular pH to fall because of excessive lactic acid accumulation. This increase in H^+ ion concentration has been shown to inhibit further the oxygen consumption in isolated tissues[9].

In ischaemia the sequence of events seems to be anoxia → increased glycolysis → lactic acid production → fall in pH → release of lysosomal enzymes into the cytoplasm. Lysosomal enzyme release can be detected within 30 min of cessation of blood flow to the tissue, but is not a uniform process. The release of these enzymes initiates the process of self-digestion within the cell. In this process the mitochondria and microsomes seem to succumb more rapidly than do nuclei. The initial effects on mitochondria are to inactivate ATPase, uncouple oxidative phosphorylation and cause the mitochondria to swell.

Although published experience of renal artery occlusion in man is rather scanty, Semb[10] suggests that the ischaemic tolerance of human kidneys lies in approximately the same range of susceptibility as that of the dog. In the unilaterally nephrectomized dog, transient impairment of function has been observed after 15 min of ischaemia and permanent damage can be expected after ischaemia lasting more than 1 h. Dogs are unlikely to survive more than

2 h of renal ischaemia without some form of premedication[11], although delayed contralateral nephrectomy may provide sufficient recovery time to allow up to 3 h of ischaemia to be tolerated. Wickham[12] constructed an approximate time scale (Table 7.1) which indicates the degree of renal functional depression which may be expected to follow specific periods of ischaemia. The simple expedient of preheparinizing the dog allows it to tolerate 60 min of renal ischaemia with minimal depression of function[11]. Washing the blood out of the kidney with normal saline at 37 °C allows the renal ischaemic tolerance to be extended up to 3 h with only mild temporary depression of function. Damage to the tubules is always more severe than to the glomeruli. It affects primarily the proximal convoluted tubule: the metabolism of the medulla, being largely anaerobic, affords some protection to the loops of Henle and the collecting system.

Table 7.1 Functional depression and recovery time after renal ischaemia

Ischaemic time (minutes)	Degree of functional depression	Time for recovery
10	none	1 h
20	40–50%	6–7 d
30	60–70%	8–9 d
60	70–80%	10–14 d
120	complete	partial recovery
180	complete	never complete

From Wickham *et al.* 1967[12]

In rats, tubular repair is usually well developed after 4 d and histologically complete by 2 weeks. A degree of atrophy commonly follows an ischaemic insult, the extent depending on the duration of the insult. After 2 h ischaemia, over three-quarters of the glomeruli show atrophic changes and failure of blood flow through the kidney is observed after 3 h ischaemia. Marked reduction in blood flow can persist for 12–18 h after restoration of the blood supply and functional ischaemia may persist unrecognized for many hours[13].

The kidney is clearly a more resilient organ than has previously been thought. Despite this resilience, efficient protection of the kidney during periods of ischaemia is obviously necessary as an integral part of every transplant procedure.

PROTECTION FROM ISCHAEMIC INJURY

Simple hypothermia

It has been known for many years that survival of isolated animal tissues can be prolonged by lowering their temperature and thereby reducing their metabolism. In so doing, the requirements for oxygen and energy-rich substrates are reduced, together with the production of harmful metabolic byproducts.

In the absence of a renal blood supply, the rate at which irreversible injury develops is significantly reduced. The technique of simple hypothermia without special arrangements to support such metabolism as remains has been explored widely.

Avramovici (1924)[14] first reported successful transplantation of dog kidneys after storage in an icebox. The kidneys were stored for up to 8 h, but he concluded that the storage interval using this technique should not exceed 12 h. Many further experiments over 40 years have confirmed these early findings.

The principal effect of hypothermia is the retardation of metabolic activity. Chemical reaction rates vary but not in a linear fashion with absolute temperature. This is an exponential function generally expressed by a factor Q10 (i.e. the numerical measurement of the change in rate of a chemical reaction induced by a temperature change of 10°). Every chemical reaction within the cell is reduced in proportion to its particular Q10. The most frequently used index of metabolic rate is oxygen consumption, the reduction of which by cold is not so much a primary effect but an ultimate consequence of the slowing of all reactions. Though slices of tissues consume less oxygen at low temperatures, they do not suddenly cease consumption at any one low temperature. This may be interpreted to mean that there is no physiological zero above freezing.

The maximum preservation time achieved by simple hypothermia falls a long way short of that theoretically attainable considering the degree of metabolic suppression at 0 °C. This relative failure of simple ice immersion to reach its full potential may be explained by two considerations:

(1) Surface cooling is an inefficient method for reducing core temperature of a large organ, and

(2) Cooling itself has adverse effects of cell physiology.

Rapid cooling of a large organ is best achieved by a combination of surface cooling and per arterial flush. Kidneys of well-hydrated donors pretreated with mannitol and a vasodilator such as phenoxybenzamine can be cooled very rapidly to below 10 °C – such kidneys blanche uniformly and their venous effluent clears rapidly suggesting minimal trapping of red cells in the microcirculation.

Many of the pathophysiological effects of cooling have now been elucidated.

Rate of cooling

A cautionary note on too rapid cooling has been issued[15]. Rabbit kidneys cooled at rates greater than 4 °C/min failed to function. Rates of cooling of this order have generally not been achieved in man or in experiments on large animal kidneys, partly because of the difficulty in keeping all of the tubing and the organ in a totally cold environment during the cooling process and also because the very size of the organ makes heat exchange slower. Nonetheless, the real possibility of thermal injury from too rapid cooling does exist.

Pathophysiology of cooling

Total body oxygen consumption at 5 °C has been shown to be 5% of normal[16]. Whilst reduction of temperature reduces the rate of accumulation of metabolic byproducts and hence autolysis it does not prevent cellular swelling which by itself may be harmful. Cell membrane reactions are accordingly reduced in proportion to the Q10. The sodium pump ceases absolutely below 10 °C. The net effect on major cations of mammalian cells should be a loss of potassium to the extra cellular fluid (ECF) and a gain of sodium and water by the cell. Experimental evidence confirms a potassium leak with hypothermia in many living systems, but not as uniformly as this hypothesis would predict. Using isotopic tracer techniques with ^{42}K and ^{24}Na in the resting anaesthetized dog, it is possible to demonstrate that hypothermia (23 °C) induces a decrease of potassium concentration and a reduction in the $[K^+]:[Na^+]$ ratio in resting skeletal muscle and beating auricular muscle. $[K^+]:[Na^+]$ ratios have also been reduced in the normothermic animal's myocardium by a 3 min period of anoxia[16].

During hypothermic storage of the kidney when metabolic activity is only 5% of normal energy production, cells lose potassium and gain sodium and water[17]. Rat kidneys perfused with normal saline under hypothermic conditions lose 66% of total potassium and 16% of total magnesium. Simple hypothermia therefore causes 'cold injury' in its own right.

Frog's muscle is capable of maintaining tissue $[K^+]$ balance even at 0 °C[18]. Studies show a proportionate reduction in inflow and efflux as temperature falls. It is also of particular interest that hibernating mammals who are able to survive for months at 5 °C without food are also able to maintain their intracellular milieu at low temperatures. In both the hamster and the ground squirrel slices of kidney cortex continue actively to extrude sodium at 0 °C[19].

Clearly simple hypothermia alone was insufficient to produce consistent 24 h storage. There was also the distinct probability that cold injury was part of the problem[17].

There were three main possibilities for improving on simple hypothermia:

(1) Reducing cold injury by manipulating the cold flush solution,

(2) Adding further metabolic blockade by physical or pharmacological means, and

(3) Lowering the temperature to subzero levels.

The role of flush solutions in simple hypothermia

Simple hypothermia alone protects the ischaemic kidney for up to 12 h. However, during this time the cold itself becomes injurious. The classical injury is an imbalance between intra- and extracellular ions, leading to a net gain in water by the cells and ultimately to cellular disruption. It was this fact that led to the idea that the precise composition of the cold flush solution might be of considerable importance[20]. The rapid loss of intracellular cations during short periods of cold perfusion might be prevented by substitution of an intracellular perfusate.

Collins first successfully applied this principle to kidney preservation[21]. He formulated a series of intracellular electrolyte solutions, C_2 to C_4 (Table 7.2). These solutions differed only in respect of the addition of procaine to C_2 to make C_3 and procaine and phenoxybenzamine to C_2 to make C_4. The technique had the immediate attractions of economy and simplicity. The kidney was immersed in crushed iced saline and flushed through its artery with approximately 200 mL of intracellular electrolyte solution from a height of 150 cm until the kidney was uniformly pale and the venous effluent clear. Twenty-four-hour storage was achieved with immediate function using all three solutions – C_2, C_3 and C_4–C_4, however, gave the best results and also allowed three survivors after 30 h storage. Collins' work has since been confirmed by many authors[22-25]. Storage time has now been extended through 48 h to 72 h using all three solutions and since C_2 is the simplest it is probably the best – a view with which Collins now concurs[27].

It has never been satisfactorily explained why such intracellular electrolyte solutions should be so successful when compared with balanced salt solutions. Increased concentrations of any impermeant solutes outside the cell minimizes cellular swelling and subsequent degeneration. This theory led to the successful introduction of hyperosmolar solutions[28] (Table 7.2) with which 72 h storage was achieved. The Eurotransplant Foundation modified Collins' C_2 solution by increasing the glucose to 35 g/L and excluding magnesium. This hyperosmolar solution is now called EuroCollins (Table 7.2).

In 1976 yet another hyperosmolar solution was introduced, this time without a basic intracellular composition. Mannitol was again used as a non-penetrant substance and citrate was added for energy. 72 h storage with this very simple solution (Table 7.3) was also achieved.

A controversy has thus developed over the relative roles of intracellular electrolyte solutions and hyperosmolar solutions. No difference in survival characteristics between the three solutions at 24 h and 48 h has been shown[24]. Several clear conclusions emerged. Balanced salt solutions were effective if their total osmolality was raised to 400 mosmol/L. Even 0.9% w.v. sodium chloride allowed 24 h storage if it was made hypertonic. Raising $[K^+]$ and $[Mg^{2+}]$ concentrations was harmful, whereas lowering $[Na^+]$ and total ionic strength

Table 7.2 Preparation and composition of Collins' intracellular flush solutions

C_2	Constituents (g/L)	EuroCollins	C_2	Composition (mmol/L)	EuroCollins
2.05	KH$_2$PO$_4$	2.05	115	K$^+$	115
9.7	K$_2$HPO$_4$.3H$_2$O	7.4	10	Na$^+$	115
1.12	KCl	1.12	30	Mg^{2+}	—
0.84	NaHCO$_3$	0.84	15	Cl$^-$	15
7.38	MgSO$_4$.7H$_2$O	—	10	HCO$_3^-$	10
25	glucose	35	30	SO$_4^{2-}$	—
			57.5	PO$_4^{2-}$	57.5
			132	glucose	195
			320	osmolality	320
			7.0	pH	7.0

From Collins et al., 1969[21]
Collins solution comprises a litre of glucose solution and an ampoule containing all of the electrolytes. The two are stored at 2°C and mixed just before use. To make Collins C_3 add procaine hydrochloride 0.1 g to C_2; to make C_4 solution add phenoxybenzamine 0.025 g to C_3

Table 7.3 Preparation and composition of mannitol-based hyperosmolar flush solutions

Sacks II	Constituents (g/L)	Hypertonic citrate	Sacks II	Composition (mmol/L)	Hypertonic citrate
4.76	KH_2PO_4	—	143	K^+	80
9.70	$K_2HPO_4.3H_2O$	—	15	Na^+	80
2.30	$KHCO_3$	—	16	Mg^{2+}	72
1.26	$NaHCO_3$	—	16	Cl^-	—
2 mEq/mL	$MgCl_2$	—	38	HCO_3^-	—
37.50	mannitol	34	120	PO_4^{2-}	—
—	potassium citrate	8.6	—	SO_4^{2-}	70
—	sodium citrate	8.2	—	citrate	162
—	HCl (2 M)	0.26 ml	206	mannitol	150
—	$MgSO_4$	10.0	430	osmolality	400
			7.0	pH	7.1

From Sacks et al.[28]; Ross et al.[26]
Both solutions can be stored indefinitely at 2 °C

had no effect. Replacing chloride by sulphate contributed significantly to the solutions' effectiveness[29].

The hypothesis that washout solutions need to mimic intracellular electrolyte composition is not supported by these data: the mechanism of action is more probably that relatively high concentrations of impermeant solutes prevent cellular uptake of water and cations. Nonetheless, the final conclusion from these experiments was that Collins' C_4 solution was superior.

Hyperbaria

This technique was first introduced in 1966[30] and produced consistent 24 h storage by a combination of hypothermia and hyperbaria. A modification using trickle perfusion 2 mL/min for the first 4 h[31] enabled dogs' kidneys to be preserved for 72 h without warm ischaemia and for 24 h after 45–60 min of warm ischaemia. Hyperbaric oxygen improves the quality of non-perfused kidneys, although there is no evidence that increasing the pressure above three atmospheres provides additional benefit.

How hyperbaric oxygen exerts its effect is unknown, but it has been postulated that it serves either to meet nutritional requirements of the cell or to depress oxidative metabolism. Oxygen, however, is apparently not essential for sustaining the viability of the organ in vitro. Hearts stored in hyperbaric nitrogen or helium maintain their viability and resume a ventricular beat when transplanted after 24 h storage at 3 atmospheres[32]. These results indicate that high pressure alone has a preservative effect either by the 'law of mass action' – compression preventing the expansion at the end of a chemical reaction and thus arresting the reaction – or possibly by closing lysosomal cell membranes. There is no doubt that hypothermia and high pressure combined influence the rate of respiration and glycolysis of cells so as to delay irreversible cell damage and death.

Organ storage by continuous hypothermic perfusion

With this method of storage the vascular bed of the kidney is continuously perfused with a cold oxygenated perfusate. This has the theoretical advantage of maintaining the patency of the microcirculation, removing any trapped debris or metabolites, and precisely controlling the oxygen tension and pH of the kidney.

Distribution of the perfusate throughout the organ presents the greatest difficulty in precisely those organs with which clinical transplantation is concerned: the kidney and the liver. A common observation of workers who have perfused kidneys with whole blood is the onset within a few minutes of a marked increase in vascular resistance with consequent changes of flow and pressure – the so-called 'outflow block'.

Dog kidneys were first successfully preserved for 24 h at 10 °C by perfusion at sub-physiological pressures, 30–40 mmHg, with oxygenated plasma or serum diluted with balanced salt solution[33]. Considerable problems continued to exist with prolonged perfusions with acellular fluids at low temperatures. The kidneys became oedematous and developed increasing vascular resistance. The oedema was reduced if albumin or dextran was added to the perfusate. Two factors contributed to the renal vascular resistance:

(1) Spasm, which could be reduced with procaine and papaverine, and

(2) The presence of a particulate material in the perfusate.

Conventional microscopic studies showed no evidence of thrombi: however, when frozen sections were taken, fat stains revealed multiple small emboli in renal arterioles and fat droplets in the tubules of intratubular cells. Rapid thawing of freeze-dried plasma caused lipoproteins to flocculate[34]: the flocculation could be removed by passing the plasma under pressure through banks of micropore filters of pore diameters 1.2, 0.45 and 0.22 μm. Perfusion of the kidney with this filtered plasma completely eliminated rise in perfusion pressure. After 72 h of perfusion, kidney function was proved by reimplantation with immediate contralateral nephrectomy. Cryoprecipitated plasma, however, was rather difficult and time-consuming to prepare. Developments to prevent precipitation of the low density groups of lipoproteins present in plasma even after microfiltration resulted in an escalation both of cost and complexity. These problems were overcome with the introduction of plasma protein fraction (PPF) as an alternative perfusate[35,22]. This solution is essentially human albumin 4.5% suspended in saline. It contains no unstable lipoproteins, no fibrinogen and no gammaglobulin. It is hepatitis-free and contains no blood group factors. Its composition has some deficiencies in that it contains no sugar, no buffer and almost no potassium. The adjustments to PPF and its final composition are shown in Table 7.4. Using plasma protein fraction, dog kidneys were stored for 24 h after up to 60 min of warm ischaemia on a simplified perfusion apparatus, and for 72 h in the absence of warm ischaemic injury.

Much effort has been expended on determining the factors which limit machine storage. A number of authors have reported successful preservation after seven[36,37,38] and eight days[38]. Despite the steady extension of storage time, little is known about the metabolic needs of the kidney during prolonged

Table 7.4 Preparation and composition of plasma protein fraction (PPF) for continuous hypothermic perfusion

Constituents		Composition	
1 PPF (Lister Institute)	400 mL	Na^+	135 mmol/L
		K^+	20 mmol/L
2 $KHCO_3$	600 mg	Mg^{2+}	3.5 mmol/L
		CA^{2+}	2.2 mmol/L
$MgCl_2$	200 mg	Cl^-	110 mmol/L
Dextrose	500 mg	HCO_3^-	25–30 mmol/L
3 Mannitol	120 mg	Total protein	45 g/L
Phenol sulphonphthalein	1–0 mL	Albumen	45 g/L
in 60 mL distilled water		Glucose	150
		Osmolality	300
4 Ampicillin	500 mg	pH at 8 °C	7.4

From Johnson et al.[22]
Constituents 2, 3 and 4 are prepared and stored separately in a refrigerator at 2°C. Each constituent is added to the PPF just before use

storage. Enzyme studies indicate that the kidney starts to decline from the start of cold storage and that continuous perfusion merely slows the rate[39]; preceding injury clearly increases the rate of decline. A most interesting observation is that the kidney can be 'recharged' by removing it from the machine and allowing 2 h of warm circulation with the host dog's blood[40]. The kidney then tolerates a further three days of storage with excellent preservation, producing a total of six days' storage with low serum creatinine concentrations. Whether this benefit is from rewarming or merely from provision of missing nutrients remains to be seen.

Providing metabolic substrates to the cold kidney is known to stimulate respiration. This may not be beneficial since it amounts to stimulating oxygen consumption; the pathway by which this is achieved is unclear and it may represent uncoupling of oxidative phosphorylation.

PRESERVATION OF ISCHAEMICALLY INJURED KIDNEYS

Twenty-four and forty-eight hour preservations have been achieved by simple hypothermia, using intracellular electrolyte solutions, hypertonic solutions, and hypertonic citrate; by a combination of hypothermia and hyperbaria; and by continuous hypothermic perfusion. It is important to test these methods in circumstances resembling the clinical situation and to determine their safety margins. Since cadaver kidneys have most often been exposed to ischaemic injury prior to preservation it is important to evaluate storage methods with ischaemically injured kidneys. Kidneys subjected to 15 min warm ischaemia failed to function after 24 h of storage using Collins' solution[41]. Kidneys subjected to up to 45 min of warm ischaemia functioned immediately after 24 h of machine preservation[23], and successful 48 h machine storage after 30 min of warm ischaemia has also been reported[39]. Kidneys do not function well after

165

warm ischaemic injury when stored by simple hypothermia with either Sacks' solution or hypertonic citrate[42,43]. This problem can be resolved by bubbling oxygen into the renal vein during storage, suggesting that it is the oxygen debt that is the problem and that this is made worse in an anaerobic environment[43]. When the pathogenesis of cold injury and ischaemic injury is considered it is not surprising that a kidney that has already acquired an oxygen debt as a result of ischaemic injury will indeed be made worse when placed in a situation where its oxygen debt cannot be corrected.

In organ preservation two factors operate which interfere with cell volume regulation: one is cooling itself, which effectively turns off the sodium pump by its effect on chemical reaction rates. The other is anoxia which reduces the synthesis of the ATP necessary to run the sodium pump. Cooling at present is unavoidable and its effects appear to be readily and completely reversible on rewarming as long as sufficient ATP is available.

The effect of anoxia is more serious because it appears to be less readily recoverable. Anoxic injury is characteristically associated with a mottled, cyanosed, vasospastic kidney. The failure of blood flow to return to a kidney that has suffered a period of warm injury is known as the 'no-reflow' phenomenon[44]. There is no doubt that this is a very important factor in determining the success of kidneys preserved after warm injury.

Changes in distribution of the kidney microcirculation in response to handling, hypovolaemic shock and warm ischaemia are well recognized. Ischaemia increases renal vascular resistance[45] but this is not due to intravascular coagulation since it is not improved by heparinization. Prevention of vascular collapse by simultaneous clamping of artery and vein was beneficial, and in one study of continuous perfusion[46] it was found that vascular resistance of ischaemically damaged kidneys decreased during perfusion until, after 12 h, it was similar to that of undamaged kidneys[23]. Pretreatment with chlorpromazine also prevents the no-reflow phenomenon[45-47]. High vascular resistance is therefore at least partly responsible for the difficulty in preserving ischaemically injured kidneys.

Pretreatment with mannitol prevents swelling of the endothelium and blockage of the vessels[48]: however, after anoxic injury mannitol alone does not improve renal blood flow whereas administration of Dextran 40 to prevent cell sludging does. This finding fits into Pegg's hypothesis[49] that it is blockage of the microcirculation by rigid anoxic red cells that causes the no-reflow phenomenon. Anoxic red cells rapidly become depleted of ATP and under these circumstances Ca^{2+}, which would normally be chelated by ATP, binds with cell membrane rendering it more rigid[50].

Direct experimental evidence for the importance of adenine nucleotide reserves and particularly ATP in warm ischaemia is strong: the adenine nucleotide content of kidneys subjected to warm ischaemia correlates with their ability to support life[51,52]. ATP levels were best maintained by continuous perfusion[53]; indeed it has recently been shown that ischaemically injured kidneys can resynthesize ATP during continuous hypothermic perfusion in the presence of oxygen, glucose and hypoxanthine[54]. Continuous perfusion has been in use since 1967 and is the method of choice in 82% of American centres[55].

Machine preservation is expensive and, despite considerable modification in design and in perfusate composition, it is a much more complex technique. Transportation on a machine is altogether more difficult. The advantages are prolonged safe storage time and the safe preservation of ischaemic kidneys. The continuous washout of metabolic byproducts, with buffering and provision of an aerobic milieu, means that oxygen debt is rapidly corrected and that energy stores are conserved. In addition patency of the microcirculation is maintained. The merits of machine storage must not be exaggerated: bad technique with machine storage is disastrous and leads to unnecessary wastage. Some centres have reserved machine storage for testing doubtful kidneys. This creates two problems: firstly, through lack of practice they are unlikely to be able to make a realistic judgement; and secondly, through inferior technique they are likely to damage the organ further. It is true that machine preservation provides an opportunity for continuous monitoring of the kidney during storage: there are, however, no reliable tests of deterioration during storage. The only tests that have been shown to be beneficial are those that indicate probability of immediate function rather than likelihood of primary non-function.

It has also been suggested that continuous perfusion with cryoprecipitated homologous plasma is associated with an increased rate of early graft loss[56]. This has been attributed to an immunological injury caused by cytotoxic IgM present in homologous plasma[57].

Albumin-based perfusates have also been widely used in clinical practice. These perfusates contain no immunoglobulins and no blood-group antibodies. There has never been any association between them and early graft failure. Excellent immediate function has been reported for human kidneys after up to 45 h of machine storage[58] with plasma protein fraction. Continuous perfusion is not for the occasional user. In practised hands it provides the highest quality of preservation for the longest period of time.

References

1. Bywaters, E. G. L. and Beall, D. (1941). Crush injuries with impairment of renal function. *Br. Med. J.*, 1, 427–32
2. Lauson, H. D., Bradley, S. E. and Cournand, A. (1944). The renal circulation in shock. *J. Clin. Invest.*, 23, 381–402
3. Carriere, S., Thorburn, G. D., O'Morchoe, C. L. and Barger, A. C. (1966). Intrarenal distribution of blood flow in dogs during haemorrhagic hypotension. *Circulat. Res.*, 19, 167–79
4. Belzer, F. O., Reed, T. W., Pryor, J. P., Kountz, S. L. and Dunphy, J. E. (1970). Cause of renal injury in kidneys obtained from cadaver. *Surg. Gynecol. Obstet.*, 130, 467–77
5. Thiel, G., de Rougemont, D., Torhorst, J., Kaufman, A., Peters-Haefeli, L. and Brunner, F. P. (1980). Importance of tubular obstruction and its prevention in ischaemic acute renal failure in the rat. In Leaf, A. (ed.) *Renal Pathophysiology.* (New York: Raven Press)
6. Carroll, R. N., Chisholm, G. D. and Shackman, R. (1969). Factors influencing early function of cadaver renal transplants. *Lancet*, 2, 551–2
7. Clegg, J. F., Kulatilake, A. E., Chisholm, G. D. and Shackman, R. (1968). The significance of ischaemia in renal allotransplantation. *Proc. Eur. Dialysis Transplant. Assoc.*, 5, 264
8. Raftery, A. T. and Johnson, R. W. G. (1979). Dopamine pretreatment in unstable kidney donors. *Br. Med. J.*, 1, 522–3
9. Enerson, D. M. and Berman, H. M. (1966). Cellular swelling II. Effects of hypotoxicity, low molecular weight dextran addition and pH on O_2 consumption of isolated tissues. *Ann. Surg.*, 163, 537–44

10. Semb, C. (1956). Partial resection of the kidney: anatomical, physiological and clinical aspects. *Ann. R. Coll. Surg. Engl.*, **19**, 137–55
11. Hoffmann, R. M., Stieper, K. W., Johnson, R. W. G. and Belzer, F. O. (1974). Renal ischaemic tolerance. *Arch. Surg.*, **109**, 550–51
12. Wickham, J. E. A., Hanley, H. G. and Joekes, A. M. (1967). Regional renal hypothermia. *Br. J. Urol.*, **39**, 727–43
13. Freidman, S. M., Johnson, R. L. and Freidman, C. L. (1954). The pattern of recovery of renal function following renal artery occlusion in the dog. *Circulat. Res.*, **2**, 231–5
14. Avramovici, A. (1924). Les transplantations du rein. *Lyon Chir.*, **21**, 734–57
15. Jacobsen, I. A., Kemp, E. and Buhl, M. R. (1979). An adverse effect of rapid cooling in kidney preservation. *Transplantation*, **27**, 135–6
16. Gollan, F. (1956). Electrolyte transfer during hypothermia. In Dripps, E. D. (ed.) *The Physiology of Induced Hypothermia.* (Washington: Nat. Acad. Sci. NRC)
17. Keeler, R., Swinney, J., Taylor, R. M. R. and Uldall, P. R. (1966). The problem of renal preservation. *Br. J. Urol.*, **6**, 653–6
18. Harris, E. J. (1952). The exchange of K^+ in frog muscle studied in phosphate media. *J. Physiol. (London)*, **117**, 278–9
19. Willis, J. S. (1964). Uptake of potassium at low temperatures in kidney cortex slices of hibernating mammals. *Nature*, **204**, 691–2
20. Keeler, R., Swinney, J. and Uldall, P. R. (1966). Effects on renal function of supercooling rat kidneys. *J. Physiol. (London)*, **184**, 69–70
21. Collins, G. M., Bravo-Shugarman, M. and Terasaki, P. I. (1969). Kidney preservation for transportation. *Lancet*, **2**, 1219–22
22. Johnson, R. W. G., Anderson, M., Flear, C. T. G., Murray, S., Swinney, J. and Taylor, R. M. R. (1972). Evaluation of a new perfusate for kidney preservation. *Transplantation*, **13**, 270–5
23. Johnson, R. W. G., Anderson, M., Morley, A. R., Taylor, R. M. R. and Swinney, J. (1972). Twenty-four hour preservation of kidneys injured by prolonged warm ischaemia. *Transplantation*, **13**, 174–9
24. Guthinger, W. P., Linke, C. A., Pranikoff, K. and Fridd, C. W. (1978). Comparison of hypertonic citrate, Collins C_2 and C_3 flushing solutions in canine cold storage kidney preservation. *Transplantation*, **25**, 279
25. Liu, W. P., Humphries, A. L., Russell, R., Stoddart, L. D. and Moretz, W. H. (1971). 48-hour storage of canine kidneys after brief perfusion with Collins' Solution. *Ann. Surg.*, **173**, 748–57
26. Ross, H., Marshall, V. C. and Escott, M. L. (1976). 72-hour canine kidney preservation without continuous perfusion. *Transplantation*, **21**, 498–501
27. Collins, G. M., Green, R. D., Boyer, D. and Halasz, N. A. (1980). Protection of kidneys from warm ischaemic injury. *Transplantation*, **29**, 83–4
28. Sacks, S. A., Petritsch, P. H. and Kaufman, J. J. (1973). Canine kidney preservation using a new perfusate. *Lancet*, **1**, 1024–8
29. Green, C. J. and Pegg, D. E. (1979). The effect of variation in electrolyte composition and osmolality of solutions for infusion and hypothermic storage. In Pegg, D. E. and Jacobsen, I. A. (eds.) *Organ Preservation II*, p. 86. (Edinburgh: Churchill Livingstone)
30. Ackermann, J. R. W. and Barnard, C. N. (1966). Successful storage of kidneys. *Br. J. Surg.*, **53**, 525–32
31. Snell, M. E., Hopkinson, W. I. and Shepherd, R. R. (1972). 72-hour preservation of canine kidneys. *Br. J. Surg.*, **59**, 307
32. Lyons, G. W., Dietzman, R. H. and Lillehei, R. C. (1966). On the mechanism of preservation with hypothermia and hyperbaric oxygen. *Trans. Am. Soc. Artif. Intern. Org.*, **12**, 236
33. Humphries, A. L. (1967). Problems of organ preservation. *Transplantation*, **5**, 1138
34. Belzer, F. O., Ashby, B. S. and Dunphy, J. E. (1967). 24- and 72-hour preservation of canine kidneys. *Lancet*, **2**, 536–9
35. Johnson, R. W. G., Anderson, M., Flear, C. T. G., Murray, S., Swinney, J. and Taylor, R. M. R. (1971). Evaluation of a new perfusate for kidney preservation. *Eur. Surg. Res.*, **3**, 215
36. Liu, W. P., Humphries, A. L., Russell, R., Stoddard, L. D., Garcia, L. A. and Serkes, K. D. (1973). 3- and 7-day perfusion of dog kidneys with human plasma protein fraction IV-4. *Surg. Forum*, **24**, 316–8

37. Woods, J. E. (1971). Successful three- to seven-day preservation of canine kidneys. *Arch. Surg.*, **102**, 614–6

38. Cohen, G. L. and Johnson, R. W. G. (1980). Perfusate buffering for 8-day canine kidney storage. *Proc. Eur. Soc. Artif. Org.*, **7**, 235–9

39. Johnson, R. W. G., Cohen, G. L. and Ballardie, F. W. (1979). The limitation of continuous perfusion with plasma protein fraction. In Pegg, D. E. and Jacobsen, I. A. (eds.) *Organ Preservation II*, pp. 18–32. (Edinburgh: Churchill Livingstone)

40. Van der Wijk, J., Sloof, M. J. H., Rijkmans, B. G. and Kootstra, G. (1980). Successful 96- and 144-hour experimental kidney preservation. *Cryobiology*, **17**, 473–7

41. Frost, A. B., Ackerman, J., Finch, W. T. and Manlove, A. (1970). Kidney preservation for transportation. *Lancet*, **1**, 620

42. Toledo-Pereyra, L. H. and Condie, R. M. (1978). Comparison of Sacks and a new colloid hyperosmolar solution for hypothermic renal storage. *Transplantation*, **26**, 166–8

43. Ross, H. and Escott, M. L. (1979). Gaseous oxygen perfusion of the renal vessels as an adjunct to kidney preservation. *Transplantation*, **28**, 362–4

44. Sheehan, H. L. and Davis, J. C. (1959). Renal ischaemia with failed reflow. *J. Pathol. Bacteriol.*, **78**, 105–20

45. Løkkegaard, H. and Bilde, T. (1972). Vascular resistance in hypothermically perfused kidneys following 1 hour of warm ischaemia. *Acta Med. Scand.*, **191**, 429–32

46. Johnson, R. W. G. (1972). The effect of ischaemic injury on kidneys preserved for 24 hours before transplantation. *Br. J. Surg.*, **59**, 765–70

47. Løkkegaard, H., Bilde, T., Gyrd-Hansen, N., Jaglicic, D., Jensen, E., Nerstrom, B. and Rasmussen, F. (1973). The effect of chlorpromazine on preservation of kidneys with one hour's warm ischaemia. *Acta Med. Scand.*, **193 (1)**, 65–72

48. Flores, J., Di Bona, D. R., Frega, N. and Leaf, A. (1972). Cell volume regulation and ischaemic tissue damage. *J. Membrane Biol.*, **10**, 331–43

49. Pegg, D. E. (1978). An approach to hypothermic renal preservation. *Cryobiology*, **15**, 1–17

50. Weed, R. I., La Celle, P. I. and Merrill, E. W. (1969). Metabolic dependence of red cell deformability. *J. Clin. Invest.*, **48**, 795–809

51. Calman, K. C. (1974). The prediction of organ viability. *Cryobiology*, **11**, 1–6

52. Calman, K. C. (1974). The prediction of organ viability. II. Testing an hypothesis. *Cryobiology*, **11**, 7–12

53. Bergstrom, J., Collste, H., Groth, C. G., Hultman, E. and Melia, B. (1971). Water, electrolyte and metabolite content of cortical tissue from dog kidneys preserved by hypothermia. *Proc. Eur. Dialysis Transplant Assoc.*, **8**, 313–20

54. Pegg, D. E., Wusteman, M. C. and Foreman, J. (1981). Metabolism of normal and ischaemically injured rabbit kidneys during perfusion for 48 hours at 10°C. *Transplantation*, **32**, 437–43

55. Belzer, F. O. and Southard, J. H. (1980). The future of kidney preservation. *Transplantation*, **30**, 161

56. Clark, E. A., Terasaki, P. I., Opelz, G. and Mickey, M. R. (1974). Cadaver kidney transplant failures at 1 month. *N. Engl. J. Med.*, **291**, 1099–102

57. Light, J. A., Annable, C., Perloff, L. J., Sulkin, M. D., Hill, G. S., Etheredge, E. E. and Spees, E. K. Jr. (1975). Immune injury from organ preservation. *Transplantation*, **19**, 511–6

58. Johnson, R. W. G., Cohen, G. L., Mallick, N. P. and Orr, W. McN. (1979). Renal function and early cadaver graft survival after continuous hypothermic perfusion with plasma protein fraction (PPF). *Transplant Proc.*, **11**, 1476

169

8
Bone Marrow Transplantation

A. K. BURNETT AND G. A. McDONALD

INTRODUCTION

Clinical bone marrow transplantation has its origin in the experimental work of Jacobson in the early 1950s[1,2,3]. His interest in rodent haemopoiesis included evaluation of hormone control. In a particular series of experiments haemopoiesis was re-established following ablative irradiation, provided one limb of the animal was shielded: subsequently intravenous spleen cell suspension was shown to be capable of restoring haemopoiesis to irradiated mice. This observation was initially interpreted as being due to a non-cellular factor in the spleen suspension, but the subsequent experiments by Lorenz established the pivotal observation that intravenous administration of haemopoietic cells was capable of re-establishing haemopoiesis[4].

These observations opened the way towards a better understanding of the cellular basis of haemopoiesis with the subsequent evolution of *in vitro* techniques of detecting progenitor cells. Techniques of demonstrating a population of pluripotent stem cells in man have not yet been developed, and this remains a matter of intensive study with important consequences for the newer developments in clinical transplantation. For practical purposes at present, it is generally accepted as an operational hypothesis that haemopoiesis is a hierarchical system of cellular development, with an ultimate haemopoietic stem cell which has the unique dual characteristics of self-renewal and the ability to feed, through committed lineage associated precursor cells, the different cell lines of haemopoiesis[5]. Pluripotent stem cells form a very small proportion of a normal bone marrow, but the assumption that only these cells are necessary for successful engraftment may be too simplistic in .the light of the recent suggestion that accessory cells, which do not have the characteristics of stem cells[6], may be required. More recent techniques involving *in vitro* treatment of bone marrow before transplantation emphasize that the cellular events taking place during the period of engraftment are complex.

The potential clinical implications of the early rodent experiments were soon recognized. Several sporadic attempts were made in clinical practice – usually unsuccessfully. Evolution of clinical transplantation to a stage where it ceased to be purely experimental has resulted from an increased understanding of the HLA system and the considerable strides which have been made in supportive care. The restriction of allogeneic transplantation to patients for whom a donor matched at HLA-A, B, D and DR loci with a non-reactive mixed lymphocyte reaction *in vitro* has permitted, in suitably conditioned patients, stable engraftment. *In vitro* tests do not, however, exclude the possibility that the immunological component of the donor's marrow may react against the host, resulting in a clinical syndrome unique to bone marrow transplantation – graft-versus-host disease (GVHD). The likeliest potential donor is a sibling and the clinical experience of transplantation within any particular disease category is virtually exclusively restricted to this relatively small subgroup of patients. Theoretically the donor pool could be expanded to include those who are phenotypically but not genotypically matched (mostly unrelated) donors. Similarly, with increased understanding of the mechanisms and prevention of the immmunobiological problems of transplantation, successful results may be possible in situations where there are degrees of non-identity at the major HLA loci. These approaches are in the early stages of clinical evaluation.

TECHNIQUE OF BONE MARROW TRANSPLANTATION

Procurement of stem cells

The vast majority of procedures involve 'harvesting' of bone marrow from the chosen donor by multiple aspirations through standard or near standard needles normally used for diagnostic taps. A sufficient number of cells can usually be obtained from the posterior iliac crests but on occasions it may be necessary to use anterior ileum and sternum. The most satisfactory technique restricts the volume of each aspirate to 5 mL: beyond this the aspirate is heavily contaminated with peripheral blood. Some groups prefer to anticoagulate the donor but this is not necessary provided the marrow can be promptly transferred into a suitable medium containing anticoagulant. The donor is usually under general anaesthetic for 30 min but it is possible to use spinal anaesthesia[7]. The procedure is remarkably well tolerated by the donor and the risks are small. The donor usually leaves hospital the next day. Complications of marrow harvesting due to infection or thrombosis, or associated with the anaesthetic are rare, with an overall incidence of 0.27% in more than 3000 procedures and no recorded fatalities[8].

Preparation of the patient

The recipient requires some form of conditioning treatment immediately prior to graft infusion, with two main objectives:

(a) To condition the immune system to accept the graft, and

172

(b) To eradicate, where relevant, residual disease.

In the fully HLA-matched situation the traditional approach has been the combination of cyclophosphamide 120 mg/kg over 2 d and total body ir- radiation (TBI). The wide variety of approaches to radiation technique between centres makes direct comparisons difficult[9], but developmental work both in dog and man suggested a midline dose of 950 cGy as the level required to achieve consistent engraftment[10]. Although considerable intercen- tre variation is inevitable because of logistic considerations, rejection is unusual in the fully matched situation.

Supportive care

A better understanding of supportive care has been a major factor in establishing bone marrow transplantation in clinical practice. In uncompplic- ated cases peripheral blood pancytopenia will last for 3–4 weeks till the new marrow establishes itself in the host. During this period the patient is at significant risk and most transplant teams make extensive arrangements to prevent problems during this phase. Blood product support is of major importance. Red cell transfusion is almost always necessary in the second week, but that is quite possibly the only red cell transfusion required. Most patients receive platelets prophylactically to keep the count above $20 \times 10^9/L$. Such support is usually required for 3–4 weeks. Our own practice is to utilize random donors initially, but on occasions HLA-matched products are required to obtain the required increase in platelet count. Granulocyte transfusions are virtually never used. All products are irradiated prior to transfusion to prevent engraftment of donor peripheral blood stem cells. It is our policy to give patients who are cytomegalovirus (CMV) seronegative pre- transplant and who have a seronegative donor, blood products exclusively from donors known to be CMV seronegative. The importance of this policy will be discussed later.

Patients are nursed in laminar air flow rooms. Selective gut decontamina- tion with non-absorbable antibiotics is attempted in order to reduce the risk of endogenous bacterial infection. Such a policy may also contribute to a reduction in the incidence of graft-versus-host disease[11]. If patients wish to eat they receive sterile food. In our experience there is no measurable benefit from indiscriminate use of parenteral nutrition. In patients who have had previous exposure to herpes simplex (type I) infection, reactivation in the first 2–3 weeks post-transplant is almost certain[12], but prompt symptomatic relief can be obtained with suitable antiviral medication (acyclovir). Since reactivation is inevitable in seropositive patients, some groups have found it of benefit to give acyclovir prophylactically[13,14].

Almost all patients become febrile and, although positive bacterial isolates are seldom obtained, most will receive broad spectrum intravenous anti- biotics. As neutrophil regeneration occurs all these measures are scaled down. Regular monitoring and medication is greatly helped by the use throughout of an indwelling right atrial catheter.

CLINICAL USES OF BONE MARROW TRANSPLANTATION

Acute leukaemia

It is fortunate that the radiobiological characteristics of haemopoietic cells and leukaemic cells appear to be similar[15]. Leukaemia eradication may thus be achieved by the same conditioning protocol required for consistent engraftment. The experimental basis of clinical transplantation was, however, originally based partially on data which suggested that residual disease could be controlled by an allogeneic or graft-versus-leukaemia effect in the host[16]. Whether such an effect is operational in clinical practice has until recently been a minor consideration to physicians treating patients, but more recent developments and the accumulated experience now available from several centres have aroused fresh interest in the contribution such an effect may make to the success of the procedure.

The development of clinical bone marrow transplantation is very much attributable to the Seattle group who conducted studies initially in patients with end-stage disease[17]. Since the technique could only be regarded as experimental in the early 1970s, it was then naturally ethically difficult to justify such an approach in an earlier stage of the disease.

The overall results of their experience showed that only a few patients became long-term survivors but a number of important factors relating to the subsequent development of bone marrow transplantation (BMT) were delineated. These studies demonstrated that lasting stable chimeric states could be established with sustained haemopoiesis and that, even in the face of resistant disease, leukaemia could be eradicated in a few patients with the chosen chemo-radiotherapeutic regimen. The major immunobiological problems were defined, namely graft-versus-host disease, pneumonitis, the consequences of immunosuppression and recurrent leukaemia; these remain the current problems.

The actuarial relapse rate in this group of patients, which comprised all types of acute leukaemia, was 60–70%, but because of the poor overall survival it was not possible to delineate a graft-versus-leukaemia effect. An important observation was made that younger patients (<40 years old), those with syngeneic donors, or those with less florid or less resistant disease had a better prospect of survival. Before BMT could find a place in clinical practice, all these problems had to be solved or ameliorated, and it appeared more useful to restrict the technique to younger patients at an earlier stage in the disease.

Transplantation in remission

Based on these early experiences the current strategy for the use of BMT in acute leukaemias became established. The current role which it fulfils in each category of leukaemia will persist only as long as alternative forms of treatment give inferior results.

Acute myeloblastic leukaemia

Over the last decade there has been a general improvement in the results of treatment designed to achieve initial remission of disease, such that this is now achieved in 60–80% of cases of all ages[18,19,20]. There has been less satisfactory progress in developing modalities of treatment to maintain remission long-term, to the extent that the operational definition of cure can be justifiably used. In most series 20% of patients appear to survive 4–5 years but there is no evidence that this survival rate can be improved by short-term consolidation at an early or late stage or by maintenance chemotherapy[21,22]. Nearly all cases eventually die from the disease. Perhaps the only subgroup in which this is not a justifiable generalization is in the paediatric subgroup of children with acute myeloblastic leukaemia (AML), where results with chemotherapy are better (around 50% five-year survival)[23].

The initial reports of the use of allograft as the definitive treatment administered with curative intent were very encouraging, both in terms of overall survival (50%) and actuarial prediction of recurrence of leukaemia (5–20%). There is now widespread experience which largely corroborates these initial studies[24-27]. The superiority of allogeneic transplantation in terms of predicted antileukaemic effect is clear. If leukaemia recurs it usually does so in the first 12–18 months post-transplant: thereafter very few relapses have been reported. Similarly those patients who succumb to the non-leukaemic causes of death usually do so within the first few months post-graft. For patients surviving one year post-transplant, the prospects of prolonged survival are excellent. Where patients are transplanted in the second or subsequent remission of disease results are poorer (30% survival), principally because of a higher incidence of recurrent leukaemia[28]. These patients, who are also likely to be less fit due to the cumulative effects of chemotherapy, probably are biologically selected in terms of having more resistant disease. There is some evidence to suggest that for patients in relapse, for whom a suitable donor is available but who were not transplanted in their first remission, it is best to proceed to transplant without attempting to gain a further remission[29]. More patients in this otherwise hopeless predicament will be salvaged by such an approach – because re-induction treatment at this point will be unsuccessful in a proportion of cases and, even if successful, will tend to increase toxicity at the subsequent transplant.

While bone marrow transplantation is an exciting and important treatment for AML, some perspective needs to be given to its overall contribution to the disease. It is restricted in its application because of the criteria of age (< 40 years) and availability of an HLA fully matched donor. Since AML incidence tends to increase with age, only about one third of all cases will be within the transplant age range, and one in three of these patients will have a suitable donor. Given that patients initially have to achieve remission, only approximately 10% of those with the disease will receive a transplant of whom half (5% of the total) appear to become long-term survivors. However, the superior antileukaemic effect achievable has given considerable incentive to the quest to apply the technique to a wider range of those with the disease.

175

Acute lymphoblastic leukaemia

The peak incidence of this disease is in children and it is here that considerable therapeutic success has been achieved over the last 15–20 years by conventional chemotherapy, such that there is currently an expectation of prolonged survival in 60–70% of cases[30]. The use of bone marrow transplantation has therefore been difficult to justify in the first remission of the disease. For those cases who fail conventional treatment, further chemotherapy offers little hope of success and it is in this setting (second or greater complete remission) that bone marrow transplantation has been used. The overall results are less good than those achieved in AML in first remission, principally because the antileukaemia effect is poorer, with the actuarial chance of recurrence being 50–60%[31,32]. The results achieved are not dissimilar from those in AML in second remission and, although only 30% will survive long-term, very few patients treated with chemotherapy at this stage of the disease would survive. With both approaches to treatment it is important to distinguish the patients who have relapsed while still on maintenance chemotherapy – whose prognosis is poor with conventional treatment–from those who have relapsed after chemotherapy has been electively discontinued. The latter group, although usually incurable, can experience useful duration of subsequent remission with conventional treatment.

While BMT may be the best available salvage procedure in patients with acute lymphoblastic leukaemia (ALL) once they have relapsed, the high relapse rate has encouraged, in recent years, the selection of subgroups who are predicted to respond poorly to first line chemotherapy. For these patients, transplantation may be used as an alternative in first remission. What constitutes 'poor prognosis' is a matter of debate but there is general recognition that patients who present with a high blast cell count, B cell disease or Philadelphia chromosome positive disease respond poorly to conventional chemotherapy and an alternative approach is justified. In addition to this could be added all adult cases of ALL, with the probable exception of teenage females for whom conventional treatment may still offer a 50% chance of survival. T cell disease is not of itself an indicator of poor prognosis. Initial clinical results of such a strategy of selection are encouraging but the experience is still small and requires longer follow-up.

Severe aplastic anaemia

The criteria for the designation of 'severe' aplastic anaemia are:

(1) Neutrophils $<200 \times 10^9/L$,

(2) Platelets $<20\,000 \times 10^9/L$,

(3) Reticulocyte count $<0.1\%$, and

(4) Greater than 70% non-myeloid cellularity in a hypocellular bone marrow biopsy confirmed from more than one site.

The prognosis for patients fitting such criteria is poor with little evidence that conservative treatment has any effect. In patients with less severe pancytopenia, i.e. mild or moderate aplasia or hypoplasia, spontaneous recovery can be observed. Bone marrow transplantation has become the treatment of choice for severe aplasia but it is inappropriate that it should be used in other less severe categories of the disease.

By the mid-seventies several groups had reported success rates of 40–50% with full haematological reconstitution[33-35]. Most protocols had adopted pregraft immunosuppression with cyclophosphamide 200 mg/kg divided over 4 d. Previous experience in syngeneic transplantation for aplasia indicated that infusion of marrow without conditioning resulted in frequent rejection, but that when immunosuppression was administered regular engraftment was achieved. In the aplastic experience a major limitation has been failure to achieve sustained engraftment in 30–50% of cases even where cyclophosphamide alone was used as conditioning.

The factors associated with rejection were delineated by the Seattle group who argued[36], on the basis of a background of experimental evidence, that prior blood transfusions may have sensitized the recipient with resultant rejection. In their series of untransfused patients given cyclophosphamide alone, rejection was 10% with an overall survival of more than 80%. Because of the nature of the disease and an inevitable pretransplant delay it is often not possible to avoid transfusion. In multiply-transfused patients rejection is less likely with a nucleated cell 'dose' of 3×10^8/kg of recipient weight. *In vitro* unidirectional reactivity between donor and host cells was found in Seattle to be predictive of rejection but such *in vitro* tests were not found to correlate when used by other centres – probably because different, and generally more intensive, preparative regimens were used[37]. Other factors have been reported by individual groups to be relevant such as male recipients, female grafts, patient age and presence of lymphocytotoxic antibodies at time of grafting, but none has been generally corroborated by other groups.

In the last decade evolution of more successful strategies to secure engraftment in multiply-transfused patients have evolved. The Seattle group routinely give unirradiated donor buffy coat in the few days immediately post-transplant[38]. The rationale is to provide additional stem cells and possibly immunocompetent cells to prevent rejection. Such an approach avoids more aggressive immunosuppression – their previous experience with additional TBI was disappointing – and has been relatively successful with a rejection rate of 13% and an overall survival rate of 71%. A disadvantage, and the major remaining cause of failure, is an increased incidence of chronic GVHD associated with the buffy coat administration[39].

Low rejection rates (5–15%) have been noted by others where some form of irradiation or chemotherapy has been added to the cyclophosphamide, but the more intensive the protocol the greater has been the incidence of GVHD[35,40]. There is sufficient anxiety about the long-term consequences of radiation for there still to be an incentive to improve the preparative regimen. The Hammersmith group[41] have found the combination of cyclophosphamide and cyclosporin to result in consistent engraftment (rejection rate 14%) with an overall success rate of greater than 70%.

In some cases where appropriate analysis has been done, autologous haemopoietic regeneration has taken place[42]. More recently it has been recognized that some successful results are from stable mixed chimeras of donor and host cells. One aspect of supportive care which has significantly affected survival of transplants for aplastic anaemia is the use of laminar air flow (LAF) rooms and gut decontamination with non-absorbable antibiotics[43]. There is experimental evidence in mice which suggests that little or no GVHD occurs in microbial free recipients of bone marrow transplants. Patients with aplasia treated in LAF have significantly less GVHD, resulting in improved survival (87% versus 69%). Such a phenomenon has not yet been demonstrated in BMT for other conditions.

For patients who do not have a suitable matched sibling donor, use has been made in a smaller number of cases of phenotypically matched, unrelated donors with some preliminary success[44]. The use of family members who are not fully matched (mismatched donors) remains a difficult approach, but wider experience of such techniques in the next few years may represent a viable option in clinical practice.

Chronic myeloid leukaemia

The clinical course of chronic myeloid leukaemia (CML) is characterized by a quiescent or chronic phase perhaps lasting 2–4 years followed in a high proportion of cases by progression of the disease to a refractory or blastic phase[45]. Progression may be rapid or gradual over a period of weeks or months, during which time clinical management of the patient becomes more difficult (accelerated phase). So, for the majority of patients, survival will not exceed four years.

There is no evidence to suggest that therapeutic intervention in the chronic phase delays progression to the blast phase[46,47]. An important disease marker of the neoplastic clone is the presence of the Philadelphia chromosome which is demonstrable at all times, indicating the presence of residual disease. The demonstration that bone marrow transplantation following ablative treatment was capable of eradicating the Ph′ positive cells in twin transplants[48], together with increasing experience with BMT, has resulted in mounting experience from several centres of allograft being the elective treatment of the disease[49-51]. The initial clinical results suggest that bone marrow transplantation will become the treatment of choice in this disease.

It is already clear that the major factor influencing outcome is the status of disease at time of transplant. In a disease with a variable quiescent period where the patient can exist virtually normally, as in the chronic phase, it is tempting to delay transplantation with its inherent risks, till there is some sign of progression of disease. Should the progression be directly into blast phase, bone marrow transplant will only salvage 10–20% of cases which, although currently the best option for patients in blast phase, is not the optimum approach. If transplantation is undertaken in the accelerating phase then survival improves to 30–40%: however, if BMT is adopted as definitive treatment of chronic phase disease, survival of 60–70% can be expected. It is of interest to note that the few cases with blastic transformation of lymphoid type who can be returned to a second chronic phase and then transplanted have good prospects of success.

Recurrence of disease following transplantation in the chronic phase, as defined by finding of Philadelphia positive cells, has been reported only in a small number of patients. The definition of relapse has emerged as an interesting consequence of this experience, since in a few cases Ph' positive metaphases have been demonstrated in the bone marrow but have subsequently disappeared – so the presence of the chromosome must persist before relapse can be finally confirmed. The eradication of the Philadelphia chromosome after allograft is the main reason for the present optimism, since the natural history of chronic phase can be several years, and only a relatively small number of patients have so far exceeded the expected median survival. It is probable that allogeneic transplantation will become widely recognized as the treatment of choice in CML with a recommendation that transplant should take place early in the course of disease.

Genetic diseases

A number of rare genetic disorders can be corrected by bone marrow transplantation. The problems associated with such cases are mostly those of GVHD, rejection, and correction of the underlying disease. In general terms it appears that early transplantation achieves better results.

Severe combined immune deficiency (SCID) is a syndrome where affected children lack T and B cell function. The phenotype of the disease varies from total lymphopenia to functional deficiency of T or B cells. In most cases life expectancy is short. Since there is no defect in other haemopoietic cell lines lymphoid engraftment is all that is required. This can be achieved in an HLA-matched transplant without any immunosuppression and with a relatively small bone marrow dose. Experience to date has indicated a 50–60% success rate[52,53], most cases having normal B and T cell function. It is of interest that non-lymphoid haemopoiesis remains of host origin post-transplant. Transplants from donors who are other than HLA genotypically matched, have been associated with a lower success rate. In recent years attempts have been made using histo-incompatible donors with poor results. In this context more recent approaches involving selective T cell depletion of the graft with monoclonal antibody or lectin separation have achieved some success[54].

Storage disorders such as Hurler's disease, Gaucher's disease and San Filippo B disease result from accumulation of the relevant substance due to lack of the appropriate metabolizing enzyme. In these and certain other disorders allogeneic leukocytes can provide a permanent source of enzyme thus preventing progression of the disease[55,56]. Biochemical and clinical improvement has been reported in these disorders but it is essential to undertake the procedure as early as possible, before the patient has suffered irreversible damage.

Isolated deficiencies of haemopoietic cell lines other than lymphoid deficiencies can be corrected by transplantation: infantile agranulocytosis, chronic granulomatous disease and osteopetrosis have all been successfully treated[57-59]. In these disorders immunosuppressive and ablative treatment is required to ensure engraftment. Numerically the most important disorder of this type is thalassaemia where recent results are encouraging[60]. Eradication of abnormal haemopoiesis in the host remains a problem, with the demonstration of persistent globin chain imbalance in 15% of cases post-transplant. Early transplantation is indicated but there is naturally anxiety about the use of TBI as the ablative treatment in such young children. Busulphan, the currently favoured alternative, results in a few additional graft failures, but seems safer in the short term. Little is yet known about its long-term toxicity.

The Wiskott–Aldrich syndrome may be correctable by transplantation of bone marrow on the basis that the underlying disorder of T lymphocytes and platelets is deficiency of membrane glycoprotein, suggesting a stem cell disorder expressing itself in T cells and platelets. This X-linked recessive disorder has been successfully treated by transplantation, provided sufficient immunosuppressive treatment is given to the recipient[61].

COMPLICATIONS OF ALLOGENEIC TRANSPLANTATION

Patients who do not survive transplantation usually die as a result of one of the immunobiological complications of the procedure itself, even when technically the underlying disease has been corrected. As previously discussed, the prospects of recurrent disease vary with the disease involved and its stage when the transplant was carried out. The major reasons for failure are:

(a) Graft-versus-host disease (GVHD),

(b) Pneumonitis, and

(c) The consequences of immunosuppression.

In practice these problems are often interrelated and it may be a matter of opinion as to which was the major component in a fatal outcome. There is in addition a proportion of patients who become long-term survivors, but who may for a period of time suffer considerable morbidity related to these problems. Much of the current development of clinical bone marrow transplantation is directed at eliminating these complications.

Graft-versus-host disease

Graft-versus-host disease (GVHD) is a major reason for failure following allogeneic transplantation, occurring to some extent in almost half of all cases, despite HLA-identity at A, B, D and DR loci and non-reactivity in mixed lymphocyte reaction. It takes two forms which can usually be distinguished clinically and histologically – acute and chronic. More general application of allograft will depend on the development of effective means of its prevention and treatment. Initial clinical studies have indicated that the severity of acute GVHD increases with age, such that most units have limited allografts to patients under forty years old.

Although most tissues express the histocompatibility antigens, acute GVHD generally restricts its clinical manifestation to skin, liver and gastrointestinal tract – usually in that order of clinical progression. The rash is typically maculopapular and sometimes difficult to distinguish from other causes – particularly a drug rash. Histological changes are described but these are difficult to distinguish from radiation changes in the early post-transplant period. Provided that the area of skin involved is small, treatment is usually not necessary but extensive involvement can result in desquamation with infective risks. In most cases a clinical response can be obtained with steroids. Liver involvement is usually manifest by bilirubin and enzyme rise, with progression to an obstructive pattern. There are usually several other possible causes of hepatic dysfunction, e.g. infection, drugs, veno-occlusive disease and parenteral nutrition: it is difficult to be confident of the cause even in the presence of a typical rash. Diarrhoea, often associated with abdominal pain, is the typical manifestation of gut involvement. In its severe form it is extremely difficult to keep up with fluid losses.

The more generalized the involvement with acute GVHD the poorer the prognosis. A clinical stage I–IV can be useful in describing the extent of the disease. Where the disease is limited to skin (stage I) or skin and mild liver involvement (stage II), steroid or antilymphocyte globulin[62] can result in a satisfactory response, but more severe involvement of liver or gut (stages III and IV) seldom responds to treatment. Overall, acute GVHD will be the main cause of death in 5–10% of transplants but, in addition, it makes a major contribution to the development of opportunistic infection which may be the principal cause of death. Even patients who develop acute GVHD and respond to treatment have reduced performance status for several weeks. Once the patient reaches the 60–70th day post-transplant the development of acute GVHD is unlikely.

Since the treatment of GVHD is unsatisfactory, most efforts have been directed at prophylaxis. Most of the initial clinical studies adopted the Seattle protocol of intermittent doses of methotrexate in the first 100 days post-graft. Such an approach was effective in the canine model but its benefits in man are less certain. Some initial reports suggested that cyclosporin A post-transplant reduced the severity of GVHD[63], and this drug gained a place in clinical practice without a great deal of evidence to suggest that it improved survival. Indeed, such comparative studies of cyclosporin and methotrexate as have been performed show no survival advantage for either group[64].

The clinical need to make allogeneic transplantation safer, to increase its application to older patients, and perhaps to transgress the strict HLA criteria to widen the donor pool give considerable incentive to the development of effective GVHD prophylaxis. The syndrome is due to immunocompetent T cells in the infused marrow. Much optimism is currently centred around techniques that selectively remove T cells in vitro by the use of monoclonal antibodies[65]. The initial clinical experience suggests that such an approach can prevent significant acute GVHD. If the risks of CMV pneumonitis and other infective complications are also reduced, this would be an important step forward. An undesirable result of such an approach has been the tendency, even in fully HLA-matched pairs, for grafts either not to take or

181

to be rejected. This rarely occurs when no *in vitro* manipulation of the marrow is performed. There is some experimental evidence to suggest that more intensive conditioning of the recipient is required to achieve consistent engraftment with T-depleted bone marrow.

A further potential disadvantage of such an approach may be loss of a theoretical graft-verus-leukaemia effect. Such an effect can be demonstrated in experimental leukaemia models[16], and is cited as the reason for the increased relapse rates in syngeneic transplants[66]. Statistical evidence has been presented to indicate a correlation between the risk of relapse and the severity of graft-versus-host disease – but such a relationship has not been demonstrated for AML transplanted in remission[67]. There is as yet no evidence to suggest an increased relapse rate in recipients of T cell-depleted marrow.

Chronic GVHD is of later onset – the risk period being from 2–15 months post-transplant. It occurs to some extent in about one third of patients and has certain well-recognized clinical manifestations in skin and buccal mucosa (most commonly a lichenoid reaction), liver, eyes, joints and rarely muscles, leading it to be compared with connective tissue diseases such as systemic lupus erythematosis, scleroderma, Sjogren's syndrome and primary biliary cirrhosis[68]. In chronic GVHD, however, there is no renal or oesophageal involvement, as forms part of lupus or scleroderma. The classic manifestations are not difficult to diagnose and skin or buccal mucosa biopsy is very useful, but there are some patients who probably have low-grade disease resulting in failure to thrive and in whom the diagnosis is more obscure. The mechanism of chronic GVHD is still poorly understood but certain immune characteristics are regularly found. Most patients have antibody and complement component deposition on skin basement membrane[69]. Non-specific suppressor T cell activity is usually demonstrable[70].

Apart from patient age as previously mentioned, administration of donor buffy coat increases the incidence of GVHD. The outcome is better for patients with disease limited to skin and probably liver, and worse for more general organ involvement. Most patients will have had preceding acute GVHD. The prognosis for patients in whom acute GVHD is successfully curtailed but who later develop chronic GVHD is better than for those who progress into chronic disease: in these latter cases it is frequently difficult to distinguish acute from chronic disease. A small proportion of cases (20%) arise *de novo* without previous acute GVHD, and this subgroup is the most responsive of all.

There is some controversy as to whether prednisolone given for several months post-graft can reduce the frequency of chronic GVHD, but there seems little doubt that immunosuppressive treatment with prednisolone and azathioprine is the treatment of choice – although this usually needs to be continued for several months[71]. Chronic GVHD can be a persistent and troublesome later complication of transplantation. Its main life-threatening implication is its own inherent immunosuppressive effect, compounded by immunosuppressive therapy. In particular these patients are at risk from zoster and pneumococcal infections, and it is important to re-introduce prophylactic penicillin or co-trimoxazole as part of the treatment.

182

Pneumonitis

Pneumonitis is one of the major threats to a patient in the first four months after transplantation. The incidence varies from centre to centre, but in major series is between 25–50%: 60–70% of these infections are fatal, giving an overall risk of death of 15–30%. Such incidents are very difficult to treat and responses to various forms of intervention are disappointing. If the patient's respiratory function deteriorates to the extent of requiring assisted ventilation the prognosis is particularly poor. The precise reasons for pneumonitis are not fully understood but information collected from large series of cases (International Bone Marrow Transplant Registry, IBMTR[72]; Seattle Transplant Group[73]; European Collaborative Group for Bone Marrow Transplantation, EBMT[74]) has delineated associated factors which appear to correlate with increased risk. In general terms, pneumonitis is either idiopathic or infective in origin, and the risk factors operate to a variable extent within this broad aetiological subdivision.

Idiopathic pneumonitis

About a third of all cases of pneumonitis are classified as idiopathic, of which two thirds are fatal. Provided adequate investigation to exclude other causes has been undertaken, the available evidence suggests that the preparative chemo-radiotherapy which the patient receives is of importance in causing the condition.

There appears to be little relationship with either patient age or disease status at the time of transplantation. However, the incidence in aplastic anaemia is relatively low (< 10%), probably because these patients do not normally receive irradiation as part of the conditioning. A less important factor may be that aplastic patients will not have had previous chemotherapy, which can be shown to produce subclinical damage to the lungs. In aplastic patients who receive a modified irradiation regimen with or without additional immunosuppressive agents, the incidence is around 25%.

There are considerable differences between centres in radiation technique. While other factors will also vary, two factors emerge as particularly important, and these are predictable on radiobiological principles:

(a) Total dose to the lungs, and

(b) Dose rate[75].

Provided the absorbed lung dose is not greater than 800 cGy the incidence of idiopathic pneumonitis will be low. The dose response curve between 800–1000 cGy to the lung is steep and most protocols are careful to limit the lung dose. Fractionation of the radiation (say 6 × 200 cGy) or single fraction to 1000 cGy at a low dose rate (less than 5 cGy/min), which is probably equivalent in radiobiological terms to hypofractionation, appears to be associated with a reduced incidence of idiopathic pneumonitis.

Idiopathic pneumonitis is essentially a diagnosis of exclusion and as such it is essential that adequate diagnostic efforts are made. The 'gold standard' in this respect is lung biopsy but broncho-alveolar lavage (BAL) has more recently been accepted as adequate for patients too ill or thrombocytopenic for biopsy to be undertaken[76]. Failure to demonstrate a causative agent by invasive techniques has raised the question of occult infective causes, due to more exotic organisms. In a study specifically designed to examine this possibility, 147 cases were carefully examined and only four revealed additional information – all due to chlamydia infections[77]. Similarly, indirect approaches such as serological demonstration of antigen (*Pneumocystis carinii*)[78] or detection of cytomegalovirus RNA by *in situ* hybridization techniques[79] do not show positive results more frequently in patients with biopsy-proven infections than in patients without pneumonia.

Infective pneumonitis

Bacterial pneumonitis is relatively uncommon in the weeks post-transplant (< 5%), particularly in patients nursed in laminar flow. Bacterial pneumonias (particularly pneumococcal) are a major risk associated with the development of chronic graft-versus-host disease. Traditionally the *Pneumocystis carinii* type is the pneumonia associated with severely immunosuppressed patients and historically this was also the case in bone marrow transplantation. However this has been largely eliminated by the prophylactic use of low-dose co-trimoxazole immediately before transplantation and for 4–6 months post-transplant.

Cytomegalovirus is the dominant infective organism in these patients[80]. The death rate in patients in whom it is diagnosed is high (90%) and historically it has been implicated as the cause of death in approximately 15% of all patients undergoing transplantation, accounting for 40–50% of all causes of pneumonitis. The period of maximum risk is 1–6 months post-transplant. There does appear to be an increased risk with age, and acute GVHD is an important predisposing factor. In situations where the recipient is seropositive pre-transplant the incidence is higher (21%) than in seronegative patients (13%). There is a trend towards increased risk with increased conditioning (e.g. aplastic patients treated with cyclophosphamide alone, 10%; leukaemic patients given additional TBI, 17%). In patients who have received methotrexate as post-graft immunosuppression the incidence is increased compared with those receiving cyclosporin. This might in part be explained by the finding that methotrexate has a detrimental effect on the alveolar macrophage for which CMV appears to have a predilection. It is of interest to note that the incidence of CMV pneumonitis has been minimal in syngeneic or autologous transplantation[81].

CMV infection arises because of either reactivation of endogenous virus or primary infection. The most likely sources of primary infection are the blood product support which these patients receive and, perhaps to a lesser extent, the donated marrow when the donor is seropositive. If seronegative status means that reactivation of endogenous virus is not a threat then it would seem logical to use blood products exclusively from seronegative donors. The logistical implications of such a policy are considerable, but in Glasgow where this policy has been in operation for three years no seronegative patient with a seronegative donor has excreted CMV or developed pneumonitis. For seropositive patients problems remain, but results of current studies using prophylactic high-titre anti-CMV immunoglobulin preparations or making prophylactic use of newer anti-viral agents are awaited with interest. Carefully designed radiotherapy technique, seronegative blood product policy, prophylaxis and effective prevention of acute GVHD can be expected to reduce the problems associated with pneumonitis in the next few years.

Immunosuppression

The technique of removing bone marrow from a donor and infusing it into the recipient is simple, but what makes bone marrow transplantation complex is the degree to which these patients are necessarily immunosuppressed. Immunosuppression is the result of the preparative protocol designed to ensure consistent engraftment and, in the case of the leukemias, to eradicate residual bone marrow. Even in straightforward cases, recovery of immune function is slow and may be further delayed by complications or post-graft infection which put the patient at significant risk.

Immune reconstitution

Despite numerical reconstitution of peripheral blood white cells which is achieved in 4–5 weeks post-graft, patients remain immunodeficient for a further 3–6 months period when opportunistic infections of bacterial, fungal or viral natures are common. By one year post-graft, measurable immune function is almost normal. This period of immunodeficiency reflects the time taken for the donor-derived immune system to mature in a balanced fashion, but it will be further prolonged if associated with graft-versus-host disease or its treatment. Several studies now indicate that repopulation of peripheral blood by T and B cells takes 3–4 months[82,83]. T cell subpopulations regenerate at different rates resulting in an imbalance. Cells with the OKT_8 phenotype recover earlier with an absolute increase in number, whereas OKT_4 cells recover more slowly. Thus during the first year the helper (OKT_4) to suppressor (OKT_8) ratio is abnormal, but it returns to normal by the end of that year. An increase in immature T cells (OKT_{10}) phenotype has been reported in the early months post-transplant, but this population falls to normal levels by 9–12 months[84].

Humoral immunity also returns at a variable rate. IgG and IgM levels are usually normal by four months but IgA remains subnormal for at least 12 months. the ability to produce an antibody response with IgM and then IgG is demonstrable at 3–4 months[85]. Cellular immunity, as measured by delayed-type hypersensitivity skin testing, may be subnormal for two years, and response to recall antigen for up to four years post-transplant.

The imbalance of T cell subsets found after BMT was initially postulated to be related to development of graft-versus-host disease, but both the pattern and pace of immune reconstitution are similar in syngeneic and autologous transplantation[86]. GVHD retards recovery of the immune system[87]. The T cell subset imbalance persists and antibody responses are subnormal with limited ability to switch from IgM to an IgG response[88]. Response to pneumococcal antibody is poor and perhaps explains the increased incidence of fatal pneumococcal infections associated with chronic GVHD in the first two years post-transplant.

The pattern of immune recovery does not appear to be substantially different in patients receiving methotrexate or cyclosporin as GVHD prophylaxis[89]. One of the hopes of T cell depletion from the graft, as a method of GVHD prevention, is that immune recovery may be more rapid and occur in a more balanced way, perhaps reducing the dangers of opportunistic infections.

Infectious complications

The pattern of infection following transplantation is related to the reconstitution of the immune system and certain pretransplant characteristics of the patient. These patients are prone to the complete spectrum of pathogenic and opportunistic infections[90]. Gram negative and positive infections are most likely to occur in the early neutropenic phase and the clinical consequences and treatment strategies for these infections are well known to physicians treating immunosuppressed patients. The pattern of bacterial frequency and sensitivity to antibiotics usually varies between institutions.

The standard practice in bone marrow transplant patients is to have an indwelling catheter (Hickman or Broviac) to facilitate sample collection and intravenous medication. This has resulted in frequent infections with *Staphylococcus epidermidis* which is often quite resistant to antibiotics but fortunately does not result in rapid clinical deterioration of the patient. As previously implied, late infections with pneumococcus are well recognized and require vigilance: the use of pneumococcal vaccine has not been scientifically assessed but would seem a rational approach for patients with restored humoral immunity. An advantage of the current practice of transplantation in remission is that patients retain some neutrophils for the first few days after transplantation. Most patients become febrile within the first 10–14 days. The yield of positive bacteriology during these episodes is low but most patients will receive empirical broad spectrum intravenous antibiotics. Within a few days the pyrexia resolves, usually as the neutrophils reappear. Since the patients are in remission there is less likelihood of their being infected pretransplant. However, if they are infected, delaying the transplant reduces the chance of clinical deterioration. In some circumstances such as aplastic anaemia deciding to delay might be difficult, but pretransplant infection is an important prognostic factor in this group of patients[91].

Fungal infections are mainly due to candida or aspergillosis and are also probably less of a problem in good risk patients who engraft promptly. Premortem diagnosis of candidal infections tends to indicate extensive infection probably beyond the capacity of antifungal therapy. There may be a role for earlier use of antifungal therapy, either almost empirically in neutropenic patients who are unresponsive to broad-spectrum antibiotic treatment, or in patients who have evidence of candidal colonisation[92].

Of the important viral infections, cytomegalovirus has already been discussed in relation to pneumonitis. Herpes simplex (type I) infection of the oropharynx and rarely of the lung or genitals is common in the first two weeks post-transplant. Patients who have had previous infections or are seropositive have a high probability of reactivating the infection[12]. These infections are seldom life-threatening but may have a major impact on patient well-being, and on compliance with oral medication or nutrition. Acyclovir is effective not only prophylactically in these patients[13,14] but also in established infections when measured by pain reduction, healing and viral shedding[93]. There is some indication that its use prevents prolongation of neutropenia.

Late infection with varicella zoster remains a threat for several months reflecting the prolonged immunosuppression. These infections are similarly amenable if treated promptly.

LATE SEQUELAE OF TRANSPLANTATION

Apart from disease recurrence and the immunobiological complications already discussed, attention must also be directed to other late effects which may be preventable by treatment modification or about which patients should be informed.

Pulmonary function

Routine monitoring of pulmonary function tests has shown that in addition to overt clinical problems – such as pneumonitis – restrictive or obstructive abnormalities can be detected[94,95]. Our own experience is that similar reductions of diffusion capacity and vital capacity occur in autologous grafts implying that such damage is directly related to the conditioning with cyclophosphamide and TBI. Many of these patients are asymptomatic. Not unexpectedly the more pronounced measurable defects were noted in patients with previous pneumonitis. In general terms restrictive changes did not progress but in some cases obstructive manifestations increased.

Cataracts

In their observation of 277 patients who received differing conditioning protocols, the Seattle group noted 86 posterior capsule cataracts occurring from one year post-transplant[96]. It has been projected that 80% of cases receiving TBI as a single fraction would go on to develop cataract, whereas the projected risk in patients receiving a fractionated approach is 19%. Other contributory factors such as drug treatment were not elucidated.

Endocrine dysfunction

Endocrine insufficiencies are known to occur in patients receiving conventional chemotherapy or radiotherapy and, although only a small number of studies have been undertaken, it is not surprising to find deficiencies after cyclophosphamide, TBI and allograft[97]. Both cyclophosphamide and TBI affect gonadal function and fertility. In the Seattle experience of aplastic anaemia (cyclophosphamide alone), prepubertal children of both sexes

187

reached puberty at the expected time with normal gonadotrophin levels. In adult females menstrual cycles returned about six months post-transplant, with normal gonadotrophin levels in those patients under 26 years old. Older women had an early menopause with elevated levels of luteinizing and follicle-stimulating hormones. In excess of 60% of males, normal gonado-trophin levels and sperm counts returned – although subnormal counts were detected in some patients. The remaining patients remained azoospermic with increased follicle-stimulating and luteinizing hormone levels.

More profound and permanent changes have been observed in leukaemic patients given additional TBI[96]. All prepubertal females had primary ovarian failure, no menstrual periods and absence of secondary sexual characteristics. In prepubertal boys a third have developed secondary sexual characteristics at the appropriate time but two thirds have experienced delayed development. In post-pubertal females ovarian failure was the rule and half the patients had menopausal symptoms. Only two patients regained fertility at three and six years post-transplant and became pregnant. Similarly azoospermia with primary gonadal failure is the rule in post-pubertal males although two out of 41 recovered spermatogenesis about six years post-graft.

It has recently been our practice to offer sperm bank storage facilities to patients about to undergo allograft or autograft. Previous chemotherapy may of course, itself have induced oligospermia.

Growth curves in children given cyclophosphamide alone do not deviate from normal, but the addition of TBI appears to decrease growth rate although bone age is equivalent to chronological age. About one third of children have subnormal growth hormone levels. Growth hormone supplementation could be considered if these studies are corroborated.

Second malignancy

Anxiety exists that some patients successfully treated by bone marrow transplantation may be at higher risk of developing malignancy some years later. The basis of this anxiety is the experimental data from dogs[98] and rhesus monkeys[99] on which radiation has been used: the data indicate the risk to be about five times that of controls. Seventeen cases of second neoplasms have been reported in humans[96]. Although several hundred bone marrow transplants have been performed, the precise incidence of neoplasia is not known. All of the reported cases have been patients who had leukaemia. In five cases leukaemia recurred in donor cells, for which phenomenon a number of explanations are possible; seven patients developed lymphomas, and five a variety of solid tumours. No second malignancy has yet been documented in patients transplanted for non-malignant disease prepared with chemotherapy.

AUTOLOGOUS BONE MARROW TRANSPLANTATION

In recent years there has been renewed interest in the therapeutic possibilities of autologous bone marrow transplantation (ABMT) in certain haemato-logical or solid tumours. The safe removal, storage and auto-administration of bone marrow creates a 'therapeutic window' during which escalated doses of chemotherapy or radiotherapy can be given without regard to the limits normally imposed by myelotoxicity. It is now well established that marrow can be safely stored, either short-term in liquid phase[100] or long-term in liquid nitrogen[101], and retain sufficient repopulative potential. Many clinical studies are underway in solid tumours where improved responses have been reported, but little evidence is yet available to demonstrate improved survival. In some respects such studies are somewhat speculative in that there is little evidence to indicate that cure may be possible. One of the areas of most activity now is in the use of ABMT in haematological neoplasms. This is a paradox in that it is questionable if the bone marrow in such conditions is free of residual disease. In acute leukaemia, however, the incentive to explore this field is the excellent antileukaemic effect demonstrated by the ablative preparative protocols employed in allogeneic transplantation.

Syngeneic transplantation has been associated with reduced mortality from pneumonitis and immunosuppression, and completely avoids the problem of graft-versus-host disease[102] – so it is a reasonable assumption that autograft using a similar ablative approach would result in acceptable toxicity. If this proves correct then such an approach might be worthy of investigation in an older group of patients who would not be offered allografts, as well as in those for whom no donor could be found. The arguments against autograft are that there would be the loss of a possible antileukaemic effect of the allogeneic graft, and that the reinfused remission marrow is likely to be contaminated by residual disease.

The early allogeneic clinical studies were partly based on the hope that the new marrow would exert immunological control over any residual disease which remained in the host after ablative treatment. There was such a demonstrable effect in rodent models[16]. The subsequent clinical evidence for such an effect has been indirect. Statistical evidence has been produced to show an inverse relationship between the severity of graft-versus-host disease and the probability of relapse[67]. But this relationship was only demonstrated for ALL in relapse and remission, or AML in relapse, but not for AML in remission. There is some evidence to suggest, however, that patients with AML who develop chronic GVHD have a reduced chance of relapse. Syngeneic transplant results in patients with AML in remission have been associated with twice the relapse rate seen in allograft – it would therefore be expected that relapse would occur in half the recipients of an autograft. If such an approach was not associated with any procedural mortality this would represent a major improvement for a substantial proportion of patients. Should reinfusion of residual clonogenic cells be a major factor, a relapse rate in excess of 50% would be expected.

Recently attention has been given to the development of techniques capable of removing residual disease from the bone marrow *in vitro*[103]. Monoclonal antibodies make such a prospect a practical proposition, assuming that the leukaemia-specific antigen is on the clonogenic leukaemic cell. Such an assumption may, however, be incorrect as antigenic differences between leukaemic blast cells and clonogenic cells have recently been demonstrated[104]. As no specific antibody is yet available in AML, alternative pharmacological methods have been devised[105]. While monoclonal antibodies may make 'cleansing' of the bone marrow possible in ALL, allogeneic experience indicates that recurrence of disease in the patient remains the major problem.

Clinical results of autologous transplantation in acute leukaemias are emerging. In poor-prognosis ALL (i.e. second or greater remission) using cleansing techniques, the major problem as predicted has been failure to eradicate disease in the patient[106,107]. In AML, either in relapse or in second remission (by which time the disease is usually resistant to conventional chemotherapy) results have been poor – as has been the experience in allograft[108]. In first remission – even where no effort has been made to remove residual disease from the graft – results from a number of groups are encouraging, with approximately half the patients remaining in remission at three years and procedural-related morbidity and mortality being low[109,110].

PROSPECTS FOR BONE MARROW TRANSPLANTATION

Enormous change has taken place in the clinical application of BMT in the last decade with several centres now established worldwide. There will be continued rapid change in several directions. The major life-threatening complications common to all forms of transplantation are well known, and most centres have in hand improved protocols which should improve survival. Greater attention to radio-therapeutic techniques, particularly fractionation and accurate dosimetry, should reduce the undesired effects of radiation on the lung without reducing antileukaemic effect. CMV pneumonitis has been a major problem but blood product policy (CMV negative donors), high-titre immunoglobulin, or new antiviral agents given prophylactically may well reduce this risk: in established cases early diagnosis and effective treatment may slowly reduce the high mortality.

Techniques of T cell depletion *in vitro* appear effective in reducing acute GVHD, with the potentially important subsidiary effects of curtailing the degree of immunosuppression given directly, or resulting from GVHD, or arising through interventional or prophylactic treatment of GVHD. T cell depletion has not been without its problems in the fully matched situation: a few graft failures have occurred, but suitable modification of the conditioning protocol may be sufficient to avoid this. There is some anxiety that reduction of GVHD, with its postulated antileukaemic effect, may result in more relapses but so far there is not enough information to assess this point. It may be that this allogeneic effect is not exclusively associated with clinical GVHD.

The antileukaemic effect of allograft is substantially better than alternative treatments, but it is possible that the conditioning normally used – cyclophosphamide and TBI – could be improved. Although higher doses of TBI have been assessed in small numbers of high-risk relapsed cases with no apparent benefit[64], there may be an enhanced effect in remission. Similarly, alternatives to cyclophosphamide[111] and irradiation[112] have resulted in lower relapse rates. In general, experience has been that results improve when the transplant is performed earlier in the natural history of the disease. It remains to be established that ALL patients deemed to be poor risks for chemotherapy are better risks for transplant. Relapse remains a serious problem in ALL, and various additional cytoreductive protocols are under evaluation but with little preliminary information available. In the meantime improvements in conventional chemotherapy can be expected.

With improved technique allograft will become safer and therefore an attractive approach for other diseases such as myeloma or certain lymphomas. Because the natural history of these diseases is so variable, transplantation will take a number of years to prove itself in these conditions.

Currently BMT is restricted to a small proportion of younger patients. Increased safety will permit inclusion of some older patients, but a more general application will depend on availability of donors. It is unclear which approach to this problem will be most fruitful. Accepting donors who are not fully HLA-matched remains beset by problems. Present results indicate that such an approach remains a major challenge[113,114]. Phenotypically but not genotypically matched donors (unrelated donor panels) represent a major logistical exercise, but there is strong incentive to pursue such an approach particularly where no alternative treatment is available (e.g. in CML and severe aplastic anaemia).

Despite the conceptual disadvantages associated with autologous transplantation, the initial results are encouraging. In view of the apparent safety of this approach – and its safe use in older patients – it may have a major impact on a high proportion of patients suffering from acute leukaemia. The future may see autograft as the vehicle for gene therapy to correct these diseases.

References

1. Jacobson, L. O. (1952). Evidence for a humoral factor (or factors) concerned in recovery from radiation injury: a review. *Cancer Res.*, **12**, 315–25
2. Jacobson, L. O., Marks, E. K. and Robson, M. J. (1949). Effect of spleen protection on mortality following X-radiation. *J. Lab. Clin. Med.*, **34**, 1538–43
3. Jacobson, L. O., Simmons, E. L., Marks, E. K. and Eldredge, J. H. (1951). Recovery from radiation injury. *Science*, **113**, 510–11
4. Lorenz, E. and Congdon, C. C. (1954). Modification of lethal irradiation injury in mice by infection of homologous and heterologous bone marrow. *J. Natl. Cancer Inst.*, **14**, 955–61
5. Till, J. E. and McCulloch, E. A. (1980). Hemopoietic stem cell differentiation. *Biochim. Biophys. Acta*, **605**, 431–59
6. Ebell, W., Castro-Malaspina, H., Moore, M. A. S. and O'Reilly, R. J. (1985). Depletion of stromal cell elements in human marrow grafts separated by soybean agglutinin. *Blood*, **65**, 1105–11
7. de Vries, E. G. E., de Meinesz, A. F., Daener, S., Mulder, W. H., Postmus, P. E., Sleijfer, D. T. and Vriesendorp, R. (1984). Bone marrow harvest without general anaesthesia for autologous bone marrow transplantation. In McVie, J. G., Dalesio, O. and Smith, I. E. (eds.) *Autologous Bone Marrow Transplantation and Solid Tumours.* pp. 1–3 (New York: Raven Press)
8. Bortin, M. M. and Buckner, C. D. (1983). Major complications of marrow harvesting for transplantation. *Exp. Hematol.*, **11**, 916–21

191

9. Serota, F. T., Burkey, E. D., August, C. S. and D'Angio, G. J. (1983). Total body irradiation in preparation for bone marrow transplantation in treatment of acute leukemia and aplastic anaemia. *Inst. J. Radiation Oncol. Biol. Phys.*, **9**, 1941–9

10. Thomas, E. D., Storb, R. and Buckner, C. D. (1976). Total body irradiation in preparation for marrow engraftment. *Transplant. Proc.*, **8**, 591–3

11. Storb, R., Prentice, R. L., Buckner, C. D., Clift, R. A., Appelbaum, F., Degg, J., Doney, K., Hansen, J., Mason, M., Sanders, J. E., Singer, J., Sullivan, K., Witherspoon, R. and Thomas E. D. (1983). Graft-versus-host disease and survival in patients with aplastic anaemia treated by marrow grafts from HLA-identical siblings. Beneficial effect of a protective environment. *N. Engl. J. Med.*, **308**, 302–7

12. Meyers, J. D., Flournoy, N. and Thomas, E. D. (1980). Infection with herpes simplex virus and cell mediated immunity after transplant. *J. Inf. Dis.*, **142**, 338-46

13. Saral, R., Burns, W. H., Lastin, O. L., Santos, G. W. and Liekman, P. S. (1981). Acyclovir prophylaxis of herpes simplex infection – a randomised double-blind controlled trial in bone marrow transplant recipients. *N. Engl. J. Med.*, **305**, 63–7

14. Hann, I. M., Prentice, H. G., Blacklock, H. A., Ross, M., Brigden, D., Clark, A., Burke, C., Noon, P. and Keaney, M. (1982). Acyclovir prophylaxis of herpes virus infections in severely immuno-suppressed patients. A randomised double-blind controlled trial. *Exp. Hematol.*, **10 (10)**, 2–4

15. Whitmore, G. F. and Till, J. E. (1964). Quantitation of cellular radiobiological responses. *Ann. Rev. Nucl. Sci.*, **14**, 347–74

16. Boranic, M. (1971). Time pattern of anti-leukaemic effect of graft-versus-host reaction in mice. *J. Natl. Cancer Inst.*, **4**, 421–32

17. Thomas, E. D., Buckner, C. D., Banajii, M., Clift, R. A., Fefer, A., Flournoy, N., Goodell, B. W., Hickman, R. O., Lerner, K. G., Neiman, P. E., Sale, G. E., Sanders, J. E., Singer, J., Stevens, M., Storb, R. and Weiden, P. L. (1977). One hundred patients with acute leukaemia treated by chemotherapy, total body irradiation and allogeneic marrow transplantation. *Blood*, **49**, 511–33

18. Rees, J. K. H., Gray, R. and Hayhoe, F. G. J. (1985). Late intensification therapy in the treatment of acute myeloid leukaemia. (Abstract). *Proc. Soc. Clin. Oncol.*, **C621**

19. Preisler, H. D., Rustum, Y., Henderson, E. S., Bjornsson, S., Creaven, P. J., Highby, D., Freeman, A., Gailoni, S. and Nasher, C. (1979). Treatment of acute non-lymphocytic leukaemia: use of anthracyclin cytosine arabinoside induction therapy and comparison of two maintenance regimens. *Blood*, **53**, 455–64

20. Gale, F. R., Foon, K. A., Cline, M. J. and Zighelboim, J. (1981). Intensive chemotherapy for acute myelogenous leukaemia. *Ann. Intern. Med.*, **94**, 753–7

21. Weinstein, H. J., Mayer, R. J., Rosenthal, D. S., Coral, F. S., Camitta, B. M. and Gelber, R. D. (1983). Chemotherapy for acute myelogenous leukaemia in children and adults: VAPA update. *Blood*, **62**, 315–9

22. Mayer, R. J., Weinstein, H. J., Coral, F. S., Rosenthal, D. S. and Frei, E. (1982). The role of intensive post-induction chemotherapy in the management of patients with acute myelogenous leukaemia. *Cancer Treatment Reports*, **66**, 1455–62

23. Creutziq, U., Ritter, J., Riehan, H. Langermann H-J., Henze, G., Kalason, H., Niethammer, D., Jurgens, H., Stollman, B., Lasson, U., Kaufmann, U., Loffler, H. and Schellozng, G. (1985). Improved treatment results in childhood acute myelogenous leukaemia: a report of the German Co-operativey Study AML-BFM-78. *Blood*, **65**, 298–304

24. Thomas, E. D., Buckner, C. D., Clift, R. A., Fefer, A., Johnson, F. L., Neiman, P. E., Sale, G. E., Sanders, J. E., Singer, J. W., Shulman, H., Storb, R. and Weiden, P. L. (1979). Marrow transplantation for acute non-lymphoblastic leukaemia in first remission. *N. Engl. J. Med.*, **301**, 597–9

25. Powles, R. L., Morgenstern, G., Clink, H. M., Hedley, D., Bandini, G., Lumley, H., Watson, J. G., Lawson, D., Spence, D., Barrett, A., Jameson, B., Lawler, S., Kay, H. E. M. and McElwain, T. J. (1980). Bone marrow ablation and allogeneic marrow transplantation in acute leukaemia. *Lancet*, **1**, 1047–50

26. Blume, K. G., Beutler, E., Bross, K. J., Chillar, R. K., Ellington, O. B., Fahey, J. L., Farbstein, M. J., Forman, S. J., Schmidt, G. M., Scott, E. P., Spruce, W. D., Turner, M. A. and Wolf, J. L. (1980). Bone marrow ablation and allogeneic marrow transplantation in acute leukaemia. *N. Engl. J. Med.*, **302**, 1041–6

27. Zwaan, F. E., Hermans, J., Barrett, A. J., Speck, B. (1984). Bone marrow transplantation for acute non-lymphoblastic leukaemia: a survey of the European group for bone marrow transplantation. *Br. J. Haematol.*, **56**, 645–53
28. Sanders, J. E., Hackman, R., Stewart, P. S., Storb, R., Sullivan, K. M., Buckner, C. D., Clift, R. A. and Thomas, E. D. (1983). Allogeneic marrow transplantation for patients with acute non-lymphoblastic leukaemia in second remission. *Leukemia Res.*, **6**, 395–9
29. Appelbaum, F. R., Clift, R. A. Buckner, C. D., Stewart, P., Storb, R., Sullivan, K. M. and Thomas, E. D. (1983). Allogeneic marrow transplantation for acute non-lymphoblastic leukaemia after first relapse. *Blood*, **61**, 949–53
30. Mauer, A. M. (1980). Therapy of acute lymphoblastic leukaemia in childhood. *Blood*, **56**, 1–10
31. Dinsmore, R., Kirkpatrick, D., Flomenberg, N., Gulati, S., Kapoor, N., Shank, B., Reid, A., Groshen, S., O'Reilly, R. J. (1983). Allogeneic bone marrow transplantation for patients with acute lymphoblastic leukaemia. *Blood*, **62**, 381–8
32. Johnson, F. L., Thomas, E. D., Clark, B. S., Chard, R. L., Hartmann, J. R. and Storb, R. (1981). A comparison of marrow transplantation to chemotherapy for children with acute lymphoblastic leukaemia in second or subsequent remission. *N. Engl. J. Med.*, **305**, 846–51
33. Camitta, B. M., Thomas, E. D., Nathan, D. G., Gale, R. P., Kopecky, K., Rappeport, J., Santos, G. E., Gordon-Smith, E. C., Storb, R. (1979). A prospective study of androgens and bone marrow transplantation for treatment of severe aplastic anaemia. *Blood*, **53**, 504–17
34. Storb, R., Thomas, E. D. Buckner, C. D., Clift, R. A., Johnson, F. L., Fefer, A., Glucksberg, H., Giblett, E. R., Lerner, K. G. and Neiman, P. (1974). Allogeneic marrow grafting for treatment of aplastic anaemia. *Blood*, **43**, 157–80
35. UCLA Bone Marrow Transplant Team. (1976). Bone-marrow transplantation in severe aplastic anaemia. *Lancet*, **2**, 921–3
36. Storb, R., Prentice, R. L., Thomas, E. D., Appelbaum, F. R., Deeg, H. J., Doney, K., Fefer, A., Goodell, B. W., Mickelson, E., Stewart, P., Sullivan, K. M. and Witherspoon, R. P. (1983). Factors associated with graft rejection after HLA-identical marrow transplantation for aplastic anaemia. *Br. J. Haematol.*, **55**, 573–85
37. Gale, R. P., Ho, W., Feig, S., Champlin, R., Tesker, A., Arenson, E., Landish, S., Young, L., Winston, D., Sparkes, R., Fitchen, J., Territo, M., Sarna, G., Wong, L., Park, Y., Bryson, Y., Golde, D., Faheyn, J. and Cline, M. (1981). Prevention of graft rejection following bone marrow transplantation. *Blood*, **57**, 9–12
38. Storb, R., Doney, K. C., Thomas, E. D., Appelbaum, F., Buckner, C. D., Clift, R. A., Deeg, H. J., Goodell, B. W., Hackman, R., Hansen, J. A., Sanders, J., Sullivan, K., Weiden, P. L. and Witherspoon, R. P. (1982). Marrow transplantation with or without donor buffy coat cells for 65 transfused aplastic anaemia patients. *Blood*, **59**, 236–46
39. Storb, R., Prentice, R. L., Sullivan, K. M., Shulman, H. M., Deeg, H. J., Doney, K. C., Buckner, C. D., Clift, R. A., Witherspoon, R. P., Appelbaum, F. A., Sanders, J. E., Stewart, P. S. and Thomas, E. D. (1983). Predictive factors in chronic graft-versus-host disease in patients with aplastic anaemia treated by marrow transplantation from HLA-identical siblings. *Ann. Intern. Med.*, **98**, 461–6
40. Devergie, A., Gluckman, E. (1982). Bone marrow transplantation in severe aplastic anaemia following cytoxan and thoraco-abdominal irradiation. *Exp. Hematol.*, **10**, (Suppl.) 10, 17–8
41. Hows, J. M., Palmer, S., Gordon-Smith, E. C. (1982). Use of cyclosporin A in allogeneic bone marrow transplantation for severe aplastic anemia. *Transplantation*, **33**, 382–6
42. Storb, R., Doney, K. (1985). Therapy of severe aplastic anaemia. *Exp. Haematol.*, **13**, (Suppl.), 17, 58–60
43. Storb, R., Prentice, R. L., Buckner, C. D., Clift, R. A., Appelbaum, F., Deeg, J., Doney, K., Hansen, J. A., Mason, M., Sanders, J. E., Singer, J., Sullivan, K. M., Witherspoon, R. P. and Thomas, E. D. (1983). Graft-versus-host disease and survival in patients with aplastic anemia treated by marrow grafts from HLA-identical siblings. Beneficial effect of a protective environment. *N. Engl. J. Med.*, **308**, 302–7
44. Gordon-Smith, E. C., Fairhead, S. M., Chipping, P. M., Hows, J., James, D. C., Dodi, A. and Bachelor, J. R. (1982). Bone-marrow transplantation for severe aplastic anaemia using histocompatible unrelated volunteer donors. *Br. Med. J. (Clin. Res.)*, **285**, 835–7

45. Sokal, J. E. (1976). Evaluation of survival data for chronic myelocytic leukemia. *Am. J. Hematol.*, **1**, 493

46. Wiernik, P. H. (1984). The current status of therapy for and prevention of blast crisis of chronic myelogenous leukemia. *J. Clin. Oncol.*, **2**, 329

47. Priesler, H. D. and Raza, A. (1982). Chronic myelocytic leukemia: comments on new approaches to therapy. *Cancer Treat. Rep.*, **66**, 1073

48. Fefer, A., Cheever, M. A., Greenberg, P. D., Appelbaum, F. R., Boyd, C. N., Buckner, C. D., Kaplan, H. G., Ramberg, R., Sanders, J. E., Storb, R. and Thomas, E. D. (1982). Treatment of chronic granulocytic leukemia with chemoradiotherapy and transplantation of marrow from identical twins. *J. Engl. J. Med.*, **306**, 63

49. Champlin, R., Ho, W., Arenson, E. and Gale, R. P. (1982). Allogeneic bone marrow transplantation in chronic myelogenous leukemia in chronic or accelerated phase. *Blood*, **60**, 1038–41

50. Clift, R. A., Thomas, E. D., Fefer, A., Singer, J., Stewart, P., Deeg, J., Buckner, C. D., Doney, K., Neiman, P. E., Sanders, J., Sullivan, K. M. and Storb, R. (1982). Treatment of chronic granulocytic leukemia in chronic phase by allogeneic marrow transplantation. *Lancet*, **2**, 621–3

51. Speck, B., Bortin, M. M., Champlin, R., Goldman, J. M., Herzig, R., McGlave, P. B., Messner, H. A., Weiner, R. S. and Rimm, A. A. (1984). Allogeneic bone marrow transplantation for chronic myelogenous leukemia. *Lancet*, **1**, 665

52. Bortin, M. M. and Rimm, A. A. (1979). Severe combined immunodeficiency disease. Characterization of the disease and results of transplantation. *J. Am. Med. Assoc.*, **238**, 591–600

53. Kenny, A. B. and Hitzig, W. H. (1979). Bone marrow transplantation for severe combined immune deficiency. *Eur. J. Pediatr.*, **131**, 155–77

54. Reisner, Y., Itsicovitch, L., Meshorer, A., Sharon, N. (1978). Hemopoietic stem cell transplantation using mouse bone marrow and spleen cells fractionated by lectins. *Proc. Natl. Acad. Sci. USA*, **75**, 2933

55. Hobbs, J. R., Hugh-Jones, K., Barrett, A. J., Byrom, N., Chambers, D., Henry, K., James, D. C., Lucas, C. F., Rogers, T. R., Benson, P. F., Tansley, L. R., Patrick, A. D., Mossman, J. and Young, E. P. (1981). Reversal of clinical features of Hurler's disease and biochemical improvement after treatment by bone marrow transplantation. *Lancet*, **1**, 709–12

56. Ginns, E. I., Rappeport, J. M. and Brady, R. O. (1982). Correction of glucocerebrosidase deficiency in Gaucher's disease by bone marrow transplantation. (Abstract). *Blood*, **60**, (Suppl.), 1, 168(a)

57. Rappeport, J. M., Parkman, R., Newburger, P., Camitta, B. M. and Chusid, M. J. (1980). Correction of infantile agranulocytosis (Kostmann's syndrome) by allogeneic bone marrow transplantation. *Am. J. Med.*, **68**, 605–9

58. Coccia, P. F., Krivit, W., Cervenka, J., Clawson, C., Kersey, J., Kim, T., Nesbit, M., Ramsay, N., Warkentin, P., Teitelbaum, S. L., Kahn, A. J. and Brown, D. M. (1980). Successful bone marrow transplantation for infantile malignant osteopetrosis. *N. Engl. J. Med.*, **302**, 701–8

59. Sorell, M., Kapoor, N., Kirkpatrick, D., Rosen, J. F., Chaganti, R. S. K., Lopez, C., Dupont, B., Pollack, M. S., Terrin, B. N., Harris, M. B., Vina, D., Rose, J. S., Goosen, C., Lane, J., Good, R. A., O'Reilly, R. J. (1981). Marrow transplantation for juvenile osteopetrosis. *Am. J. Med.*, **70**, 1280–7

60. Thomas, E. D., Buckner, C. D., Sanders, J. E., Papyannopoulou, T., Pagnatti, C. B., Stephano, P., Sullivan, K., Clift, R. A. and Storb, R. (1982). Marrow transplantation for thalassaemia. *Lancet*, **2**, 227–9

61. August, C. S., Hathaway, W. E. and Githens, J. H. (1973). Improved platelet function following bone marrow transplantation in an infant with the Wiskott–Aldrich syndrome. *J. Pediatr.*, **82**, 58–64

62. Storb, R., Gluckman, E., Thomas, E. D., Buckner, C. D., Clift, R. A., Fefer, A., Glucksberg, H., Graham, T. C., Johnson, F. L., Lerner, K., Neiman, P. and Ochs, H. (1974). Treatment of established human graft-versus-host by anti-thymocyte globulin. *Blood*, **44**, 57–75

63. Powles, R. L., Clink, H. M., Spence, D., Morgenstern, G., Watson, J. G., Selby, P. J., Woods, M., Barrett, A., Jameson, B., Sloane, J., Lawler, S. D., Kay, H. E. M., Lawson, D., McElwain, T. J. and Alexander, P. (1980). Cyclosporin A to prevent graft-versus-host disease in man after allogeneic bone marrow transplantation. *Lancet*, **1**, 327–9

64. Irle, C., Deeg, H. J., Buckner, C. D., Kennedy, M., Clift, R., Storb, R., Appelbaum, F. R., Beatty, P., Bensinger, W., Doney, K., Cheever, M., Fefer, A., Greenbert, P., Hill, R., Martin, P., McGuffin, R., Sanders, J., Stewart, P., Sullivan, K., Witherspoon, R. and Thomas, E. D. (1985). Marrow transplantation for leukemia following fractionated total body irradiation. A comparative trial of methotrexate and cyclosporin. *Leuk. Res.*, **9**, 1255–61

65. Prentice, H. G., Blacklock, H. A., Janossy, G., Gilmore, M. J., Price-Jones, L., Tidman, W., Trejdosiewicz, L. K., Skeggs, D., Parrjwarie, D. and Ball, S. (1984). Depletion of T lymphocytes in donor marrow prevents significant graft-versus-host disease in matched allogeneic leukaemia marrow transplant recipients. *Lancet*, **1**, 472–6

66. Gale, R. P. and Champlin, R. E. (1984). How does bone marrow transplantation cure leukemia? *Lancet*, **2**, 28–30

67. Weiden, P. L., Flournoy, N., Thomas, E. D., Prentice, R., Fefer, A., Buckner, C. D. and Storb, R. (1979). Antileukemic effect of graft-versus-host disease in human recipients of allogeneic-marrow grafts. *N. Engl. J. Med.*, **300**, 1068–73

68. Sullivan, K. M., Shulman, H. M., Storb, R., Weiden, P. L., Witherspoon, R. P., McDonald, G. B., Schubert, M. M., Atkinson, K. and Thomas, E. D. (1981). Chronic graft-versus-host disease in 52 patients: adverse natural course and successful treatment with combination immunosuppression. *Blood*, **57**, 267–76

69. Tsoi, M. S., Storb, R., Jones, E., Weiden, P. L., Shulman, H., Witherspoon, R., Atkinson, K. and Thomas, E. D. (1978). Deposition of IgM and complement at the dermo-epidermal junction in acute and chronic graft-versus-host disease in man. *J. Immunol.*, **120**, 1485–92

70. Reinherz, E. L., Parkman, R., Rappeport, J., Rosen, P. S. and Schlossman, S. F. (1979). Aberrations of suppressor T cells in human graft-versus-host disease. *N. Engl. J. Med.*, **300**, 1061–8

71. Sullivan, K. M., Storb, R. and Flournoy, N. (1982). Preliminary analysis of a randomised trial of immunosuppressive therapy of chronic graft-versus-host disease. *Blood*, **60** (Suppl. 5), 173a (abstract)

72. Bortin, M. M., Kay, H. E. M., Gale, R. P. and Rim, A. A. (1982). Factors associated with interstitial pneumonitis after bone marrow transplantation for acute leukaemia. *Lancet*, **1**, 437–9

73. Buckner, C. D., Meyers, J., Springmeyer, S. C., Sullivan, K. M., Hackman, R. C., Flournoy, N., Clift, R., Storb, R., Witherspoon, R. P., Peterson, F. B. and Thomas, E. D. (1984). Pulmonary complications of marrow transplantation: review of the Seattle Experience. *Exp. Hematol.*, **12** (Suppl. 15), 1–5

74. Barrett, A. (1982). Total body irradiation (TBI) before bone marrow transplantation in leukaemia: a co-operative study from the European Group for Bone Marrow Transplantation. *Br. J. Radiol.*, **55**, 562–7

75. Bortin, M. M., Gale, R. P., Kay, H. E. M. and Rimm, A. A. (1983). Bone marrow transplantation for acute myeloid leukaemia. Factors associated with early mortality. *J. Am. Med. Assoc.*, **249**, 1166–75

76. Leskinen, R., Tukiainen, P., Taskinen, E., Volin, L., Renkonen, R., Ruutin, T. and Hayry, P. (1984). Bronchoalveolar lavage in the diagnosis of pulmonary complications in bone marrow transplant recipients: preliminary experience. *Exp. Hematol.*, **12**, (Suppl. 15), 24–5

77. Meyers, J. D., Hackman, R. C. and Stamm, W. E. (1983). Chlamydia trachomatis infection as a cause of pneumonia after human marrow transplantation. *Transplantation*, **36**, 130–4

78. Meyers, J. D., Pifer, L. L., Sale, G. E. and Thomas, E. D. (1979). The value of Pneumocystis carinii antibody and antigen detection for diagnosis of Pneumocystis carinii pneumonia after marrow transplantation. *Am. Rev. Resp. Dis.*, **120**, 1283

79. Medeiros, E. R., Neiman, P. E., McDougall, J. K. and Thomas, E. D. (1980). Detection of cytomegalovirus RNA in lung tissue from patients with interstitial pneumonia following bone marrow transplantation. (Abstract). *International Conference on Human Herpes Viruses*. Atlanta, GA, March 17–21, 1980

80. Meyers, J. D., Flournoy, N., Wade, J. C., Hackman, R. C., McDougall, J. K., Neiman, P. E. and Thomas, E. D. (1983). Biology of interstitial pneumonia after marrow transplantation. In Gale, R. P. (ed.) *Recent Advances of Bone Marrow Transplantation*, pp. 405–23. (New York: Alan R. Liss)

81. Appelbaum, F. R., Meyers, J. D., Fefer, A., Flournoy, N., Cheever, M. A., Greenberg, P. D., Hackman, R. and Thomas, E. D. (1982). Non-bacterial non-fungal pneumonia following marrow transplantation in 100 identical twins. *Transplantation*, 33, 265–8

82. Atkinson, K., Hansen, J. A., Storb, R., Goehle, S., Goldstein, G. and Thomas, E. D. (1982). T-cell subpopulations identified by monoclonal antibodies after human marrow transplantation. I. Helper–inducer and cytotoxic-suppressor subsets. *Blood*, 59, 1292–8

83. Bacigalupo, A., Mingari, M. C., Moretta, L., van Lint, M. T., Piaggio, G., Raffo, M. R., Poesta, M., Marmont, A. M. (1980). T cell subpopulations after allogeneic bone marrow transplantation. In Thierfelder, S., Todt, H. and Kolb, H. J. (eds.) *Immunobiology of Bone Marrow Transplantation*, pp. 135–140. (Berlin: Springer-Verlag)

84. Forman, S. J., Nocker, P., Gallagher, M., Zaia, J., Wright, G., Bolen, J., Mills, R., Hecht, T. and Blume, K. (1982). Pattern of T cell reconstitution following allogeneic bone marrow transplantation for acute hematological malignancy. *Transplantation*, 34, 96–8

85. Halterman, R. H., Graw, R. G. Jr. and Fuccillo, D. A. (1972). Immunocompetence following allogeneic bone marrow transplantation in man. *Transplantation*, 14, 689–97

86. Singer, C. R. J., Tansey, P. J. and Burnett, A. K. (1982). T lymphocyte reconstitution following autologous bone marrow transplantation. *Clin. Exp. Immunol.*, 51, 455–60

87. Noel, D. R., Witherspoon, R. P., Storb, R., Atkinson, K., Doney, K., Mickelson, E. M., Ochs, H., Warren, R. P., Weiden, P. and Thomas, E. D. (1978). Does graft-versus-host disease influence the tempo of immunologic recovery after allogeneic human marrow transplantation? An observation on 56 long-term survivors. *Blood*, 51, 1087–105

88. Witherspoon, R. P., Storb, R., Ochs, H. D., Flournoy, N., Kopecky, K., Sullivan, K. M., Deeg, H. J., Sosa, R., Noel, D., Atkinson, K. and Thomas, E. D. (1983). Recovery of antibody production in human allogeneic marrow graft recipients: influence of time posttransplantation, the presence or absence of chronic graft-versus-host disease, and antithymocyte globulin treatment. *Blood*, 58, 360–8

89. Witherspoon, R., Lum, L., Storb, R. and Thomas, E. D. (1984). Transplant-related immune deficiency in man. In Gale, R. P. (ed.) *Recent Advances in Bone Marrow Transplantation*. pp. 473–482 (New York: Alan R. Liss)

90. Watson, J. G. (1983). Problems of infection after bone marrow transplantation. *J. Clin. Pathol.*, 36, 683–92

91. Gluckman, E., Barrett, A. J., Arcese, W., Devergie, A. and Degoulet, P. (1981). Bone marrow transplantation in severe aplastic anaemia: a survey of the European Group for Bone Marrow Transplantation (EGBMT). *Br. J. Haematol.*, 49, 165–73

92. Hann, I. M., Prentice, H. G., Corningham, R., Blacklock, H. A., Keaner, M., Shannon, M., Noone, P., Gascoigne, E., Fox, J., Boesen, E., Szawatkowski, M. and Hoffbrand, A. V. (1982). Ketoconazole versus nystatin plus amphotericin B for fungal prophylaxis in severely immunocompromised patients. *Lancet*, 1, 826–9

93. Meyers, J. D., Wade, J. C., Mitchel, C. D., Saral, R., Lietman, P. S., Durack, D. T., Levin, M. J., Segreti, A. C. and Balfour, H. H. (1982). Multicenter collaborative trial of intra-venous acyclovir for the treatment of mucocutaneous herpes simplex virus infection in the immunocompromised host. *Am. J. Med.* (Acyclovir Symposium) 229–35

94. Springmeyer, S. C., Flournoy, N., Sullivan, K. M., Storb, R. and Thomas, E. D. (1983). Pulmonary function changes in long-term survivors of allogeneic marrow transplantation. In Gale, R. P. (ed.) *Recent Advances in Bone Marrow Transplantation*. pp. 343–353 (New York: Alan R. Liss)

95. Depledge, M. H., Barrett, A. and Powles, R. L. (1983). Lung function after marrow grafting. *Int. J. Radiat. Oncol. Biol. Phys.*, 9, 145–51

96. Deeg, H. J., Storb, R. and Thomas, E. D. (1984). Bone marrow transplantation: a review of delayed complications. *Br. J. Haematol.*, 57, 185–208

97. Sanders, J. E., Buckner, C. D., Leonard, J. M., Sullivan, K. M., Witherspoon, R. P., Deeg, H. J., Storb, R. and Thomas, E. D. (1983). Late effects on gonadal function of cyclophosphamide, total body irradiation and marrow transplantation. *Transplantation*, 36, 252–5

98. Deeg, H. J., Prentice, R., Fritz, T. E., Sale, G. E., Lombard, L. S., Thomas, E. D. and Storb, R. (1983). Increased incidence of malignant tumours in dogs after total body irradiation and marrow transplantation. *Int. J. Radiat. Oncol. Biol. Phys.*, 9, 1505–11

99. Broerse, J. J., Hollander, C. F. and van Zwieten, M. J. (1981). Tumour induction in rhesus monkeys after total body irradiation with X-rays and fission neutrons. *Int. J. Radiat. Biol.*, **40**, 671–6

100. Burnett, A. K., Tansey, P., Hills, C., Alcorn, M. J., Sheehan, T., McDonald, G. A. and Banham, S. W. (1983). Haematological reconstitution following high-dose and supralethal chemo-radiotherapy using stored, non-cryopreserved autologous bone marrow. *Br. J. Haematol.*, **54**, 306–16

101. Schaeffer, U. W., Dicke, K. A. (1973). Use of frozen bone marrow cells for restoration of haemopoiesis. (Abstract). *Int. J. Radiat. Biol.*, **23**, 195

102. Fefer, A., Cheever, M. A., Thomas, E. D., Appelbaum, F. R., Buckner, C. D., Clift, R. A., Glucksberg, H., Greenberg, P. D., Johnson, F. L., Kaplan, H. G., Sanders, J. E., Storb, R. and Weiden, P. L. (1981). Bone marrow transplantation for refractory acute leukemia in 34 patients with identical twins. *Blood*, **57**, 421–30

103. Ritz, J., Bast, R. C., Takvorian, T. and Sallan, S. E. (1984). Clinical applications of monoclonal antibodies in acute leukemia. *Ann. NY Acad. Sci.*, **428**, 308–17

104. Sabbath, K. D., Ball, E. D., Larcom, P., Davis, R. B. and Griffin, J. D. (1985). Heterogeneity of clonogenic cells in acute myeloblastic leukaemia. *J. Clin. Invest.*, **75**, 746–53

105. Yeager, A. M., Kaizer, H., Braine, H. G., Colvin, M., Rowley, S., Saral, R. and Santos, G. W. (1985). Autologous bone marrow transplantation (ABMT) in acute leukaemia: phase I and II studies of *ex-vivo* marrow treatment with 4-hydroperoxycyclophosphamide (4HC). *Int. J. Cell Cloning*, **3**, 237–8

106. Anderson, K. C., Sallan, S., Takvorian, T., Bast, R. C. and Ritz, J. (1985). Monoclonal antibody (MA) purged autologous bone marrow transplantation (ABMT) for relapsed non-T acute lymphoblastic leukemia (ALL). *Int. J. Cell Cloning*, **3**, 239–40

107. Ramsay, N. Le Bien, T., Nesbit, M., McGlave, P., Weisdorf, D., Kenyon, P., Hurd, D., Goldman, A., Kimm, T. and Kersey, J. (1985). Autologous bone marrow transplantation for patients with acute lymphoblastic leukemia in second or subsequent remission: results of bone marrow treated with BA-1, BA-2 and BA-3 plus complement. *Blood*, **66**, 508–13

108. Gorin, N. C. (1984). Autologous bone marrow transplantation for acute leukaemia in Europe. *Exp. Hematol.*, **12**, (Suppl. 15), 123–5

109. Burnett, A. K., Tansey, P., Watkins, R., Alcorn, M., Maharaj, D., Singer, C. R. J., McKinnon, S., McDonald, G. A. and Robertson, A. G. (1984). Transplantation of unpurged autologous bone-marrow in acute myeloid leukaemia in first remission. *Lancet*, **2**, 1068–70

110. Gorin, N. C., Herve, P., Aegerter, P., Goldstone, A., Maraninchi, D., Burnett, A., Helbig, W., Meloni, G., Ver Doinck, L. F., Rizzoli, V., Parlier, Y., Auvert, B. and Goldman, J. (1985). Autlogous bone marrow transplantation for acute leukemia in remission. *J. Cell Cloning*, **3**, 248 (Abstract)

111. Goss, G. D., Powles, R. L., Barrett, A., Millar, J., Gore, M., Porta, F., Pimentel, P., Bagnub, S. and Hernandez, F. (1985). Melphalan plus total body irradiation versus cyclophosphamide prior to bone marrow transplantation in acute myeloid leukaemia in first remission. *Exp. Haematol.*, **13**, (Suppl. 17), 12–3

112. Santos, G. W., Tutschka, P., Brookmeyer, R., Saral, R., Beschorner, W. E., Bias, W. B., Braine, H. G., Burns, W. H., Elfenbein, G. J., Kaizer, H. Mellits, D., Sensenbrenner, L. L., Stuart, R. K. and Yeager, A. M. (1983). Marrow transplantation for acute non-lymphocytic leukemia after treatment with bisulphan and cyclophosphamide. *N. Engl. J. Med.*, **309**, 1347–53

113. Powles, R. L., Morgenstern, G. R., Kay, H. E. M. McElwain, T. J., Clink, H. M., Dady, P. J., Barrett, A., Jameson, J., Depledge, M. H., Watson, J. G., Sloane, J., Leigh, M., Lumley, H., Hedley, D., Lawler, S. D., Filshie, J. and Robinson, B. (1983). Mismatched family donors for bone marrow transplantation as treatment for acute leukaemia. *Lancet*, **1**, 612–5

114. Beatty, P. G., Clift, R. A., Mickelson, E. M., Nisperos, B. B., Flournoy, N., Martin, P., Sanders, J. E., Stewart, P., Buckner, C. D., Storb, R., Thomas, E. D. and Hansen, J. A. (1985). Marrow transplantation from related donors other than HLA-identical siblings. *N. Engl. J. Med.*, **313**, 765–71

9
Liver Transplantation

P. McMASTER, R. M. KIRBY AND B. K. GUNSON

INTRODUCTION

There have now been over 1000 liver transplant operations since the first attempt in man in March 1963[1]. Until the late 1970s the procedure was beset by major technical difficulties which frequently led to graft failure and overwhelming infection. Knowledge of the many aspects involved has improved slowly; the graft can now be stored for up to six hours quite safely, the post-operative period is less complicated and a more coordinated evaluation of hepatic function can be made. While it remained true in the early phase that overwhelming hepatic rejection was much less common than had been observed in renal transplantation, the difficulty in the precise diagnosis of hepatic rejection often caused high doses of steroids to be given in the critical post-operative phase. This immunosuppressive approach in the critically ill patient with technical complications meant that the initial results were extremely disappointing, with rates of survival rarely approaching 30% at one year. It was the advent of a more realistic appraisal of patients suitable for transplantation, combined with the introduction of refined technical management, that heralded the new era in transplantation of the liver. Nevertheless, had it not been for improved diagnostic techniques for rejection and the introduction of the non-steroidal immunosuppressive agent cyclosporin A[2], the overall success rates currently being achieved would not have been possible.

In experienced centres over 75% of all children and 55% of adults coming to transplantation will be alive and well at one year[3]. It is the purpose of this review to highlight current approaches to clinical practice and to outline areas of difficulty which are still being experienced.

CURRENT PATIENT SELECTION

While liver replacement might, in theory, be thought possible for any patient with overwhelming hepatic disease or failure, in practice there are increasingly

199

more clearly defined categories of patients. The absolute and relative contra-indications for liver transplantation are set out in Table 9.1. It will be seen that active alcoholic disease, one of the commonest causes of major hepatic disorders, is still considered by most centres to be a relative contraindication to transplantation because of the inevitable difficulties of post-operative management and follow-up control. Nevertheless, an alcoholic who has discontinued drinking for at least two years may well be considered for transplantation.

In clinical practice those coming to liver transplantation fall into the two categories of paediatric and adult patients.

Adult patients

Primary hepatocellular malignancy

Primary hepatocellular malignancy may appear to be the most obvious indication for liver replacement but there are formidable problems associated with the assessment and management of such patients. Although the patients are usually young, i.e. 20–35 years old, the majority of tumours are associated with cirrhosis and the patients may also be hepatitis B antigen positive. The clinician faced with such a patient has not only to ensure that the primary diagnosis is indeed correct rather than the more common secondary hepatic tumour, but also that the disease has extended throughout both lobes of the liver, making a conservative resection impracticable[4]. It is then important to exclude extra-hepatic spread of tumour to ensure that patients are not subjected to the major surgical procedure of hepatic replacement with little realistic hope of rehabilitation. At the present time, even with the help of many investigations such as CAT scanning, ultrasound and laparoscopy, the involvement of lymph nodes adjacent to the liver and coeliac axis can often only be determined at laparotomy. A high incidence of recurrent disease has occurred in patients with positive nodes transplanted for primary liver cancer, and many centres would now question the value of transplantation in this group of patients. Patients with cholangiocarcinoma of the liver are rarely suitable candidates as tumours almost invariably reoccur.

Hepatic cirrhosis

The patient with advanced cirrhosis presents a very different problem. The ideal candidate would be 2–50 years old, be free of active infection, and would not have undergone previous upper abdominal surgery. Previous

Table 9.1 Current absolute and relative contraindications for liver transplantation

Absolute contraindications	Active alcoholism
	Tumour beyond the liver
Relative contraindications	Active sepsis
	Age $>60\,y$
	HB_sAg^+

surgery such as portacaval shunting or splenectomy is a major adverse factor leading to technical problems and bleeding from adhesions at the time of transplantation[5]. Whenever possible these procedures should not be undertaken in patients with advanced cirrhosis, not only because of the poor results but because it may jeopardize the patient's chance of subsequent successful transplantation. It is now often possible to forecast the rate of clinical deterioration in patients with chronic active hepatitis or primary biliary cirrhosis (Table 9.2), although this may be accelerated by active infection or haemorrhage from oesophageal varices. Secondary biliary cirrhosis or sclerosing cholangitis is often associated with active biliary infection and may be further complicated by previous surgery.

Common indications for liver transplantation in adults are set out in Table 9.3. One condition which should not be overlooked is that of the acute Budd–Chiari syndrome, resulting in fulminant deterioration of hepatic function and intractable ascites. While the chronic variant of this disease may allow relatively good health for 1–2 years, the acute fulminant form invariably causes death within 3–4 months and the 'window' for transplantation may therefore be small.

Table 9.2 Features associated with increased risk of death in liver transplantation

↑ Ascites
↑ Biochemistry
Encephalopathy
Recurrent bleeding or infection

Table 9.3 Common indications for liver transplantation in adults

Primary biliary cirrhosis
Chronic active cirrhosis
Sclerosing cholangitis
Budd–Chiari syndrome
Idiopathic cirrhosis

Acute and subacute hepatic failure

In acute hepatic failure events may move quickly with the development of severe coagulopathy, renal failure, increasing cerebral oedema and coma. In spite of prodigious medical efforts, mortality remains high in patients who develop grade IV coma. In the Kings College series of acute hepatic failure consisting of 453 patients, 49% of patients had fulminant failure due to paracetamol overdose, 38% viral hepatitis, 4% halothane and less than 5% were in coma due to hepatic failure produced by other drugs, lymphoma and the Budd–Chiari syndrome[6]. The speed with which clinical events develop, combined with their uncertain prognosis in the initial phase, makes the time available for finding a suitable liver replacement short.

201

The picture in subacute hepatic failure is however somewhat different. Progressive deterioration occurs over a 6–8 week period, often due to toxins or non-A non-B hepatitis. Not only is there time to make a more accurate evaluation and diagnosis, but the window in which liver transplantation may realistically be expected to succeed is greater.

Paediatric indications

Liver transplantation has a high rate of success in children. Inevitably, detailed consideration has been given to the selection of the most suitable cases. Biliary atresia occurs in most western countries and affects approximately 1–2 per 100 000 live births. In over a third of these children, satisfactory biliary drainage can be achieved by one of the reconstructive types of intestinal drainage. However, such procedures need to be performed at under eight weeks of age if longstanding cirrhosis and portal hypertension are to be avoided; even when successful, many children suffer from recurrent cholangitis and infection. When biliary reconstruction is not undertaken early in infancy, or cannot successfully achieve a bile flow of more than 150 mL a day, progressive hepatic cirrhosis and dysfunction occur with death by the age of 2 or 3 years. Such children in many ways represent ideal candidates for liver replacement provided repeated surgical intervention is not undertaken, and transplantation can be avoided during episodes of active infection. The advent of cyclosporin A has meant that many of these children can be treated with low doses of steroids or no steroids at all, thus ensuring that adequate growth and maturation will occur.

In addition to the child with biliary atresia, children with inborn errors of metabolism such as α_1-antitrypsin deficiency, Gaucher's disease, Nieman–Pick and glycogen storage disease type IV, may be suitable for liver replacement. In the children who have developed advanced cirrhosis with portal hypertension it is important to ensure that the portal vein is patent, so that adequate vascular reconstruction is possible.

TECHNICAL ASPECTS

Donor procurement

It is now common practice for multiple organ harvesting to be undertaken so that many kidney donors could also be suitable hepatic donors. The size of the donor liver is important, however, because insertion of an excessively large liver would lead to splinting of the diaphragm and major pulmonary complications. Although a discrepancy of 10–15 kg in overall body weight between recipient and donor produces few problems in adults, there may be major difficulty in finding a suitable organ sufficiently small for implantation in a child. A discrepancy of up to 25% in body weight between recipient and donor may be acceptable. Unfortunately neonatal livers have proved unsuitable for transplantation because of their immaturity and inability to tolerate ischaemia and the procurement procedure.

At present there is no indication that tissue typing plays any role in the outcome of liver grafts. Indeed, there is evidence that livers can be successfully transplanted not just across a positive cytotoxic crossmatch, but also across major ABO blood group incompatibility. While few centres would take this step lightly, there can be no doubt that replacement of the liver by an ABO-incompatible donor in the patient with rapid clinical deterioration offers a reasonable prospect of success[7].

Liver transplantation remains a formidable surgical procedure, frequently undertaken in the critically ill patient at very short notice. Inevitably a coordinated team of surgeons, physicians, nurses and technicians is needed to mount such an operation, and any hospital accepts a considerable responsibility when setting up such a programme. The practical clinical measures relating to liver replacement are detailed below and give a broad indication of the scope and range of problems encountered.

Pre-operative management

Once a patient has been accepted on the 'active' transplant list the only limiting factor is the availability of a suitable liver. Depending on the clinical status, the patient will either need to be supported in hospital with intensive nursing as in the case of acute or chronic liver failure, or may be allowed home.

Once a suitable organ donor is available, the patient is immediately readmitted and medically reassessed to exclude active infection. Pre-operative liver function tests, urea and electrolytes and clotting profile are all repeated, together with a chest X-ray and both sputum and urine specimens for microscopy and culture.

The logistics of liver transplantation are complicated by the need to coordinate a major surgical procedure with the timing and requirements of the donor hospital. Theatre operating time must be coordinated at the two hospitals. Transport has to be arranged for the harvesting team travelling between the hospitals, and the ancillary and biochemical services must be alerted in the transplantation centre. Liver transplantation requires the time and coordinated efforts of haematology departments, blood bank technicians, transfusion services and biochemistry staff. Thirty units of HTLV-screened blood, which are less than 48 h old, are made available along with fresh frozen plasma and platelet concentrates. The premedication includes vitamin K, 10 mg intravenously, amphotericin lozenges orally, nystatin orally and, cefotaxime, 2 g intravenously. Diazepam is given as a sedative.

Donor and recipient operation

A detailed account of the surgical techniques involved in both donor and recipient operation[8] would be inappropriate in this text. Yet the extent and the magnitude of the procedure does need to be highlighted. Harvesting of the donor, normally involving the removal of liver, kidneys and other organs, takes $1\frac{1}{2}$ h. The liver is cooled *in situ* using a hypertonic citrate solution at 4 °C, infused via both the portal vein and the coeliac axis. This perfusion technique leads to a liver which can be adequately stored for 4–6 h and, less predictably, beyond 8 h. Few centres are satisfied with longer ischaemic preservation periods and failure of donated grafts has occurred when there has been inadequate preservation.

The transplant operation begins as soon as the liver has been harvested. In orthotopic liver transplantation the most difficult part of the procedure is the preparation and mobilization of the grossly diseased recipient liver. This liver is frequently shrunken, cirrhotic and associated with dense vascular adhesions made worse by previous upper abdominal surgery. The complete identification of structures in the porta hepatis is essential, with dissection of the hepatic artery, portal vein and common bile duct. During this phase of dissection, as the liver is becoming increasingly ischaemic and therefore less metabolically effective, there may be significant blood loss requiring transfusion. The use of the automated transfusion cell saver apparatus (Haemonetics), ensures that blood lost during this phase can be washed and then returned to the patient in the form of red blood cell concentrates. Such an auto-transfusion apparatus has significant benefit when it is appreciated that blood loss during dissection of the recipient liver is 2–15 L. Transfusion of stored blood, with relatively high potassium and citrate concentrations, can lead to a progressive accumulation of citrate and a fall in ionized calcium levels[9]. While this is partially corrected by the exogenous administration of ionized calcium, the need to re-establish primary hepatic function by implanting the new liver is sometimes paramount.

After this difficult first phase of dissection the venous return to the heart is discontinued by cross-clamping of the inferior vena cava and removal of the diseased liver. The resultant sharp fall in cardiac output and blood pressure may diminish perfusion of vital organs such as the kidneys.

A venous bypass system was used in the early attempts at liver replacement but this was frequently associated with technical problems and thrombosis. The introduction of the Biomedicus centrifugal pump and heparin bonding tubing has meant that bypass from the portal vein and inferior vena cava to the superior vena cava is now possible without heparinization, and most major centres now use this technique. However, control data are not yet available to demonstrate whether this technique results in significant benefit: the one comparison so far showed no significant reduction in mortality at 3 months[10].

Post-operative management

Following surgery, patients are electively ventilated for at least 12 h in an Intensive Therapy Unit (ITU), but isolation or barrier nursing is not usually necessary. In the first few hours following transplantation haemodynamic and biochemical factors may change from one minute to the next and it is therefore essential that there is close monitoring of the patient. Depending on liver function, blood glucose levels are usually elevated in the early stages following transplantation but this rarely requires treatment with insulin. Serum potassium levels may be low as the hepatocytes of the new liver take up potassium. Ionized calcium levels continue to be monitored post-operatively. Blood gases are measured in order to control the necessary inspired oxygen concentrations and the degree of ventilatory support.

Post-operative immunosuppression

Immunosuppression is started within 12 h of transplantation. In adults, once the patient is haemodynamically stable and good renal function has been demonstrated both in terms of urine production and serum biochemistry (stable or decreasing serum urea and creatinine concentrations), treatment with cyclosporin A 5 mg/kg intravenously twice daily and hydrocortisone 100 mg twice daily is commenced. Cyclosporin A is witheld in patients who develop impaired renal function (approximately 20%). If renal impairment continues and acute tubular necrosis (ATN) develops, azathioprine 1.5 mg/kg/day is given. Intravenous cefotaxime is continued for at least 48 h in the absence of infection. The antifungal agents are continued and every patient receives an H_2 blocker (ranitidine in this unit), given intravenously, to protect against stress peptic ulceration.

Oral immunosuppressive agents are introduced as soon as possible: prednisolone 20 mg daily and cyclosporin A 10 mg/kg daily. Some units use higher steroid regimes (prednisolone 200 mg per day reducing by 2.5 mg each 5th day), and azathioprine continues to be used in some programmes.

Cyclosporin A is monitored by measuring whole blood (trough) levels by radioimmunoassay (300–600 ng/mL). Monitoring blood levels has proved important because the reduced clearance of metabolites in hepatic dysfunction increases the risk of nephrotoxicity[11].

Post-operative complications

Major haemorrhage during surgery may continue into the post-operative period and result in an unstable situation with high blood product requirement. Prolonged bleeding may result in hypotension which may lead to hepatic ischaemia and damage.

If major ischaemia occurs, gross biochemical abnormalities (especially marked elevation of aspartate transaminase), coagulation defects and fulminant hepatic failure develop rapidly. Death invariably ensues unless retransplantation is undertaken.

Biliary complications may result from leakage or obstruction to bile flow or by the production of 'sludge' within the bile duct. The latter has been shown to be the result of prolonged cold ischaemia on biliary epithelium causing necrosis and sloughing[12], and is now relatively rare if adequate perfusion of the biliary system has been achieved at the time of harvesting. Bile leaks which were seen so frequently in earlier years are now rarely encountered with meticulous microvascular techniques of biliary reconstruction.

One of the more common complications after liver transplantation is *liver rejection*. Acute rejection is initially suggested by biochemical changes, with elevation of serum bilirubin, liver transaminases and alkaline phosphatatase, although it may also be associated with both pyrexia and tenderness over the liver. Unfortunately the biochemical changes are non-specific and can be caused by hepatic dysfunction induced by other factors such as ischaemia, cytomegalovirus infection or cholangitis: at present the diagnosis of rejection is often initially one of exclusion. Indeed ischaemia, obstruction and also cholangitis often occur at the same time as rejection. The diagnosis of rejection should therefore be confirmed by needle biopsy before steroid treatment is initiated. Histological features indicative of rejection include portal tract inflammatory infiltration with both lymphocytes and polymorph neutrophils, cholestasis, and damage to the small bile ducts[13]. In severe rejection there is hepatocyte damage, areas of infarction and disappearance of bile ducts. Large blood vessels are not usually seen on this type of biopsy, but 'endothelialitis' has been described as an early event in rejection, with complete occlusion in the final stages[14]. The treatment of acute rejection is by increased corticosteroid dosage for three days (either 200 mg prednisolone orally or 1 g methyl prednisolone intravenously), and may need to be repeated. Both anti-thymocyte globulin (ATG) and anti-lymphocyte globulin (ALG) and, more recently, monoclonal antibodies (CAMPATH 1 and OKT3 antibody) have been used to treat acute rejection but no control data are yet available.

Chronic rejection may not respond to steroid therapy and in the past has been a major cause of late death in liver transplant patients. Re-operation and regrafting of these patients is now regarded as being the only realistic treatment, and in the Pittsburg series 25% of liver transplants undertaken are now regrafts[15].

Cholangitis may present in a similar fashion to rejection and whereas increased immunosuppression is the optimal treatment for rejection, it is ideally avoided in the severely infected patient with cholangitis. Bile cultures are therefore necessary before high dose steroids are commenced, even though complete sterility is rare after two weeks with an indwelling biliary T-tube. Most of the organisms cultured are merely colonizing organisms and do not necessarily indicate active infection. When pus cells are present and there is clinical evidence of an ascending cholangitis, the appropriate antibiotics should be administered and the biliary tract drained by allowing the biliary T-tube to drain freely.

Other complications occur following liver transplantation, as in other major abdominal procedures. Right-sided pleural effusions are very common but usually need no treatment; pulmonary collapse and consolidation, although less common, usually require active physiotherapy or occasionally bronchial aspiration. More widespread infections usually occur some weeks after transplantation and are most frequently seen when repeated steroid courses have been given. Infection may be bacterial, viral or fungal although the latter is usually a preterminal event with aspergillosis and candidiasis promoted by the injudicious use of antibiotics. Viral infections may be hepatic as with cytomegalovirus (CMV) hepatitis, or systemic as with herpes simplex infection. Careful viral screening is important and CMV hepatitis may be diagnosed histologically. Recurrent hepatitis resulting in fulminant hepatic failure has been noted on two occasions, and hepatitis B carrier and delta postitive status must now be considered a relative contraindication to liver transplantation.

Renal failure is seen in 20% of liver transplant patients. When it is associated with massive haemorrhage and large transfusion requirements it is a poor prognostic sign: it may, however, simply be an indication of the extent of pre-operative disease, as renal impairment is commonly encountered in the agonal phase of liver failure. Nephrotoxic drugs such as the aminoglycosides and cyclosporin A must be used with care and carefully monitored.

RESULTS

Overall survival has shown a significant improvement (in the major units) since 1980, averaging in excess of 75% one-year graft and patient survival in children, and over 50% in adults. Survival rates depend on not only the proportion of the different diseases requiring surgery but also the proportion of patients with concomitant relative contraindications, such as active infection, previous upper abdominal surgery and major systemic disorders. These patients have a survival rate of less than 40% at one year. Whenever, possible, infection is therefore eradicated before surgery and injudicious surgical intervention, particularly in the upper abdomen, is best avoided in patients with marked impairment in liver function. One of the major advantages of liver transplantation when compared with other forms of transplantation, is that significant morbidity is usually restricted to the first three months after surgery and thereafter most patients grafted for chronic liver disease enjoy excellent rehabilitation for many years. Nearly half of all patients currently transplanted in the Pittsburgh programme are expected to live for more than five years.

Patients transplanted for primary hepatocellular carcinoma, on the other hand, tend to develop recurrences 18 months to two years after transplantation, although patients with the fibrolamellar variant of hepatocellular carcinoma achieve slightly better results[16]. The best survival after transplantation for malignant disease is achieved by those patients undergoing transplantation for cirrhosis in whom an incidental primary hepatocellular carcinoma is found. In these patients no recurrent disease develops (Table 9.4).

Quality of rehabilitation is just as important as survival after such major surgical procedures and clearly children undergo the most successful rehabilitation after transplantation. Nearly 90% of children will be able to go to school and are free of major medical problems, with natural growth and psychological development occuring in the majority. This catch up

Table 9.4 Overall incidence of tumour recurrence following liver transplantation for primary hepatic cancer

Reason for transplantation	Tumour recurrence rate
Hepatocellular carcinoma:	
non-fibrolamellar	82%
fibrolamellar	54%
Cirrhosis + tumour (incidental)	0%
Bile duct cancer	80%

phenomenon, both in growth and maturation, is impressive and even those children who have had to undergo retransplantation because of chronic rejection still achieve excellent rehabilitation with over 50% alive and well at two years[17].

The quality of rehabilitation for adults is also impressive with over 85% of surviving adults returning to occupation or full-time activities and women having normal pregnancies and families. Psychosocial and neuropsychiatric evaluations suggest consistent improvement following hepatic replacement.

The role of liver transplantation in the treatment of subacute hepatic necrosis or acute fulminant hepatic failure has yet to be fully established. The outcome for patients with subacute hepatic necrosis, progressing inexorably over a 6–8 week period, is poor with less than 5% of patients suffering from a non-A non-B hepatitis subacute hepatic failure surviving. Isolated reports are now appearing of patients successfully transplanted in this phase. Because these patients deteriorate rapidly, developing neurological and cerebral signs within a short period, there is only a very small window during which transplantation may be undertaken before irreversible cerebral damage occurs. To date, very few acute fulminant hepatic failures have been transplanted making evaluation of this group difficult.

One other group of patients deserves careful consideration: the young patients with extensive secondary metastatic hepatic disease. Recent studies have shown that conservative resection, when one area of the liver is affected by colorectal metastatic cancer, can result in nearly a third of patients being alive and disease-free at five years[18]. It would therefore be tempting to consider transplantation when both lobes of the liver are involved with secondary metastatic tumour, although initial reports suggest that tumour has often spread beyond these confines.

A small number of patients with secondary metastases due to colorectal cancer have undergone liver replacement. Transplantation has also been performed for other tumour metastases in which the cancer might be considered chemosensitive – breast cancer, testicular tumours, ovarian and small cell bronchial cancer. The Innsbruck group have recently reported their experiences with liver replacement for metastatic disease followed by radical chemotherapy and autologous bone marrow rescue: recurrent disease was common although extended periods of good rehabilitation were achieved. These initial attempts clearly indicate a growing need to evaluate further the role of liver replacement in metastatic disease.

CONCLUSIONS

The first twenty years of liver transplantation were those of major technical struggles in critically ill patients who were then often over-immunosuppressed. Improvements in results followed the development of new techniques and a greater appreciation of the need to reduce immunosuppression in the postoperative period. This was combined with a more realistic evaluation of the patients accepted for transplantation. With most groups now showing more than 50% of patients alive and well at the end of one year, and 75% of good risk candidates surviving, there can be little doubt that liver transplantation has a growing role to play in the treatment of patients with advanced liver disease.

References

1. Starzl, T. E. (1969). *Experience in Hepatic Transplantation*. (Philadelphia: W. B. Sunders)
2. Calne, R. Y. and White, D. G. (1982). The use of cyclosporin A in clinical organ grafting. *Ann. Surg.*, **196**, 330–7
3. Starzl, T. E., Iwatsuki, S., Shaw, B. W., Van Thiel, D. H., Gartner, J. C., Zitelli, B. J., Malatack, J. J. and Schade, R. R. (1984). Analysis of liver transplantation. *Hepatology*, **4**, 47S–49S
4. Iwatsuki, S., Gordon, R. D., Shaw, B. W. and Starzl, T. E. (1985). *Ann. Surg.*, **202**, 401–7
5. Bontempo, F. A., Lewis, J. H., Van Thiel, D. H., Spero, J. A., Ragni, M. V., Butler, P., Israel, L. and Starzl, T. E. (1985). The relation of post-operative coagulation findings to diagnosis, blood usage and survival in adult liver transplantation. *Transplantation*, **39**, 532–6
6. Williams, R. and Gimson, A. E. S. (1984). An assessment of orthotopic liver transplantation in acute liver failure. *Hepatology*, **4**, 22S–24S
7. Starzl, T. E., Porter, K. A., Putnam, C. W., Halgrimson, R., Weil, R., Hoelscher, M. and Reid, H. K. (1976). Orthotopic liver transplantation in 93 patients. *Surg. Gynecol. Obstet.*, **142**, 487–505
8. Calne, R. Y. and Williams, R. (1977). Orthotopic liver transplantation: the first 60 patients. *Br. Med. J.*, **1**, 471–6
9. Gray, T., Buckley, B. M., Sealey, M., Smith, S. C. H., Tomlin, P. and McMaster, P. (1985). Is calcium important for haemodynamic stability during liver transplantation? *Transplant. Proc.*, **17**, 290–3
10. Shaw, B. W., Martin, D. J., Marquez, J. M., Kang, Y. G., Bugby, A. C., Iwatsuki, S., Griffiths, B. P., Hardesty, K. L., Bahnson, H. T. and Starzl, T. E. (1984). Venous bypass in clinical liver transplantation. *Ann. Surg.*, **200**, 524–34
11. Burckhart, G., Starzl, T. E., Williams, L., Sangvhi, A., Gartner, C., Venkataramanan, R., Zitelli, B., Malatack, J., Urbach, A., Diven, W., Ptachcinski, R., Shaw, B. W. and Iwatsuki, S. (1985). Cyclosporin monitoring and pharmocokinetics in paediatric liver transplant patients. *Transplant. Proc.*, **17**, 1172–5
12. McMaster, P., Herbertson, B., Cusick, C., Calne, R. Y. and Williams, R. (1978). Biliary sludging following liver transplantation in man. *Transplantation*, **25**, 56–62
13. Hubscher, S. G., Clements, D. G., Elias, E. and McMaster, P. (1985). Biopsy findings in cases of rejection of liver allograft. *J. Clin. Pathol.*, **38**, 1366–73
14. Snover, D. C., Sibley, R. K., Freese, D. K., Sharp, H. L., Bloomer, J. H., Najarian, J. S. and Ascher, N. L. (1985). A pathological study of 63 serial liver biopsies from 17 patients with specific reference to the diagnostic features and natural history of rejection. *Hepatology*, **4**, 1212–22
15. Shaw, B. W., Gordon, R. D., Iwatsuki, S. and Starzl, T. E. (1985). Hepatic retransplantation. *Transplant. Proc.*, **17**, 264–271
16. Starzl, T. E., Iwatsuki, S., Shaw, B. W., Nalesnik, M. A., Farhi, D. C. and Van Thiel, D. H. (1986). Treatment of fibrolamellar hepatoma with total hepatectomy and liver transplantation. *Surg. Gynecol. Obstet.*, **162**, 145–8
17. Starzl, T. E., Iwatsuki, S., Shaw, B. W. and Gordon, R. D. (1985). Orthotopic liver transplantation in 1984. *Transplant. Proc.*, **17**, 264–71
18. Soreide, O., Czerniak, A. and Blumgart, C. H. (1985). Large hepatocellular cancers: hepatic resection or liver transplantation. *Br. Med. J.*, **291**, 853–7

risk candidates surviving the long wait, it is doubtful that liver transplantation has a growing role to play in the treatment of patients with advanced liver disease.

References

1. [illegible]

10
Cardiac and Cardiopulmonary Transplantation

C. G. A. McGREGOR

INTRODUCTION

Cardiac transplantation has evolved from preliminary animal experiments in the early part of this century to an accepted form of treatment for terminal heart disease in the 1980s. The major advances in cardiac transplantation originated in the empirical surgical application of new techniques and drugs, rather than from basic discoveries in immunology. These advances include better donor management and organ preservation, more refined recipient selection, and improvements in immunosuppression and the management of infection. The advent of cyclosporin A in 1980, enabling a reduction or discontinuation of steroid therapy, has allowed the development of cardiopulmonary transplantation and introduced the possibility of isolated lung transplantation. Cardiopulmonary transplantation is in an earlier state of its evolution but promising results in the last five years will lead to its more widespread application.

CARDIAC TRANSPLANTATION

History

Carrel described the first heart transplant in the literature in 1905[1]. A heart transplanted from one dog into the neck of another dog continued to beat for two hours. This technique was refined by Mann[2] in the 1930s to allow physiological studies of the beating, perfused transplanted heart. In the late 1940s and early 1950s Demikhov[3] performed intrathoracic cardiac transplantation with the transplanted heart supporting the circulation for fifteen hours. The development of cardiopulmonary bypass in the mid-1950s made orthotopic cardiac transplantation feasible and led to the landmark paper by Lower and Shumway[4] in 1960 from Stanford University: five out of eight dogs survived 6–21 days. This report laid the foundations for future clinical development, with description of the surgical technique of excision and implantation of the heart at mid-atrial level and the use of topical cold saline for myocardial preservation. Further progress in the Stanford laboratory in the 1960s included the demonstration that cardiac rejection produced a reduction in summated electrocardiographic voltages.

In 1964 Hardy[5] performed the first human cardiac transplant using a chimpanzee as a donor: this attempt failed as the donor heart was unable to maintain the circulation. In 1967 Barnard[6] performed the first human to human cardiac transplant on Louis Washkansky, who died of pneumonitis after 17 days. This case elicited worldwide media and medical interest, and, within a year, 101 cardiac transplants had been performed by 64 surgical groups in 24 countries. Most of these patients died so that within the next 12-month period fewer than 20 cardiac transplants were undertaken, most of these at Stanford by Shumway and Stinson. The Stanford group persevered with clinical and laboratory research throughout the 1970s and the one-year survival of patients following cardiac transplantation increased from 22% in the first year of the programme (1968) to 67% by 1979 (Table 10.1). Advances achieved at Stanford during this period included the use of endomyocardial biopsy for the diagnosis of cardiac rejection[7] and the clinical application of anti-thymocyte globulin (ATG)[8]. As the Stanford results improved, a re-crudescence of interest in cardiac transplantation occurred in the late 1970s and further centres such as Papworth and Harefield in the UK initiated new cardiac transplant programmes.

Cyclosporin A was first used for immunosuppression following cardiac transplantation at Stanford in December 1980, and it caused both an increase in patient survival and further application of the technique worldwide. More than 400 cardiac transplants were performed in 1984, and by 1985 80 units in the USA had each performed at least one heart transplant. In the UK the number of cardiac transplants performed increased from three in 1979 to 137 in 1985.

Table 10.1 Stanford cardiac transplantation: One-year survival

1968	22%
1969	44%
1970	50%
1971	42%
1972	54%
1973	47%
1974	62%
1975	67%
1976	70%
1977	58%
1978	60%
1979	67%

Recipient selection

The major indication for heart transplantation is end-stage cardiac failure with New York Heart Association class IV symptoms and no alternative effective conventional therapy. Most patients have either cardiomyopathy or terminal ischaemic heart disease. Rarer indications for heart transplantation have included terminal valvular disease, myocarditis, cardiac tumour, some forms of congenital heart disease, coronary emboli, and post-traumatic cardiac aneurysm.

A list of contraindications is shown in Table 10.2. Irreversible pulmonary vascular hypertension of more than 6 Wood units remains an important contraindication, as this would result in acute right ventricular failure of the donor heart which would be unable to produce, acutely, an adequate cardiac output against the elevated pulmonary vascular pressure.

In essence, any condition that would compromise the success of the transplant is a contraindication. In recent years, since the introduction of cyclosporin A, some relaxation of selection criteria has occurred so that patients with non-insulin-dependent diabetes mellitus, recently healed pulmonary infarcts or recently controlled infections can now be considered heart transplant candidates.

There is now no lower age limit for heart transplantation and the upper age limit has been extended to 55 years. Patients should be psychosocially stable and fully informed of the implications of the procedure. Estimates of the number of potential cardiac recipients in the UK has varied from 450 to 900[9,10] although these estimates presume stricter selection criteria than now apply.

Table 10.2 Contraindications to cardiac transplantation

Fixed elevated pulmonary vascular hypertension
  (>6 Wood units)
Cancer
Active infection
Diabetes mellitus
Severe hepatic or renal dysfunction
  (creatinine clearance <40 mL/min)
Recent pulmonary embolism
Collagen vascular disease
Age >55 years

Donor selection and management

Donor availability remains and is likely to remain the major limiting factor in the expansion of cardiac transplantation both in the UK and the USA[11]. Potential cardiac donors must have satisfied the brain death criteria of the Royal Colleges[12]. An active minority opposed to the concept of brain death can cause a dramatic reduction in the number of donors referred to the transplant services. As many as a third of patients die on the waiting list for cardiac transplantation, and so programmes of education and awareness are necessary in the medical and lay communities to avoid the wastage of many valuable organs. The positive aspects of organ donation, in terms of the salvage of life and the provision of some solace to the relatives of deceased patients, have tended to be overshadowed by intermittent media attention to unorthodox views seeking to undermine public confidence in the accepted brain death criteria.

Potential cardiac donors should be less than 35 years old if male, and less than 40 years if female, and free from current or previous cardiac disease. Long periods of external cardiac massage or severe hypotension contra-indicate cardiac donation. Potential donors should have no active systemic infection, although many will have purulent sputum and lung infiltrates. Diabetes insipidus is treated by intermittent vasopressin administration and insulin therapy may be required to control hyperglycaemia.

Careful assessment of the cardiovascular system is important as marked cardiovascular changes occur in brain-dead patients. Central venous pressure measurement is helpful to optimize fluid replacement and thus enable inotropic drugs, which are often used, to be discontinued. If significant inotropic support is required in the presence of an adequate cardiac filling pressure then the heart is not suitable for donation.

Donor and recipient matching

The donor and recipient are matched for ABO blood group compatibility without rhesus matching. The donor should be within 20% of the body mass of the recipient, although if the recipient has an elevated pulmonary vascular resistance, the use of a larger donor, with as short an ischaemic time as possible, is necessary to avoid donor right heart failure.

All potential recipients have their serum tested against a panel of lymphocytes from normal individuals (usually from around 50 individuals) for the presence of cytotoxic antibodies. If a patient demonstrates a positive lymphocytotoxicity against any member of the panel, which is representative of the major histocompatibility antigens in the community, then a direct crossmatch between the recipient and intended donor is required. In normal circumstances, such a direct crossmatch between the recipient and actual donor is performed retrospectively after the transplant has been performed.

There is some suggestion that mismatching at the HLA-A2 locus between donor and recipient may result in an increased incidence of accelerated coronary artery disease in the recipient, but this is based on retrospective historical data, and may not apply to the current methods of immunosuppression. Prospective matching is not in general practicable for heart transplantation.

Distant procurement of the heart is now common with simultaneous removal of kidneys, liver, heart and corneas. The maximum acceptable ischaemic time of the heart is around 4 h and this allows procurement at a maximum distance of around 1000 miles from the recipient hospital, using air transportation. Transportation can often account for the major part of the total ischaemic time and careful coordination of donor and recipient operations and transport therefore is critical.

214

Operative techniques

Donor operation

The surgical technique for distant organ procurement is straightforward, does not require cardiopulmonary bypass and can be performed in any standard hospital theatre. A median sternotomy incision is used and after careful inspection of the heart and dissection of the great vessels, the patient is fully heparinized. Venous inflow occlusion is achieved by tying or clamping the venae cavae, following which the aorta is cross-clamped and cold potassium cardioplegic solution is infused into the aortic root. During this infusion the inferior pulmonary veins as well as the inferior vena cava are divided to allow decompression of the heart. Topical cooling with cold saline at 4 °C is performed. When the cardioplegic infusion is complete the heart is excised by dividing the aorta, the venae cavae, the remaining pulmonary veins and the right and left pulmonary arteries. The heart is placed in a cold saline (4 °C) solution within a laparotomy bag which is then placed in a plastic suction container to be transported surrounded by ice in a standard cooler box.

Recipient operation

Orthotopic cardiac transplantation is the technique of choice in most centres and the technical aspects of the operation are little changed since the original description by Lower and Shumway[4]. A median sternotomy incision is used and the patient placed on cardiopulmonary bypass. The recipient heart is excised by dividing the aorta and pulmonary artery close to valvular level. The right atrium is then excised close to the atrioventricular ring leaving most of the interventricular septum behind. The left atrium is then excised leaving a generous cuff behind, including the pulmonary veins.

The donor heart is then prepared by opening the left atrium between the pulmonary veins and the left atrial anastomosis is performed first (Figure 10.1). When this is complete, an incision is made in the donor right atrium in a curvilinear fashion towards the base of the right atrial appendage avoiding the sino-atrial node, allowing for maintenance of sinus rhythm in the heart after transplantation. The right atrial anastomosis is then carried out (Figure 10.2), followed by aortic and pulmonary arterial anastomoses (Figure 10.3). After de-airing of the transplanted heart, cardiopulmonary bypass is discontinued.

Heterotopic cardiac transplantation (piggyback transplant) is performed less commonly, usually when the size of the donor is significantly smaller than the recipient and where the donor heart would not be expected to be able to maintain the recipient circulation. Proponents of this technique describe the potential for the recipient's own heart to maintain the circulation during acute rejection of the transplanted heart and advocate its use in the presence of severe pulmonary vascular hypertension, but this remains a doubtful indication. Disadvantages of the technique include thrombo-embolic complications, the need for anticoagulation, persistent angina pectoris in

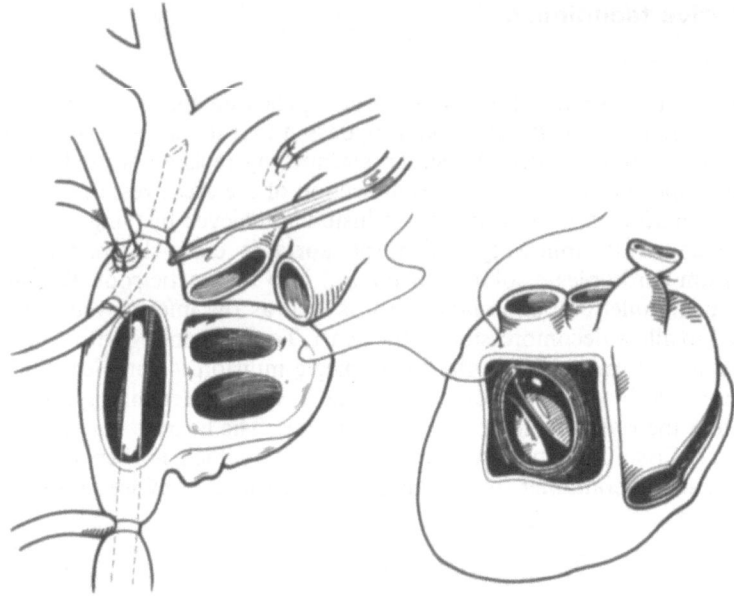

Figure 10.1 Left atrial anastomosis beginning at the base of the left atrial appendage in the donor and adjacent to the left superior pulmonary vein in the recipient

patients with ischaemic heart disease and the risk of infection in the prosthetic graft material used to join the donor and recipient pulmonary arteries. The actual techique has been described in detail elsewhere[13] (Figure 10.4).

Post-operative management

At the completion of the operation the patient is transferred to a single cubicle in the intensive care unit where he or she is reverse barrier nursed for up to one week. A constant infusion of isoprenaline is required for some days following cardiac transplantation to overcome the effects of acute denervation and optimize cardiac output. Circulatory management is otherwise similar to that for general cardiac surgical patients. Post-operative arrhythmias are rare but are treated in a way similar to that in non-transplant patients. Patients are extubated as early as possible (usually on the morning following surgery) and removal of all indwelling lines and catheters is carried out as soon as practicable. Early ambulation is encouraged. Reverse isolation can be discontinued as soon as the patient is on baseline maintenance immunosuppression, but is often reintroduced during augmented immunosuppression for treatment of cardiac rejection.

Immunosuppression

Immunosuppressive techniques have continued to evolve over the 18 years of clinical heart transplantation. Although nearly all the immunosuppressive regimes used currently are based on the use of cyclosporin A, no consensus

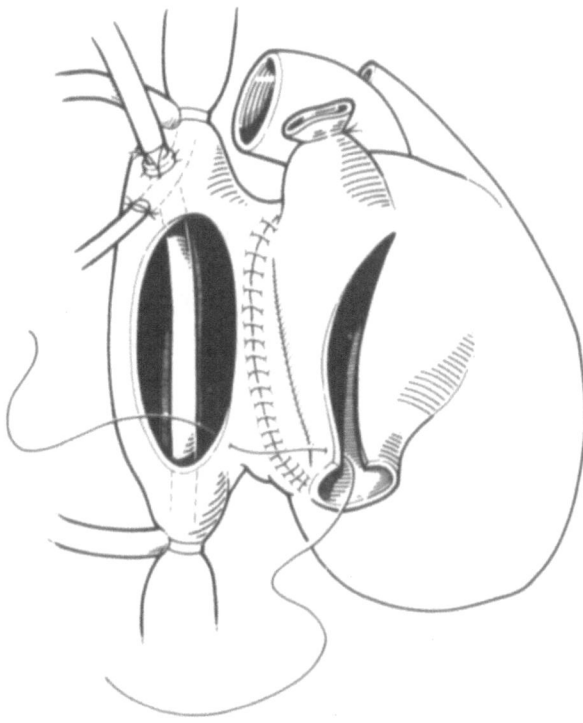

Figure 10.2 Right atrial anastomosis. Note curvilinear incision in donor right atrium to avoid donor sinoatrial node

exists as to the optimal use of this agent. Most major units have adjusted immunosuppressive protocols over recent years. To understand this evolution it is helpful to examine the history of immunosuppression for cardiac transplantation at Stanford University and to outline the reasons for their changes in protocol.

Immunosuppression begins pre-operatively with a single oral dose of cyclosporin A of 4–14 mg/kg according to pre-operative renal function. In theatre, after discontinuation of cardiopulmonary bypass, intravenous methylprednisolone in a dose of 500 mg is given intravenously, and further doses of 125 mg are given every 12 h for 36 h. Thereafter maintenance immunosuppression is begun as discussed below.

The 'conventional' pre-cyclosporin A regime used at Stanford is illustrated in Table 10.3. This was used in 99 consecutive patients undergoing heart transplantation between 1974 and 1980 and was representative of therapy used throughout the world at that time.

Following impressive results from the animal laboratory, cyclosporin A was introduced to clinical practice in December 1980. The first cyclosporin A protocol (Table 10.4) was used in the next 28 consecutive heart transplant patients. Cyclosporin A was given in a standard dose regime starting at 18 mg/kg/d reducing to 10 mg/kg/d at 2 months. Rabbit ATG (2.5 mg/kg/d)

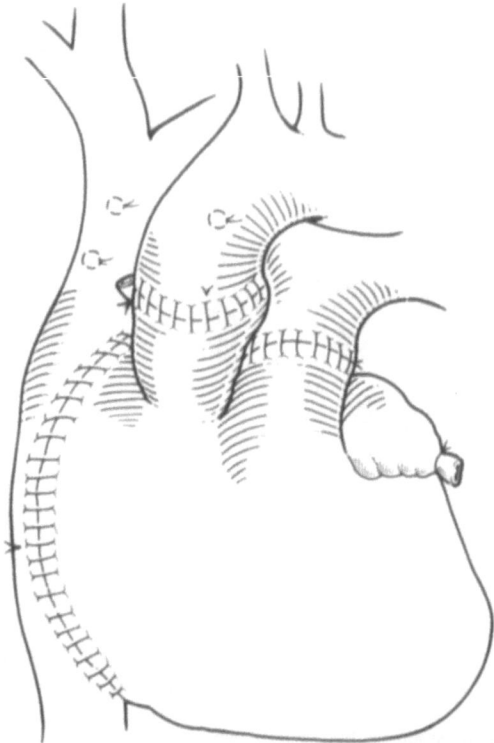

Figure 10.3 Completed aortic and pulmonary arterial anastomoses

was given pre-operatively and for 2–4 d post-operatively according to the circulating T lymphocyte count. Prednisolone was administered initially at 1 mg/kg/d and reduced using a tapering schedule to 0.2 mg/kg/d at 2 months.

In this initial group of cyclosporin A-treated patients there were four cases of malignant lymphoma in the first 6 months. Early nephrotoxicity was noted. The mean number of rejection episodes per patient in this group was 0.89 in the first 60 days compared with 1.22 episodes in the previous 'conventionally' treated group. There was also an increase in the number of patients free from all rejection and there appeared to be a reduction of overall infection. The high incidence of lymphoma indicated over-immunosuppression and so a further protocol was introduced in January 1982 (Table 10.5).

The prophylactic use of ATG was discontinued with this regime and the cyclosporin A dose reduced to achieve targeted trough serum levels of 200–300 ng/mL. Seventy-four consecutive patients received this therapy which resulted in an overall reduction in cyclosporin A dosage. Lymphoma developed in only two of the 74 patients in the first year, an incidence comparable to other transplant groups. Again nephrotoxicity was noted, as before, although later follow-up indicated that this was not completely reversible as had initially been thought. Several patients from this group

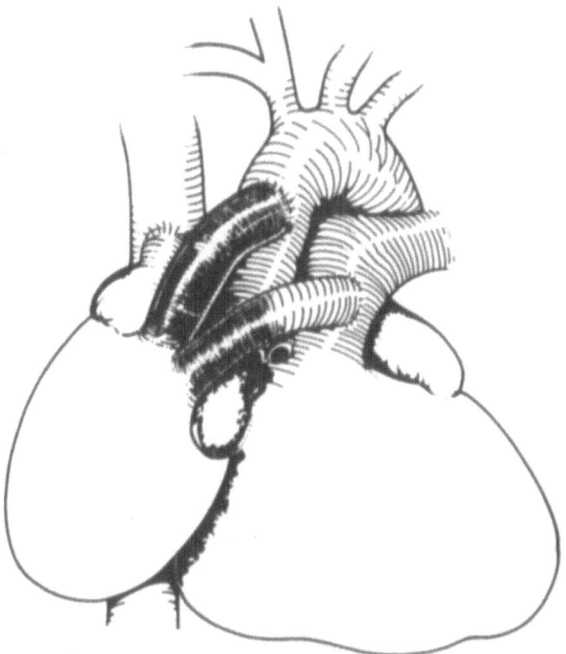

Figure 10.4 Completed heterotopic cardiac transplant

Table 10.3 Conventional immunosuppression: treatment of 99 patients at Stanford, January 1974–December 1980

(A)	Azathioprine	1–2 mg/kg/d
(B)	Prednisone: initial dose 2 months 1 year	 1.5 mg/kg/d 1 mg/kg/d 0.3 mg/kg/d
(C)	Rabbit ATG	14-day course

Table 10.4 Initial cyclosporin A regime: treatment of 28 patients at Stanford, December 1980–January 1982

(A)	Cyclosporin A: initial dose 2 months	 18 mg/kg/d 10 mg/kg/d
(B)	Prednisone: initial dose 2 months	 1 mg/kg/d 0.2 mg/kg/d
(C)	Rabbit ATG	2–4-day initial course

Table 10.5 Modified cyclosporin A regime: treatment of 74 patients at Stanford, January 1982 – May 1984

(A)	Cyclosporin A:	
	initial dose	18 mg/kg/d
	Thereafter dosage adjusted to maintain	
	trough serum level	200–300 ng/mL (radioimmunoassay)
(B)	Prednisone:	
	initial dose	1 mg/kg/d
	1 month	0.5 mg/kg/d
	2 months	0.2 mg/kg/d
(C)	Prophylactic ATG discontinued	

have required cessation of cyclosporin A therapy because of chronic renal failure. In addition most patients from this group required multiple drug therapy for hypertension. As a result of the nephrotoxicity and hypertension a third cyclosporin A protocol was introduced in May 1984 (Table 10.6).

Targeted trough cyclosporin A levels were lowered to 50–150 ng/mL after the first month and patients were treated with 'low dose' steroids (0.2 mg/kg/d of prednisolone) or no steroids. With this overall reduction in immunosuppression, azathioprine was reintroduced in doses to maintain the white blood cell count at 4–6000 mm^{-3}. ATG was also given for one week postoperatively. It is interesting that all patients who were randomized to the no steroids group eventually required low dose steroid therapy because of recurrent rejection.

These changes have resulted in the evolution of the currently commonly used low dose triple therapy of cyclosporin A, azathioprine and prednisolone or prednisone. Improved patient survival has been maintained with each cyclosporin A protocol and it appears that complications such as nephrotoxicity can be reduced while maintaining excellent patient survival. Patients require immunosuppressive therapy for life. It is important that any changes

Table 10.6 Third cyclosporin A regime: (May 1984 onwards)

(A)	Cyclosporin A	16–18 mg/kg loading dose Thereafter dosage adjusted to maintain trough serum level 100–300 ng/mL for 1 month; 50–150 ng/mL after 1 month
(B)	Azathioprine	4 mg/kg loading dose Thereafter 1–3 mg/kg/d to maintain WBC 4–6000 mm^3
(C)	Equine ATG	7-day course: 10 mg/kg/d according to T cell rosette count
(D)	Prednisone	Randomized: (a) 0.2 mg/kg/d (b) no corticosteroids

in immunosuppression should be based on careful assessment of clinical results in well-defined patient populations of a size suitable to allow reliable statistical analysis.

Rejection

Histological examination of endomyocardial biopsy specimens remains the 'gold standard' for the diagnosis of cardiac rejection. This technique, pioneered by Caves[7], is performed under local anaesthesia, using a per-cutaneous Seldinger technique under fluoroscopic control, and takes around 20 min (Figure 10.5). Three to five biopsies are taken and the operation can be performed on an out-patient basis. There has been no mortality from endomyocardial biopsy in over 5000 cases at Stanford. Cardiac biopsies are performed weekly for 6 weeks, every second week for a further 6 weeks, once a month for three months and thereafter three-monthly for life. Continuing investigations into various non-invasive methods for the diagnosis of cardiac

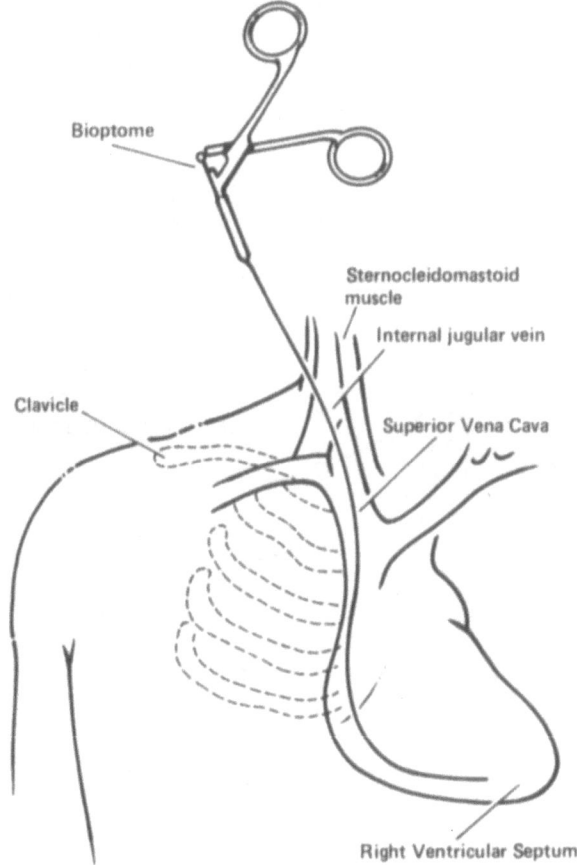

Figure 10.5 Technique of cardiac biopsy

rejection including nuclear medical techniques, echocardiography and immunological monitoring have so far failed to supercede cardiac biopsy. The measurement of summated electrocardiographic voltages, which was useful for the detection of rejection in 'conventionally' treated patients, seems to be unhelpful in cyclosporin A-treated patients.

The histological appearances and grading of rejection have been described[14], and the indication for augmented antirejection therapy is the presence of myocyte necrosis. The presence of a mild infiltrate does not require additional antirejection therapy.

In the first 6 weeks after transplantation the treatment of rejection episodes, as diagnosed by the presence of myocyte necrosis on cardiac biopsy, is by 'pulse' therapy with 1 g of methylprednisolone intravenously each day for three days. Severe rejection in the first biopsy, failure of resolution of rejection after two pulse therapies of methylprednisolone or impaired haemodynamics associated with rejection indicate the need for concomitant ATG therapy. If rejection continues despite repeated pulse therapy then cardiac retransplantation is required.

After the first six weeks following transplantation, rejection episodes can be treated by temporary increases in oral prednisolone dosage to 100 mg daily for 3 days, reducing by 5 mg daily until a level of 5 mg per day greater than the previous maintenance dose is achieved. If the patient is well this treatment can be on an out-patient basis.

Survival

Actuarial survival of cardiac transplant recipients treated at Stanford University, over three time frames, is shown in Figure 10.6. The calculated one- and five-year survival figures (Cutler–Ederer life table method) for

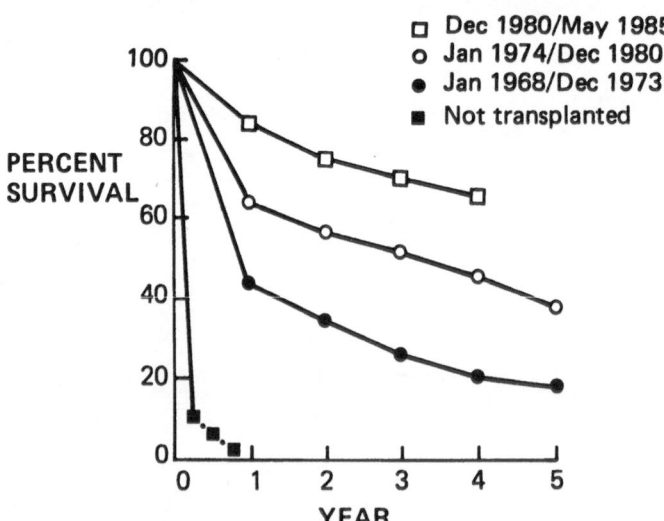

Figure 10.6 Actuarial survival of cardiac transplant recipients over three time frames (Stanford University)

222

Table 10.7 Cause of death during first post-operative year

	Cyclosporin A (125 patients)	Conventional (99 patients)
Rejection	4	7
Infection	9	28
Graft arteriosclerosis	—	—
Graft failure	4	—
Lymphoma	2	—
Non-lymphoid malignancy	—	—
Pulmonary embolus	—	—
Pulmonary hypertension	—	2
CVA	1	—
Other	1	—
Total	21	37

cyclosporin A-treated patients beginning in December 1980 are 83% and 60% respectively.

The improvements in results from the initial time frame (January 1968 to December 1973) to the second time frame (January 1974 to December 1980) can be principally attributed to the application of endomyocardial biopsy and the introduction of the ATG for the treatment of rejection. The improvements in results from the second time frame (January 1974 to December 1980) and during the most recent time frame (December 1980 onwards) is principally due to the introduction of cyclosporin A and improved methods for the diagnosis and treatment of infection.

The causes of death after heart transplantation at Stanford during and after the first post-operative year in 'conventionally' treated patients and cyclosporin A-treated patients are shown in Tables 10.7 and 10.8. The introduction of cyclosporin A can be seen to have resulted in a dramatic reduction in death from infection. The incidence of infection is the same between the groups, so that infections are easier to treat and have a lower mortality in cyclosporin A-treated patients.

Table 10.8 Cause of death after first post-operative year

	Cyclosporin A (125 patients)	Conventional (99 patients)
Rejection	1	4
Infection	1	15
Graft arteriosclerosis	4	2
Graft failure	—	—
Lymphoma	1	3
Non-lymphoid malignancy	—	—
Pulmonary embolus	—	1
Pulmonary hypertension	—	—
CVA	—	—
Other	1	5
Total	8	30

Table 10.9 Organisms in cyclosporin A-treated patients (Stanford 1980–1984)

Bacterial	74
Viral	77
Fungal	20
Protozoan	3
Nocardia	3

The principal causes of death are rejection and infection. The relative proportions of death from rejection and infection will vary from unit to unit depending on the particular immunosuppressive protocol used. If the balance is towards over-immunosuppression then more patients will die of infection whereas if the balance is towards under-immunosuppression the major cause of mortality will be rejection. It is interesting that beyond the first year after transplantation in cyclosporin A-treated patients, the principal cause of death is accelerated graft arteriosclerosis.

Infection

Peri-operative antibiotic cover is given and continued until the chest drains and urinary catheter are removed, usually within 48 h. Aggressive investigation of any post-operative fever is carried out. The intravascular lines are removed and the tips cultured. Sputum and urine cultures are performed daily, as well as 8-hourly aerobic and anaerobic blood cultures. In the presence of a pulmonary infiltrate and a non-diagnostic sputum, transtracheal aspirate is performed and if this fails to elicit a diagnosis, transbronchial biopsy or transthoracic needle biopsy is carried out. Serological investigation for cytomegalovirus, herpes virus, toxoplasma, coccidioides and cryptococcus is performed.

'Blind' antibiotic therapy is not given without a specific bacteriological diagnosis unless life-threatening infection is present. Routine surveillance cultures of sputum and urine are carried out three times each week as well as weekly serology. The types of organism and infectious episodes in cyclosporin A-treated patients in the Stanford series are shown in Tables 10.9 and 10.10.

Complications of cardiac transplantation

Accelerated graft arteriosclerosis

The development of this complication is now the major cause of death after the first year following cardiac transplantation. This occurs whether the pre-operative condition was cardiomyopathy or ischaemic disease and may develop within months of transplantation. Almost half the patients examined angiographically five years after cardiac transplantation exhibit this form of arteriosclerosis which is different from the more common type seen in ischaemic heart disease in that it tends to be diffusely concentric, and therefore not amenable to coronary artery surgery. The transplanted heart is denervated

Table 10.10 Infectious episodes in cyclosporin
A-treated patients (Stanford 1980–1984)

Pulmonary	40
Septicaemia	18
Urinary tract	23
Mediastinum	8
Herpes simplex	35
Herpes zoster	12
CMV	30
Retinitis	2
Empyema	1
CNS	1

and therefore angina pectoris is not present, so that such patients present with acute cardiac failure secondary to a silent myocardial infarction, or with sudden death. The presence of this complication in both main coronary arteries is an indication for retransplantation. There is some experimental evidence that administration of aspirin and dipyridamole reduces the incidence of this complication, and so most patients are placed on these medications. The incidence of this complication has not fallen since the introduction of cyclosporin A and may, in fact, have increased. The cause of accelerated arteriosclerosis remains unknown but it has been attributed to chronic, immunologically-mediated blood vessel injury.

Malignant disease

Neoplasia is known to complicate immunosuppressive therapy for any cause and a small number of cyclosporin A-treated patients have developed lymphoma, often of the diffuse histiocytic type with central nervous system involvement. The presence of Epstein–Barr virus has been implicated in its development, and the use of prophylactic acyclovir therapy has been used in several centres.

Other complications

Hypertension requiring therapy has been a common complication of cyclosporin A usage although its severity has been reduced by lowering dosage levels. The problems of nephrotoxicity have resulted in changes in immunosuppressive protocols and it remains to be seen if these will reduce long-term renal complications. Other complications such as hirsutism, gum hypertrophy, hepatic dysfunction, tremor and convulsions have not proved major problems.

Constant alertness is required regarding the drug interactions between cyclosporin A and other medications used in cardiac transplant recipients, such as the aminoglycoside antibiotics.

Costs of cardiac transplantation

The cost of cardiac transplantation has fallen by approximately a third since the introduction of cyclosporin A. This reduction in cost has continued as greater experience with this medication has been achieved, with fewer complications, and a reduction in hospital in-patient time.

A detailed analysis of the cost of transplantation has been performed by the Brunel University Group at the request of the Department of Health and Social Security (DHSS)[10]. The cost of the first year of treatment including operation is £17 000, and the subsequent annual cost is around £4500. These costs compare favourably with those for the treatment of other terminal diseases, dialysis for chronic renal failure and intravenous feeding.

Summary

A sustained improvement in the results of cardiac transplantation has occurred since its inception in 1967 with a current 1 year survival in excess of 84% and a 5 year survival in excess of 60%. It is important to note that 80% of these survivors are able to select the lifestyle of their choice, and are thus well rehabilitated as well as having the benefits of increased longevity. Most patients can return to employment and lead active lives, although they do require to be on life-long medication.

There remains a gulf between the need for heart transplantation and available resources. An expansion of cardiac transplant services and active measures to increase organ donation are indicated.

History

Initial research into cardiopulmonary transplantation was performed in the dog. In the 1940s Demikhov[15] achieved survival of 5 days in 2 out of 67 animals, and in 1953 Neptune[16] using systemic hypothermia and circulatory arrest, reported survival of 6 hours. In 1957 Webb and Howard[17] obtained 22-hour survival using cardiopulmonary bypass. In 1961 Lower and Shumway[18] obtained 6-day survival and Grinnan[19] reported a 10-day survivor in 1970.

Nakae demonstrated that pulmonary denervation in dogs results in abnormal respiration with absence of the Hering–Breuer reflex[20]: thus these animals died of respiratory failure. The primate did not have such abnormal respiration following denervation and Castaneda achieved long-term survival after cardiopulmonary transplantation in primates in 1972[21]. Reitz and associates at Stanford achieved long-term survival in baboons after cardiopulmonary transplantation in 1980 using cyclosporin A[22] and this experience was the forerunner for the successful clinical programme.

The first human cardiopulmonary transplant was performed by Cooley in 1968 on a 2½-year-old child who died 14 hours after operation[23]. In 1969 Lillihei performed a cardiopulmonary transplant on a 43-year-old man with emphysema who died of pneumonitis eight days after transplantation[24]. Pneumonitis was the cause of death in the third human cardiopulmonary transplant performed by Barnard in 1971[25].

Based on more than 20 years of laboratory research, including long-term survival in primates and the use of cyclosporin A in the clinical heart transplant programme, cardiopulmonary transplantation was begun at Stanford in March 1981. The first patient, a 45-year-old woman with primary pulmonary hypertension, survived five years and died of non-transplant related pathology.

Recipient selection

Up to this time, the majority of patients accepted for cardiopulmonary transplantation have suffered from either primary pulmonary hypertension[26] or pulmonary hypertension secondary to Eisenmenger's syndrome[27]. A small number of patients have undergone this procedure for terminal lung diseases such as cystic fibrosis or emphysema, and these conditions may be an increasing indication for cardiopulmonary transplantation in the future. The disadvantage of cardiopulmonary transplantation for primary lung conditions is that a healthy heart may be removed from the recipient with the diseased lungs, and the replacement heart, transplanted with the lungs, will be open to all the complications of transplantation. The possibility of newer operations such as isolated lung transplantation for the treatment of pulmonary fibrosis[28] and the use of double lung transplantation for the treatment of emphysema and the septic pulmonary diseases, may limit the indications for cardiopulmonary transplantation in the future to those patients with concomitant heart and lung disease.

Recipient selection criteria are similar to those for heart transplantation although a priority has been given to younger patients with end-stage disease and a deteriorating course, as there is a very limited supply of suitable donors. Previous major intrathoracic surgery is a relative contraindication to cardiopulmonary transplantation as this appears to increase the early operative mortality secondary to haemorrhage from adhesions. The number of patients who could benefit from cardiopulmonary transplantation is unknown and will be determined by future indications, but clearly the numbers could be considerable if various types of lung transplantation proved effective for the treatment of terminal lung disease.

Donor selection and management

Distant organ procurement for cardiopulmonary transplantation has been applied only in the last two years. The optimum method of preserving the lungs is not yet known and several methods are currently in clinical use. These include cooling the body on cardiopulmonary bypass, the use of a ventilated beating heart-lung preparation and the administration of various solutions, crystalloid and colloid, to preserve the lungs. The majority of potential cardiopulmonary donors will be found to be unsuitable as pulmonary complications such as aspiration, pneumonitis or oedema are often present in the brain-dead patient, thus contraindicating cardiopulmonary donation. The cardiopulmonary donor should have normal blood gases and it is necessary to match donor and recipient thoracic cage size such that the donor is of similar size to, or smaller than, the potential recipient. Careful cardiovascular management of these donors is required in order to maintain satisfactory haemodynamics with a low central venous pressure.

The availability of donor organs will continue to be the limiting factor in the expansion of cardiopulmonary transplantation, and this problem is even more acute than in the case of the heart, as donor selection criteria are stricter.

Operative technique

Donor operation

Cardiopulmonary bypass is not required and lung preservation is achieved by the methods described above. Topical cooling of both organs is employed during transportation.

Recipient operation

The operative technique for cardiopulmonary transplantation has been described elsewhere[29]. Essential aspects of the procedure include preservation of the vagus, phrenic and recurrent laryngeal nerves and meticulous haemostasis, as many patients have large bronchial collateral channels in the mediastinum.

The tracheal anastomosis is performed first using a continuous polypropylene suture followed by the atrial and aortic anastomoses. Peri-operative immunosuppressive techniques are similar to those for heart transplantation.

Post-operative management

Post-operative immunosuppression is similar to that following heart transplantation, except that the use of steroids after the first 36 hours is avoided for 2 weeks, to allow healing of the tracheal anastomosis. Immunosuppression during this period is based on cyclosporin A, azathioprine and ATG.

There is still no reliable method for the diagnosis of lung rejection, and the previously accepted concept that cardiac and pulmonary rejection occur together and therefore that lung rejection could be diagnosed by cardiac biopsy has been shown to be no longer acceptable: isolated pulmonary rejection has been demonstrated clinically[30]. Haemodynamic management of the cardiopulmonary transplant recipient is similar to that after heart transplantation. High inspired oxygen concentrations are avoided and more aggressive diuresis sought to maintain a low normal central venous pressure and reduce the likelihood of pulmonary oedema. Early extubation is sought and active chest physiotherapy initiated.

Survival

A review of the results of the Stanford programme of cardiopulmonary transplantation between March 1981 and August 1985 has recently been published[31]. Twenty-eight cardiopulmonary transplants were performed at Stanford during this period including one patient who underwent retransplantation. There were eight peri-operative deaths, with adhesions from previous intrathoracic surgery implicated in the majority.

Rehabilitation has been excellent, and essentially normal early cardiopulmonary function has been demonstrated in operative survivors. Late cardiorespiratory function has continued to be near normal in half the patients[31]. Actuarial survival at one, two, three and four years has been 65, 54, 54 and 54% respectively (Figure 10.7).

Complications

The major long-term complication following cardiopulmonary transplantation has been the development of late respiratory failure in ten of the twenty long-term survivors. Patients complain of cough, often productive, and progressive shortness of breath. Chest radiography has shown interstitial infiltrates and variable pleural thickening. Respiratory function tests have demonstrated a progressive obstructive physiology with superimposed restriction in half of the patients[32]. All of these patients have shown the features of obliterative bronchiolitis on open lung biopsy or autopsy. The cause of this complication remains unknown but potential factors include chronic lung rejection, the effects of pulmonary denervation such as the absence of the cough reflex and altered-sputum rheology, chronic respiratory infection and the effects of pulmonary ischaemia. The condition of the ten patients who developed obliterative bronchiolitis continued to deteriorate and four died. More recently, two patients with this complication have been treated with high dose corticosteroids early in the course of their deterioration, and both have shown significant improvement in symptoms and in pulmonary physiology[33]. Obliterative bronchiolitis does not appear uniformly after cardiopulmonary transplant and a greater understanding of its cause is required to improve long-term results. Other complications are similar to those following cardiac transplantation alone, such as cyclosporin A nephrotoxicity and accelerated graft arteriosclerosis.

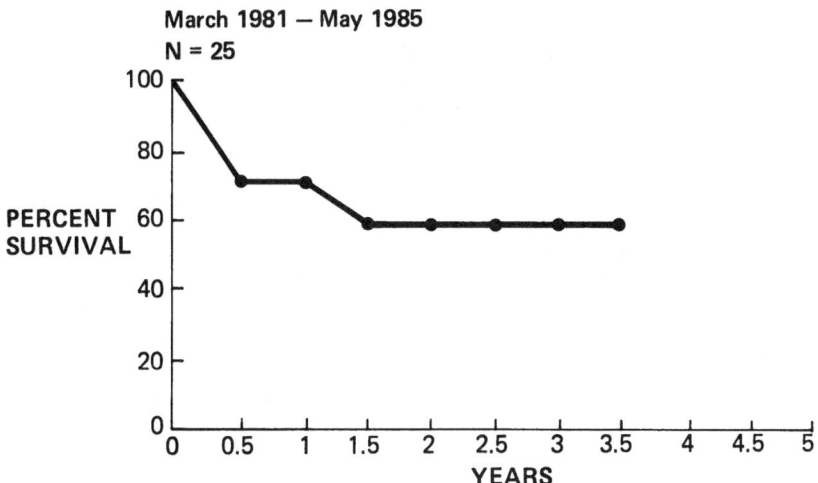

Figure 10.7 Actuarial survival of cardiopulmonary transplant recipients (Stanford University)

229

Summary

Cardiopulmonary transplantation remains at an experimental stage in its development in relation to recipient selection, optimal pulmonary preservation and the diagnosis of pulmonary rejection.

The recent report of successful isolated lung transplantation for pulmonary fibrosis[28] and the successful demonstration of double lung transplantation (without the heart) in the laboratory will modify the indications for cardiopulmonary transplantation in the future. Thoracic medicine and surgery are entering one of the most exciting periods over the last 50 years, with the potential for treating many hundreds of patients with terminal lung disease for whom there is no other form of treatment.

References

1. Carrel, A. and Guthrie, C. C. (1905). Transplantation of veins and organs. *Am. Med.*, **10**, 1101
2. Mann, F. C., Priestley, J. T., Markowitz, K. and Yater, W. M. (1933). Transplantation of the intact mammalian heart. *Arch. Surg.*, **26**, 219–44
3. Demikhov, V. P. (1960). *Some Essential Points of Techniques of Transplantation of the Heart, Lungs and Other Organs.* (Moscow: Medgiz State Press for Medical Literature)
4. Lower, R. R. and Shumway, N. E. (1960). Studies on orthotopic transplantation of the canine heart. *Surg. Forum*, **11**, 18–9
5. Hardy, J. D., Kurrus, F. D., Chavez, C. M., Neely, W. A., Eraslan, S., Turner, M. D., Fabian, L. W. and Labecki, J. D. (1964). Heart transplantation in man: developmental studies and report of a case. *J. Am. Med. Assoc.*, **188**, 1132–40
6. Barnard, C. N. (1967). The operation. *S. Afr. Med. J.*, **41**, 1271–4
7. Caves, P. K., Stinson, E. B., Billingham, M. E., Rider, A. K. and Shumway, N. E. (1973). Diagnosis of human cardiac allograft rejection by serial cardiac biopsy. *J. Thorac. Cardiovasc. Surg.*, **66**, 461–6
8. Bieber, C. P., Griepp, R. B., Oyer, P. E., Wong, J. and Stinson, E. B. (1976). Use of rabbit antithymocyte globulin in cardiac transplantation: relationship of serum clearance rates to clinical outcome. *Transplantation*, **22**, 478–88
9. British Cardiac Society (1984). Report on cardiac transplantation in the United Kingdom. *Br. Heart J.*, **52**, 679–82
10. Buxton, M., Acheson, R. M., Caine, N., Gibson, S. and O'Brien, B. (1985). *Costs and Benefits of the Heart Transplant Programmes at Harefield and Papworth Hospitals.* Research Report No. 12 (Brunel Report). (London: HMSO)
11. Evans, R. W., Manningen, D. L., Garrison, L. P. and Maier, A. M. (1986). Donor availability as the primary determinant of the future of heart transplantation. *J. Am. Med. Assoc.*, **255**, 1892–8
12. Conference of the Medical Royal Colleges and their Faculties in the United Kingdom. (1976). Diagnosis of brain death. *Br. Med. J.*, **2**, 1187–8
13. Novitsky, D., Cooper, D. K. C. and Barnard, C. N. (1983). The surgical technique of heterotopic heart transplantation. *Ann. Thorac. Surg.*, **36**, 476–82
14. Billingham, M. E. (1986). Histological diagnosis of rejection in conventional and cyclosporine treated patients. *Heart Transplant.* (In press)
15. Demikhov, V. P. (1962). Experimental transplantation of vital organs. Trans. Basil Haigh, New York Consultants Bureau. pp. 126
16. Neptune, W. B., Cookson, B. A., Bailey, C. P., Appler, R. and Rajkowski, F. (1953). Complete homologous heart transplantation. *Arch. Surg.*, **66**, 174–8
17. Webb, W. R. and Howard, H. S. (1957). Cardiopulmonary transplantation. *Surg. Forum*, **8**, 313–7
18. Lower, R. R., Stofer, R. C., Hurley, E. J. and Shumway, N. E. (1961). Complete homograft replacement of the heart and both lungs. *Surgery*, **50**, 842–5

19. Grinnan, G. L. B., Graham, W. H., Childs, J. W. and Lower, R. R. (1970). Cardiopulmonary homotransplantation. *J. Thorac. Cardiovasc. Surg.*, **60**, 609–15
20. Nakae, S., Webb, W. R., Theodorides, T. and Gregg, W. L. (1967). Respiratory function following cardiopulmonary denervation in dog, cat and monkey. *Surg. Gynec. Obstet.*, **125**, 1285–2
21. Castaneda, A., Zamora, R., Schmmidt-Habelman, P., Horung, J., Murphy, W., Ponto, D. and Moller, J. H. (1972). Cardiopulmonary autotransplantation in primates (baboons). Late functional results. *Surgery*, **72**, 1064–70
22. Reitz, B. A., Burton, N. A., Jamieson, S. W., Bieber, C. P., Pennoch, J. L., Stinson, E. B. and Shumway, N. E. (1980). Heart and lung transplantation. Autotransplantation and allotransplantation in primates with extended survival. *J. Thorac. Cardiovasc. Surg.*, **80**, 360–71
23. Cooley, D. A., Bloodwell, R. D., Hallman, G. L., Nora, J. J., Harris, G. M. and Leachman, R. D. (1969). Organ transplantation for advanced cardiopulmonary disease. *Ann. Thorac. Surg.*, **8**, 30–46
24. Lillehei, C. D., Wildevuur, C. R. H. and Benfield, J. R. (1970). Review of 23 human lung transplantations by 20 surgeons. *Ann. Thorac. Surg.*, **9**, 515
25. Losman, J. G., Campbell, C. D., Replogle, R. L. and Barnard, C. N. (1982). Joint transplantation of the heart and lungs. Past experience and present potentials. *J. Cardiovasc. Surg.*, **23**, 440–52
26. Jamieson, S. W., Stinson, E. B., Oyer, P. E., Reitz, B. A., Baldwin, J., Modry, D., Dawkins, K., Theodore, J., Hunt, S. and Shumway, N. E. (1984). Heart–lung transplantation for irreversible pulmonary hypertension. *Ann. Thorac. Surg.*, **38**, 554–62
27. McGregor, C. G. A., Jamieson, S. W., Baldwin, J. C., Burke, C. M., Dawkins, K. D., Stinson, E. B., Oyer, P. E., Billingham, M. E., Zusman, D. R., Reitz, B. A., Morris, A., Yousem, S., Hunt, S. A. and Shumway, N. E. (1986). Combined heart and lung transplantation for end-stage Eisenmenger's syndrome. *J. Thorac. Cardiovasc. Surg.*, **91**, 443–50
28. Toronto Lung Transplant Group. (1986). Unilateral lung transplantation for pulmonary fibrosis. *N. Engl. J. Med.*, **314**, 1140–5
29. Jamieson, S. W., Stinson, E. B., Oyer, P. E., Baldwin, J. C. and Shumway, N. E. (1984). Operative technique for heart–lung transplantation. *J. Thorac. Cardiovasc. Surg.*, **87**, 930–5
30. McGregor, C. G. A., Baldwin, J. C., Jamieson, S. W., Billingham, M. E., Yousem, S. A., Burke, C. M., Oyer, P. E., Stinson, E. B. and Shumway, N. E. (1986). Isolated rejection after combined heart–lung transplantation. *J. Thorac. Cardiovasc. Surg.*, **91**, 443–50
31. Burke, C. M., Theodore, J., Baldwin, J. C., Tazelaar, H. D., Morris, A. J., McGregor, C. G. A., Shumway, N. E., Robin, E. D. and Jamieson, S. W. (1986). An evaluation of the results of human heart–lung transplantation. *Lancet*, **1**, 517–9
32. Burke, C. M., Morris, A. G., McGregor, C. G. A., Theodore, J., Stinson, E. B. and Jamieson, S. W. (1985). Late airflow obstruction following clinical heart–lung transplantation. *J. Heart Transpl.*, **4**, 437–40
33. Allen, M. D., Burke, C. M., McGregor, C. G. A., Baldwin, J. C., Jamieson, S. W. and Theodore, J. (1986). Steroid responsive bronchiolitis following human heart–lung transplantation. *J. Thorac. Cardiovasc. Surg.* (In press)

231

11
Pancreatic and Islet Cell Transplantation

K. ROLLES

INTRODUCTION

Since the observation by Joseph Von Mering and Oscar Minkowski in 1889 that extirpation of the pancreas of the dog resulted in diabetes mellitus[1], attempts have been made to ameliorate diabetes both in the experimental animal and latterly in man by providing the afflicted individual with normal functioning pancreatic tissue. Prior to his epochal discovery of 'isletin' (insulin) in 1922, even the thoughts of Frederic Banting seemed to feature pancreas transplantation as a likely option in the management of diabetes[2].

As the prognosis for a child newly diagnosed as diabetic was approximately one year before the discovery of insulin, R. D. Lawrence in 1925 was clearly justified in commenting, 'Now modern discoveries such as insulin have changed the outlook for the diabetic patient'[3]. However, as has been the case with so many major advances in science, the advent of insulin effectively abolished early mortality from diabetes to reveal a second generation of long-term complications which are frequently severe, progressive and life-shortening. In a cohort study in 1978, Deckert showed that 56% of an insulin-dependent diabetic population had died over a 40-year period compared with 10% of a matched non-diabetic group: 30% of these diabetics died of renal failure and 25% of myocardial disease[4].

Great improvement in the short-term results of kidney transplantation in the diabetic in renal failure has been observed and reported by several groups over the last five years. The Minneapolis group now sees no difference between diabetics and non-diabetics receiving kidney transplants over the first two years, but the problem of recurrent diabetic nephropathy in the transplant of the poorly controlled diabetic has not been overcome[5]. Compared to renal transplantation, which is merely a means of treating one established secondary complication of diabetes, pancreas transplantation is both more profound and logical. Pancreas transplantation is one approach

233

to the treatment of diabetes mellitus whereby prevention, arrest or reversal of the long-term complications of diabetes including nephropathy, retinopathy and microangiopathy is sought.

Transplantation of pancreatic tissue has been performed, both clinically and experimentally, by two different approaches. These are transplantation of the whole or part of the pancreas as a solid vascularized organ graft, which clearly includes both exocrine and endocrine components of the graft, or transplantation of the functioning insulin-producing tissue only – the islets of Langerhans.

WHOLE OR SEGEMENTAL PANCREAS TRANSPLANTATION

After almost 20 years of clinical pancreas transplantation there is still no agreement as to the optimal technique. The basic question of whether whole organ grafting is better than segmental organ grafting is still unresolved. In 1966 Kelly reported a human segmental pancreas transplant comprising body and tail of the pancreas, using the proximal splenic artery and vein as the vascular pedicle[6]. The graft functioned for six days. In 1970 Lillehei reported a series of pancreatico-duodenal grafts using the whole organ and duodenum[7]. Most of the grafts functioned briefly but morbidity and mortality were high.

Although the vast majority of vascularized pancreas grafts performed subsequently have been segmental (Figure 11.1), recently interest in whole organ grafting has arisen once again, but now usually without the duodenum. Arguments in favour of the whole organ graft seem to be currently based on the impression that there is a lower incidence of vascular thrombosis with

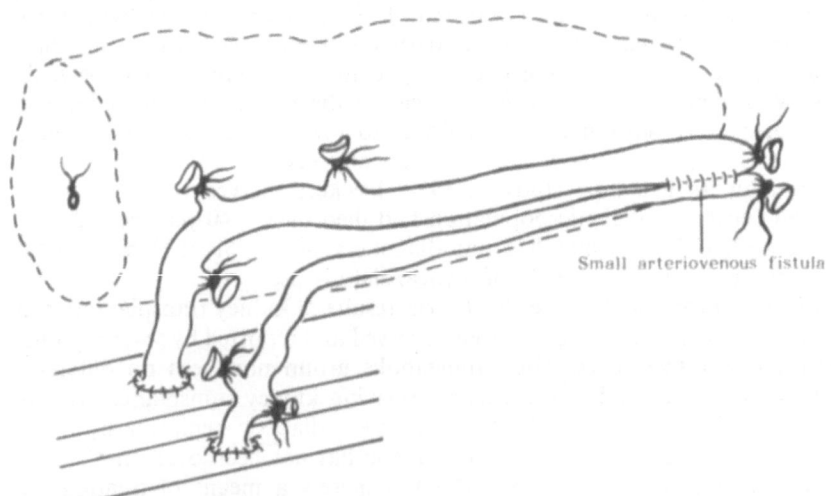

Figure 11.1 Segmental pancreas graft consisting of body and tail of the pancreas with a splenic artery and vein as the vascular pedicle

this preparation, and that the transplantation of a larger functional mass of islet tissue may be an advantage for the long-term success of the allograft in controlling carbohydrate metabolism[8].

In support of the segmental preparation is the fact that no difference has been seen in metabolic studies between whole organ and segmental grafts to date[9], and also the consideration that use of the whole organ graft currently precludes use of the donor liver for transplantation.

The main problem areas in vascularized solid organ pancreas grafting remain, as always:

(a) Thrombosis of the graft;

(b) How to deal with the exocrine secretion, and

(c) The diagnosis and treatment of rejection.

Graft thrombosis

The Pancreatic Transplant Registry, supervised by Dr Sutherland of Minneapolis, reports a technical failure rate due to graft thrombosis of approximately 20%[10], a four- or five-fold increase when compared to graft thrombosis in renal transplantation.

Following experimental studies in the dog which demonstrated that blood flow to the pancreas constituted only 18% of the coeliac artery total blood flow, the Cambridge group have created a small arteriovenous fistula between the splenic artery and splenic vein at the tail of the pancreas in order to increase the blood flow through the major vessels and across the anastomoses[11]. Despite this innovation, the graft thrombosis rate in the Cambridge series is 20%. Other workers have used subcutaneous heparin, systemic anticoagulation[12] and anti-platelet preparations such as dipyridamole and aspirin, in an attempt to reduce the incidence of vascular thrombosis, but no reports of significant improvements have appeared.

The exocrine secretion

The number of different techniques described in the management of the pancreatic duct and exocrine drainage of the pancreas graft suggests that none have proved entirely satisfactory in either the short- or the long-term post-operatively. These techniques include:

 duct ligation
 duct open (draining into peritoneal cavity)
 duct injection/occlusion
 enteric drainage (Roux loop or stomach)
 urinary drainage (ureter or bladder).

Duct ligation

This is the simplest approach and has been successful in a variety of animal models, but clinically the technique has been associated with exocrine leakage and peritonitis, and very poor early graft survival. Of 12 reported cases no graft functioned beyond four months[10]. Most workers now regard this approach as obsolete.

Open duct drainage

Open duct drainage into the peritoneal cavity has fared a little better in clinical practice. Of 15 cases, three grafts were reported functioning at 4.6–5.8 y by Sutherland, but four patients developed severe pancreatic ascites and so this technique is also regarded as obsolete[13].

Duct injection

Duct injection with neoprene to occlude the major exocrine ducts and promote atrophy of the exocrine element of the gland was popularized by Dubernard in Lyon in 1977[14]. This method has been used extensively by many other workers over the last eight years, leading to a total world experience in excess of 260 cases, more than with any other technique. Most reported series feature a high incidence of cutaneous pancreatic fistulae and wound infections, usually of a temporary nature. More recently doubts have been expressed about the long-term effects of duct injection on graft function[15]. Intense and progressive fibrosis of the gland has been linked to the duct injection technique, leading to slow failure of endocrine function at 6–24 months post-transplant or sudden graft failure due to late thrombosis. Nevertheless the early graft survival of duct-injected grafts at 30% one-year actuarial is similar to other currently used methods of duct management.

A number of different synthetic or semi-synthetic polymers have been used for duct injection as alternatives to neoprene. These include latex rubber solution, prolamine (Ethiboc, an absorbable biological glue), polydimethylsiloxane, a silicone rubber and acrylate glue. All have been associated with good early graft function both experimentally and in man, but all are also associated with subsequent fibrosis.

Enteric drainage

Early attempts to drain the exocrine secretion of pancreatico-duodenal grafts, whole organ pancreas grafts with only the papilla of Vater retained, and segmental pancreas grafts into a Roux en Y loop of recipient jejunum were disappointing and accompanied by a high morbidity and mortality.

The use of high dose steroids to prevent rejection undoubtedly had an adverse effect on enteric anastomosis healing, and in those cases where donor bowel was transplanted it is likely that this tissue was rejection more aggressively than donor pancreatic tissue.

The advent of the non-steroidal immunosuppressive cyclosporin A has led to a revival of interest in exocrine duct drainage techniques with lower morbidity and mortality and improved early results. Sutherland (1985) reports 41% (55 out of 156) one-year actuarial graft survival of segmental grafts with enteric drainage[10]. Calne has recently described duct drainage into the stomach as part of his paratopic segmental graft technique[16] (Figure

11.2) and has reported a one-year actuarial graft survival of 60% in his 14-patient series[17].

Experimentally, despite occasional evidence of mild to moderate fibrosis, histological preservation of the pancreas graft with successful duct drainage has been extremely good when compared to duct-injected grafts at similar times post-transplant.

Urinary drainage

Merkel reported end-to-side anastomosis of pancreatic duct to recipient ureter in 1973[18]. Subsequently others have advocated end-to-end duct to ureter anastomosis necessitating removal of the ipsilateral kidney[19]. More recently some groups have described direct implantation of the duct into the urinary bladder[20]. One-year actuarial graft survival for grafts with urinary tract exocrine drainage is 29% (16 out of 47) according to Sutherland (1985)[10].

There is little doubt that the short-term results of pancreas transplantation

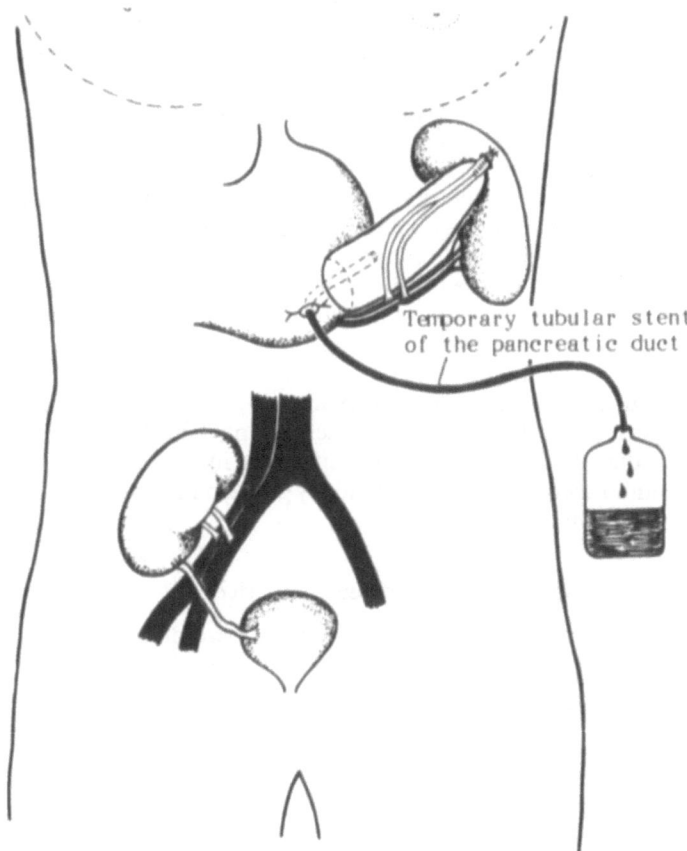

Temporary tubular stent of the pancreatic duct

Figure 11.2 'Paratopic' segmental graft (Calne, 1985) and heterotopic kidney graft

237

are slowly improving in terms of both patient and graft survival, largely irrespective of the technique of pancreatic duct management, but in securing better long-term graft survival the technique of duct management may prove crucial. It may well transpire that for continuing long-term endocrine function (> 10 y), free exocrine drainage through a permanently patent duct system will be a fundamental requirement.

The diagnosis and treatment of rejection

In clinical practice the diagnosis of rejection in the pancreatic allograft has frequently been difficult. Serum amylase estimations are of no practical value and may be elevated or low in rejection, in pancreatitis or in other intra-abdominal pathology. Percutaneous biopsy may be impractical in some cases as the graft is not as easily palpable as a kidney graft is situated in the left or right iliac fossa, and other organs or underlying large blood vessels may be at risk.

Allograft rejection histologically appears as oedema, interstitial haemorrhage and round cell infiltration, but usually there is also a significant representation of polymorphonuclear leukocytes such that rejection could be confused with infection, pancreatitis or preservation injury. The Cambridge group has found interpretation of biopsies particularly difficult in duct-injected pancreases where a vigorous 'foreign body reaction' to the polymer is occurring.

From a purely clinical standpoint we have noted in some cases that by the time glucose homeostasis has become deranged on account of immunological rejection, the damage already sustained by the grafts may be irreversible by antirejection treatment. Thus, hyperglycaemia is a late sign of allograft rejection. Consequently, it has been felt by ourselves and others that combined transplantation of kidney and segmental pancreas graft from the same organ donor may be advantageous for the diabetic in renal failure, as monitoring of renal graft function would be easier and might serve as an 'immunological barometer' for the pancreas graft. However, in the most recent report of the International Pancreas and Islet Registry, Sutherland points out that there is no significant difference in graft survival at one year between simultaneous pancreas and kidney grafts, pancreas alone, or pancreas after kidney grafts[10].

Pancreas transplantation – does it work?

This all-important question can be answered at two different levels. In terms of glucose homeostasis, it has been conclusively shown that a patient with a well-functioning pancreas allograft will have:

(a) Good control of blood glucose excursions without dietary restrictions. Twenty-four-hour blood glucose profiles will be normal or near normal.

(b) Abnormal glucose tolerance curves and an abnormal pattern of insulin release leading to a slower return of blood glucose to basal levels. We have found the glucose tolerance curves of patients with segmental pancreas grafts to be identical to those of patients who have survived a Whipple's pancreatico-duodenectomy. Thus, the minor abnormalities of glucose control may reflect a reduced islet cell mass in both these groups of patients. Glucose tolerance tests are similar whether the pancreatic graft venous effluent is drained into the systemic circulation or into the portal circulation, but plasma insulin levels are at least twice as high in those with systemic venous drainage.

(c) Return of glycosylated haemoglobin values (Hb AIC) to the normal range.

The effectiveness of pancreas transplantation in altering the natural history of the secondary complications of diabetes has to be judged according to the severity of these complications prior to transplantation.

Experimentally, the earlier changes of diabetic nephropathy in rats were shown to be reversible by Lee[21] when these kidneys were transplanted into non-diabetic animals. Conversely, normal kidneys transplanted into diabetic rats rapidly developed diabetic glomerulopathy. Pancreas transplantation has been shown to reverse or arrest kidney and eye lesions in diabetic rats.

In man, Abouna reported disappearance of early diabetic lesions from the kidneys of a young diabetic donor, when these kidneys were transplanted into non-diabetic recipients[22]. Sutherland has recently reported no progression of diabetic lesions in the transplanted kidneys of diabetics also bearing pancreas grafts, in contrast to those bearing kidney grafts alone[23].

Reports of improvement in peripheral nerve conduction times in diabetics following pancreas transplantation have emerged from the Lyon[24] and Genoa[25] groups. From the Cambridge group, Black[26] reported objective improvement in retinopathy in two patients receiving grafts, but most patients with eye problems have found a marked improvement in acuity.

Overall results

In a recent report of the International Pancreas and Islet Transplant Registry, Sutherland provided an update including cases registered in 1984[10]. Sixty institutions have reported 561 pancreas transplants in 525 patients between the years 1966 and 1984. In the last two years of the registry 295 cases have been reported, reflecting the increased worldwide interest in pancreas grafting. Current patient survival rates of 77% at one year, with graft survival of 40% at one year, represent a significant improvement in graft survival when compared to 206 cases performed in the years 1977–82 (one-year survival 20%). However, this encouraging trend has to be tempered by the fact that long-term function of a pancreas graft, i.e. $>5\,y$, has seldom been achieved. Hopefully the recent improvement in short-term survival will hold up and yield more long-term survivors, which would be a real cause for optimism.

Quite clearly, to achieve its maximum effect on the natural history of the secondary complications of diabetes mellitus, long-term function of the pancreas graft is essential. In the event of a long-term graft survival becoming easy to achieve it could be argued that, for true potential to be fulfilled, the insulin-dependent diabetic should receive a pancreatic graft very early in the course of the disease at the first sign of secondary complications. Under such circumstances, pancreas grafting would certainly be breaking new ground, as never before in the field of organ transplantation have organs been grafted prophylactically.

Graft failure

At present 60% of pancreas grafts performed will have ceased to function within the first 12 months. Twenty per cent will be early graft failures with clear evidence of graft thrombosis. Of the remaining 40%, surprisingly little will be known of the underlying causes of failure in the majority[10]. Grafts which have failed after several months of good function are frequently not surgically removed from the recipient because of the accompanying operative risk, and so complete histological studies of this large proportion of pancreas transplants are rare. Thus, the causes of graft failure are often a matter of speculation. Presumably some of these failures are attributable to immunological rejection, either acute or chronic, but the incidence is unknown. The extent to which graft fibrosis is responsible for failure is unknown as is the relationship of this fibrosis to chronic rejection, the non-patency of the ductal system, or possibly even the use of cyclosporin A as an immunosuppressant–this drug has been linked with interstitial fibrosis in kidneys, both allografts and native, and a severe fibrotic pleural reaction in some heart–lung graft recipients.

Invocation of the autoimmune mechanisms responsible for the development of diabetes mellitus in the recipient originally leading to destruction of the graft islet mass and 'recurrent disease' has been demonstrated by Sutherland in three living related segmental grafts donated by non-diabetic identical twins[27]. It may be significant that the recipients of these grafts did not receive immunosuppression, and immunosuppression might have prevented the 'recurrence'. Once more, the extent to which such factors may contribute to graft failure is unknown.

ISLET TRANSPLANTATION

As two of the major problems affecting the outcome of vascularized pancreas grafts are vascular thrombosis and exocrine duct management, the attraction of transplantation of the islets of Langerhans alone becomes only too apparent! However, although attractive in theory, the concept of islet grafting has been beset by several major problems of its own. So far, the only successful grafting of pancreatic tissue in man has been achieved using the vascularized solid organ graft.

The major problems to be overcome in islet transplantation include:

(1) Separation of islet tissue,

(2) Preservation of separated islets,

(3) Site of implantation of islet preparation, and

(4) Rejection of islet grafts.

Separation of islets

There is a marked species difference in the amount of fibrous tissue contained in the pancreas and this has a direct effect on the ease of separation of islets from the rest of the pancreatic tissue. In the rat, there is little fibrous tissue and islets are generally quite large and easily identifiable making separation relatively easy. In man, there is much more fibrous tissue and islets tend to be smaller and of variable size, making islet separation much more difficult.

Simple mechanical mincing of the whole donor pancreas results in a very impure islet preparation contained in small pancreatic fragments. Transplantation of these fragments, containing substantial quantities of exocrine tissue, has not been successful except in one report using fetal pancreata from more than 20 donors in a rat isograft model[28]. The associated exocrine enzymes tended to digest the transplant tissue and injure the recipient.

Better separation of islets from exocrine tissue can be achieved by subsequent collagenase digestion of the pancreatic fragments and implantation after thorough washing[29]. Approximately 30% of islets are recoverable by this technique. A variation on this approach is injection of the ductal system of the whole gland with collagenase solution, followed by mechanical disaggregation of the gland and repeated sieving[30]. Yields are approximately the same. These collagenase-digested preparations are usually referred to as dispersed pancreas.

A more purified preparation of 'isolated islets' can be separated from the collagenase-digested or dispersed preparation by hand-picking under the microscope or separation on a Ficoll density gradient. This preparation, with little associated exocrine tissue, is most likely to achieve engraftment when autografted or allografted, but only 5–10% of the original islet tissue is recovered necessitating multiple donors to accumulate enough islet tissue for a successful transplant.

For widespread application of islet transplantation in the clinical field, a requirement for multiple organ donors to produce a single islet graft would be impractical and better methods of islet separation are needed. A promising report from the Newcastle upon Tyne group, using one third of dispersed pancreas for each diabetic recipient in a canine autograft model gives some grounds for optimism[31].

Preservation

Preservation of islet preparations for more than 20 days can be achieved in organ culture, but functional capacity of the tissue decreases as the culture period is increased.

Methods of successful cryopreservation are emerging and cryopreservation techniques may be of assistance in improving separation of islets from unwanted pancreatic exocrine tissue.

Site of implantation

Much of the knowledge gained and obstacles identified in islet grafting have resulted from work with the rat. In the rodent many different sites of islet transplantation have been used successfully including subcutaneous, intraperitoneal, intrathoracic, under the kidney capsule, in the testis, into the portal vein, and into the spleen. Intraportal infusion seemed to be the most successful. Complete amelioration of diabetes was not possible with the subcutaneous or intramuscular sites[32].

Rejection

Using the rat isograft model, Ballinger and Lacy have demonstrated that 400–600 isolated islets can permanently ameliorate diabetes[32]. Later Mirkovitch and Campiche showed that, following total pancreatectomy, dogs could be rendered normoglycaemic by autotransplantation to the spleen of a single collagenase-digested (dispersed) pancreas[33]. In man, pancreatectomy for chronic pancreatitis followed by islet autotransplantation has been performed by a number of workers. Most successful grafts have functioned adequately for only a few months but some long-term successes are emerging[34]. However, islet tissue allografts in higher mammals have so far been extremely disappointing. The International Pancreas and Islet Transplant Registry reported 169 human islet allografts up until mid-1983. None of the recipients are currently insulin independent[10]. By extrapolation from work in animal models, the persistent failure of human islet transplantation has been attributed to rejection, phagocytosis, inadequate islet cell mass, and the possibility of recurrent disease. Rat allograft experiments have shown that isolated islets are rejected more quickly than whole organ or segmental pancreas grafts performed in the same strain combinations[35]. Macrophages clearly have an important role in the rapid destruction of the islet allograft, as poisoning of the host reticulo-endothelial system has been shown to be more effective than any other post-transplant immunosuppressive drug regimen in prolonging the survival of islet allografts in the rat[36].

The concept of reducing the immunogenicity of potential islet allografts has now been established by Lacy[37], Lafferty[38], Scharp[39] and other workers and raises hope for the future of clinical islet transplantation. Several methods have been described which have the common end result of eliminating those cells in the donor preparation which provide the allogeneic stimulus to the host immune system. These 'dendritic' cells and possibly other unidentified cell types could be selectively destroyed by donor pretreatment with cyclophosphamide, by prolonged organ culture in an oxygen-rich atmosphere, pretreatment of the donor graft with anti-Ia serum and complement, or ultraviolet irradiation of donor tissue. In many of these fascinating experiments, functional islet allografts have survived without any post-transplant immunosuppression and donor specific tolerance has been observed. The preoccupation of many workers worldwide is the translation of these remarkable achievements in the rodent to the field of clinical application.

References

1. Von Merin, J. and Minkowski, O. (1890). Diabetes mellitus nach pancreasextirpation. *Arch. Exp. Pathol. Pharmacol.*, **26**, 371–87
2. Bliss, M. (1982). *The Discovery of Insulin*, p. 52 (Edinburgh: Paul Harris)
3. Lawrence, R. D. (1925). *The Diabetic Life*. 1st Edn. (London: J. A. Churchill)
4. Deckert, T., Poulsen, J. E. and Larsen, M. (1978). Prognosis of diabetics with diabetes onset before the age of 31. *Diabetologia*, **14**, 363–77
5. Sutherland, D. E. R., Fryd, D. S., Payne, W. D., Ascher, N., Simmons, R. L. and Najarian, J. S. (1985). Renal transplantation in diabetics at the University of Minnesota. *Diab. Nephrop.*, **4**, (No. 3), 123–6
6. Kelly, W. D., Lillehei, R. C., Merkel, F. K., Idezuki, Y. and Goetz, F. C. (1967). Allotransplantation of pancreas and duodenum along with the kidney in diabetic nephropathy. *Surgery*, **61**, 827–33
7. Lillehei, R. C., Simmons, R. L. and Najarian, J. S. (1970). Pancreaticoduodenal allotransplantation: experimental and clinical experience. *Ann. Surg.*, **172**, 405–36
8. Sutherland, D. E. R., Chinn, P. L., Elick, B. A. and Najarian, J. S. (1984). Maximisation of islet mass in pancreatic grafts by near total or total whole organ excision without the duodenum from cadaver donors. *Transplant. Proc.*, **16**, 115–9
9. Sutherland, D. E. R., Goetz, F. C. and Najarian, J. S. (1984). One hundred pancreas transplants at a single institution. *Ann. Surg.*, **200**, 414–38
10. Sutherland, D. E. R. and Kendall, D. (1985). A report of the International Pancreas and Islet Registry: cases submitted through 1984. *Diab. Nephrop.*, **4** (No. 3), 154–8
11. Calne, R. Y., McMaster, P., Rolles, K. and Duffy, T. J. (1980). Technical observations in segmental pancreas allografting: observations on pancreatic blood flow. *Transplant. Proc.*, **12** (Suppl. 2), 51–7
12. Groth, C. G., Lundren, G., Wilczek, H., Klintmalm, G., Tyden, G., Gunnarsson, R. and Ostman, J. (1984). Segmental pancreas transplantation with duct ligature or enteric diversion: technial aspects. (No effect of Warfarin on graft thrombosis.) *Transplant. Proc.*, **16** (No. 3), 724–8
13. Sutherland, D. E. R., Goetz, F. C. and Najarian, J. S. (1985). Experience with pancreas transplants at the University of Minnesota. *Diab. Nephrop.*, **4**, 149–53
14. Dubernard, J. M., Traeger, J. and Neyra, P. (1978). A new method of preparation of segmental pancreatic grafts for transplantation: trials in dogs and in man. *Surgery*, **84**, 633–9
15. Liu, T., Sutherland, D. E. R., Heil, J., Dunning, M. and Najarian, J. S. (1985). Beneficial effects of establishing pancreatic duct drainage into a hollow organ (bladder, jejunum, stomach) compared to free intraperitoneal drainage or duct injection. *Transplant. Proc.*, **17** (No. 1), 366–71
16. Calne, R. Y. and Brons, I. G. M. (1985). Observations on paratopic pancreas grafting with splenic venous drainage. *Transplant. Proc.*, **17** (No. 1), 340–1
17. Brons, I. G. M., Calne, R. Y., Rolles, K., Olczak, S. and Evans, D. B. (1986). Paratopic segmental pancreas with simultaneous kidney transplantation in man: a one year follow up study. *Transplant. Proc.*, (In press)
18. Merkel, F. K., Ryan, W. G. and Armbrusler, K. (1973). Pancreatic transplantation for diabetes mellitus. *Illinois Med. J.*, **144**, 477–9
19. Gliedman, M. L., Trellis, V. A., Sobermann, R. (1978). Long term effects of pancreatic transplantation in patients with advanced juvenile onset diabetes mellitus. *Diab. Care*, **1**, 1–9
20. Sollinger, H. W., Kalayoglu, M., Hoffman, R. M. and Belzer, F. O. (1985). Results of segmental and pancreaticosplenic transplantation with pancreaticocystostomy. *Transplant. Proc.*, **17**, (No. 1), 360–2

21. Lee, C. S., Mauer, S. M. and Brown, D. M. (1974). Renal transplantation in diabetes mellitus in rats. *J. Exp. Med.*, **139**, 793–800

22. Abouna, G. M., Kremer, G. B. and Daddaw, S. K. (1983). Reversal of diabetic nephropathy in human cadaveric kidneys after transplantation into non-diabetic recipients. *Lancet*, **2**, 1274–76

23. Sutherland, D. E. R., Najarian, J. S. and Greenberg, B. I. (1981). Hormone and metabolic effects of a pancreas endocrine graft. *Ann. Intern. Med.*, **95**, 537–41

24. Traeger, J., Dubernard, J. M., Ruitton, A. M., Malik, M. C. and Touraine, J. L. (1981). Clinical experience with 15 neoprene injected pancreatic allografts in man. *Transplant. Proc.*, **13**, 298–304

25. Valente, U., Barabino, C. and Barocci, S. (1985). Segmental pancreatic transplantation in diabetics: follow up of eight patients. *Transplant. Proc.*, **17**, 349–52

26. Black, P. D. (1981). Visual studies of diabetic patients after pancreatic transplantation. *Trans. Ophthalmol. Soc. UK*, **101**, 100–4

27. Sutherland, D. E. R., Sibley, R. K. and Chinn, P. L. (1984). Identical twin pancreas transplants: reversal and recurrence of pathogenesis of Type I diabetes. *Clin. Res.*, **32**(2), 561A

28. Usadel, K. H., Schwedes, U. and Lenacker, U. (1974). Development of isologous transplants of cell suspensions of the fetal pancreas in the rat. *Acta Endocrinol. (Copenhagen)*, **84** (Suppl. 205), 97

29. Moskalewski, S. (1965). Isolation and culture of the Islets of Langerhans of the guinea pig. *Gen. Comp. Endocrinol.*, **5**, 342

30. Lacy, P. E. and Kostianovsky, M. (1967). Method for the isolation of intact Islets of Langerhans from the rat pancreas. *Diabetes*, **16**, 35

31. Griffin, S. M., Alderson, D. and Farndon, J. R. (1986). An improved harvesting technique for pancreatic islet transplantation. *Transplant. Proc.*, (In press)

32. Ballinger, W. F. and Lacy, P. E. (1972). Transplantation of intact pancreatic islets in rats. *Surgery*, **72**, 175–86

33. Mirkovitch, V., Campiche, M. (1977). Intrasplenic allotransplantation of canine pancreatic tissues. Maintenance of normoglycaemia after total pancreatectomy. *Eur. Surg. Res.*, **9**, 173–90

34. Valente, U., Arcuri, V. and Barocci, S. (1985). Islet and segmental pancreatic autotransplantation after pancreatectomy: follow up of 25 patients for up to 5 years. *Transplant. Proc.*, **17**, 363–5

35. Perloff, L. J., Naji, A. and Silvers, W. K. (1980). Whole pancreas vs isolated islet transplantations: an immunological comparison. *Surgery*, **88**, 222–30

36. Bell, P. R., Wood, R. F., Peters, M. and Nash, J. R. (1980). Comparison of various methods of chemical immunosuppression in islet cell transplantation. *Transplant. Proc.*, **12**, 291–3

37. Lacy, P. E., Davie, J. M. and Finke, E. H. (1979). Prolongation of islet allograft survival following *in vitro* culture (24°C) and a single dose of ALS. *Science*, **204**, 312–3

38. Lafferty, K. J., Prowse, S. J. and Simeonovic, C. J. (1984). Current status of experimental islet transplantation. *Transplant. Proc.*, **16**, 813–9

39. Scharp, D. W. (1984). Clinical feasibility of Islet transplantation. *Transplant. Proc.*, **16**, 820–5

12
Problems of the Immunosuppressed Patient

S. C. GLOVER

Since the early 1950s renal transplantation has evolved from an experimental procedure into an acceptable and effective treatment for irreversible or end-stage renal disease. The one-year patient survival rate for recipients from living related donors is greater than 95% and greater than 90% for recipients from cadaveric donors. The one-year graft survival rates are greater than 85% and 65% respectively. These excellent results have been attained by a variety of advances in a number of different areas (Table 12.1).

Notwithstanding these advances in the management of renal transplant

Table 12.1 Factors influencing the outcome of renal transplantation

(1) Accurate tissue typing and matching of donor kidney to potential recipient:
    effect – reduced incidence of acute kidney rejection.

(2) Pretransplant recipient care including treatment of urinary tract infection, screening for helminthic infection and pretransplantation blood transfusion.

(3) Careful selection of donor kidney, preferably from CMV seronegative donor. Optimum donor organ preservation.

(4) Improved surgical techniques.

(5) Changes of immunosuppressive therapy:
    less anti-thymocyte globulin, more use of cyclosporin A.

(6) Prevention, prompt investigation and specific therapy of opportunistic infection.

recipients, infections are still a major cause of morbidity and mortality occurring in more than 80% of patients[1].

Cardiac, liver, pancreas and heart–lung transplantation are less well established procedures but advances can be expected in patient and graft survival rates using the experience gained from both renal and bone marrow transplantation programmes. This chapter addresses the major infections complicating renal transplantation and makes some reference to those infections also occurring in bone marrow transplant recipients.

RENAL TRANSPLANTATION

General principles

There are four major factors which contribute to the pathogenesis of infection in renal transplant recipients:

(1) The transplant operation itself with potential contamination of the renal tract;

(2) The need for post-operative catheterization of the bladder;

(3) The need for immunosuppressive therapy to prevent kidney rejection; and

(4) The patient's presence in a hospital environment with potential exposure to multi-resistant Gram negative bacilli and other environmental opportunistic pathogens.

Immunosuppressive therapy with corticosteroids and azathioprine has a profound effect on the efficiency of the *cell-mediated* arm of the patient's immune defences[2], in particular impairing the T lymphocyte–macrophage interaction. This results in an increased susceptibility to infection with intracellular pathogens as summarized in Table 12.2. Cyclosporin A has a subtle effect on cell-mediated immunity by inhibiting T cell-dependent B cell activation, expansion of unprimed T helper and cytotoxic T cell subsets and gamma interferon production.Whether the incidence of post-transplant opportunistic infection is reduced in patients maintained on cyclosporin A remains to be evaluated.

Table 12.2 Common intracellular pathogens associated with impaired cell-mediated immunity and therapeutic immunosuppression

Bacteria	Protozoa	Fungi	Viruses
Mycobacterium tuberculosis	Pneumocystis carinii	Aspergillus spp.	Cytomegalovirus
Atypical mycobacteria	Toxoplasma gondii	Candida spp.	Herpes simplex,
Nocardia asteroides		Phycomycetes	I and II
Listeria monocytogenes		Cryptococcus	Herpes varicella
Legionella pneumophila		neoformans	zoster
Legionella micdadei			Epstein–Barr virus
Salmonella spp.			

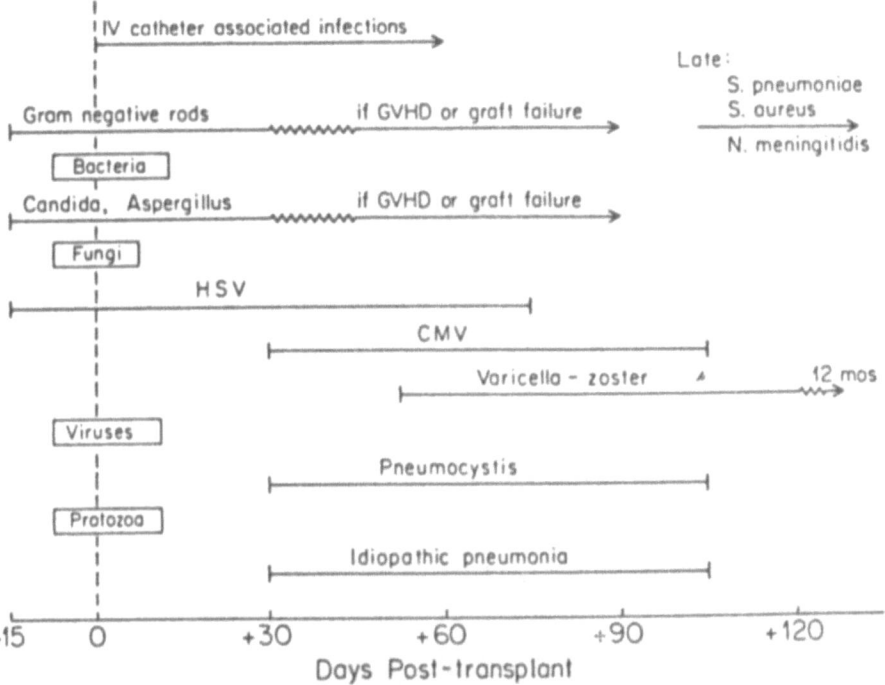

Figure 12.1 Timetable for the occurrence of infection in the renal transplant patient. From Young[91], with kind permission of the author and Academic Press

Taking these four factors into consideration it is possible to construct a dynamic timetable or pattern of opportunistic infections arising around and after both renal and bone marrow transplantation. These timetables (Figures 12.1 and 12.2) serve as a useful aide-memoire for the multiple potential infections which arise at varying intervals after transplantation. It can be seen from this temporal chart that the major causes of infection occurring in the first month of renal transplantation are bacterial wound, pulmonary, urinary tract or intravenous access site related infections. Nosocomial hospital-acquired infection also occurs at this stage but opportunistic fungal and protozoal infections are rare. Between one and six months post-transplant, the risks of life-threatening opportunistic fungal, viral, bacterial and protozoan infections are increased, occurring at a time when the therapeutic immunosuppression is at its most intense and cytomegalovirus (CMV) infection, itself a potent immunosuppressive agent, is most frequent. Beyond 6 months, when immunosuppressive therapy is at a low and maintenance level, the infection problems are the chronic virus infections such as virus hepatitis, chronic CMV retinitis, the occasional *Cryptococcus neoformans* infection and a continuing risk of the more banal, everyday chance infections such as pneumococcal pneumonia, influenza A virus and Gram negative urinary tract infection.

Although this timetable is a useful differential diagnostic index for the

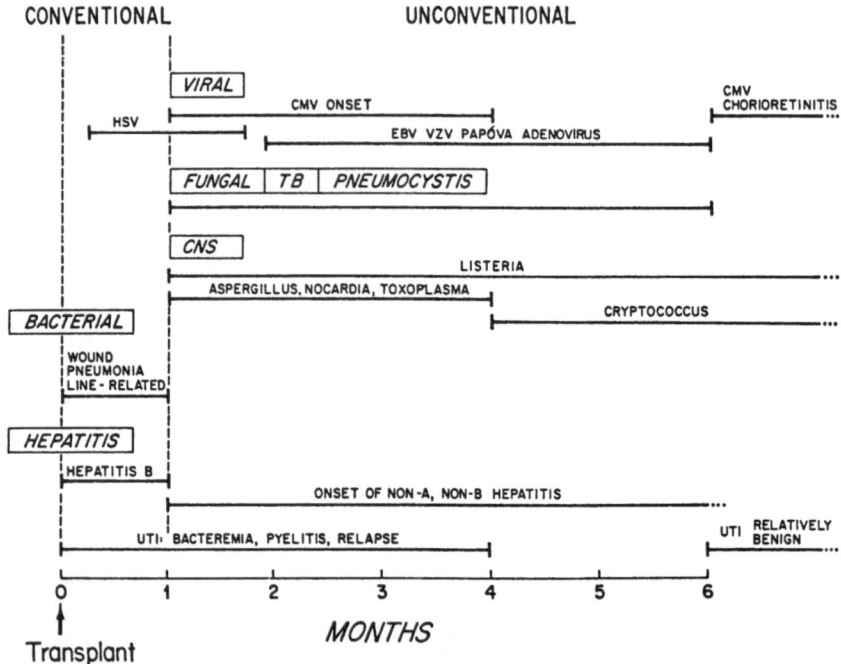

Figure 12.2 Timetable for the occurrence of infection in the bone marrow transplant recipient, with kind permission of the Editor, *American Journal of Medicine.*

clinician facing a febrile or a non-febrile but ill patient at any time post-transplantation, it must be remembered that the immunosuppressive therapy may itself attenuate and mask the clinical signs and symptoms of potentially lethal infection. A 'high index of suspicion' and the courage to investigate such patients aggressively will allow an early diagnosis and prompt initiation of specific therapy. It should also be remembered that fever in the immunosuppressed patient post-transplant may not be an indicator of active infection but a clue to some other non-infective pathological process such as acute graft rejection or malignancy.

A further set of factors must be carefully considered in the febrile or ill post-transplant patient, namely the patient's immediate environment. Major differences exist between various transplantation units regarding the frequency and type of surgical wound, urinary tract and respiratory tract infections. Such differences are influenced by the local surgical techniques and expertise, the type of peri-operative and post-operative antimicrobial chemoprophylaxis employed within the unit, and the microbiological milieu of the hospital at large. For example, an unusually high rate of *Pseudomonas aeruginosa* bronchopulmonary infection was recorded in a group of renal transplant patients on the same floor as patients with serious burns complicated by *Pseudomonas aeruginosa* infection. Removal of the transplant patients to a separate site and away from the burns patients stopped this

248

nosocomial spread of pseudomonas infection to the transplant patients[3]. Similarly, colonization and subsequent infection with troublesome antibiotic resistant gram negative bacilli such as *Klebsiella* spp. *Serratia marcescens* and *Acinetobacter* remain a potential and serious threat to the immunosuppressed patient.

Legionella pneumophila infection, originating from water sources and appliances within the transplant unit, has recently been described and eradicated by attention to water temperature and chlorination levels[4-7]. It is highly likely that *Pneumocystis carinii* pneumonia[8] and *Legionella micdadei* infections have also occurred nosocomially on transplant units[9]. The early occurrence of Aspergillus infection within the first month should alert the clinician to the likelihood of an environmental source of this pathogenic fungus[10,11].

Types of infection encountered in renal transplant recipients

Systemic infections

Certain types of infection commonly present in the post-transplant patient with systemic symptoms such as fever, malaise and general deterioration without any focal clues or signs to help specify the aetiology. Both polymicrobial bacteraemia and fungaemia may present in this way with dissemination to multiple internal organs and skin occurring later. The most common cause of fever and malaise in the 1st to 6th months post-transplant is cytomegalovirus disease[12].

Cytomegalovirus (CMV) infection is the most common cause of systemic infection after renal transplantation when up to 60% of seronegative recipients and 90% of seropositive recipients show serological or clinical evidence of CMV infection at any time between 2 weeks and 6 months post-transplant[13]. There are two main epidemiological patterns of CMV disease:

(1) *Reactivation* of latent CMV is the more common, occurring among patients who were seropositive before receiving their renal transplant. This type of CMV disease is less severe than the primary infection, only 20–25% of patients requiring hospital admission[14].

(2) *Primary cytomegalovirus infection* occurs in recipients who were known to be CMV seronegative before transplantation. Since primary CMV infection is rare in seronegative recipients given kidneys from seronegative donors, it is inferred that, in primary CMV infection, the source of the virus is the donor kidney[15]. More convincing evidence of this mode of transmission has been reported by Orsi who isolated virus from donor kidneys[16], whilst Wertheim and colleagues, using DNA restriction enzyme analysis, showed that two recipients of kidneys from the same donor excreted CMV strains with identical DNA profiles[17]. Primary CMV infection is a more severe illness, 65–75% of patients requiring in-patient hospital care.

CMV infection may be *covert* (asymptomatic) especially in reactivation of latent infection. All these patients will excrete CMV in the urine and exhibit a rise in CMV antibody titres. Patient to patient spread of this virus is very rare despite cytomegalovirus viruria. *Overt* CMV infection may be classified into three groups:

(1) CMV infection with fever, interstitial pneumonitis, hepatitis, leukopenia, thrombocytopenia, pancreatitis, gastrointestinal ulceration and haemorrhage, retinitis and adrenalitis;

(2) CMV-induced immunosuppression and leukopenia which compounds the therapeutic immunosuppression. This may be associated with a reduction of the T helper/inducer lymphocyte to T suppressor/cytotoxic lymphocyte ratio[18,19].

(3) Impairment of renal allograft function, the renal impairment being due to a diffuse glomerulopathy with interstitial changes[20]. These patients have CMV viraemia, may have a reduced T helper lymphocyte to T suppressor lymphocyte ratio and may require a reduction in the degree of immunosuppressive therapy.

As CMV infection causes considerable morbidity and mortality, steps must be taken to prevent it. Careful matching of donor and recipient is the ideal and whenever feasible, kidneys from seropositive donors should not be transplanted to seronegative recipients. In reality, there is a shortage of donor kidneys in the UK and as many as 50% of UK donors are seropositive for CMV. This places a finite limit on the primary prevention of CMV infection post-transplantation.

Because CMV infections are secondary to immunosuppression, it may be possible to reduce the intensity of therapeutic immunosuppression and thus the incidence of this infection. In a randomized, controlled trial of high-dose prednisolone and azathioprine versus low-dose prednisolone with azathioprine over two years, Morris showed that patient and graft survival were identical but that there was a significant reduction of the steroid-associated infection rate[21]. Many transplant centres now use cyclosporin A with or without corticosteroids as a first-line immunosuppressive agent but the European Multicentre Trial Group have not shown any difference in the prevalence of bacterial, fungal or viral infection between patients treated with cyclosporin A and azathioprine–corticosteroid treated patients[22]. In the Canadian Transplant Study Group's trial of 69 patients who received cadaveric renal allografts, the one-year cumulative graft survival was 88% in patients treated with cyclosporin A alone and 84% in those given additional corticosteroids, although the incidence of opportunistic infection was not significantly different[23]. Cyclosporin A immunosuppression has also been associated with the development of malignant tumours – usually lymphoproliferative lesions in association with Epstein–Barr virus infection. Starzl and colleagues have described 17 such lymphoproliferative tumours in recipients of renal, liver, heart and heart–lung transplants. These lesions respond poorly to IV acyclovir but have regressed on reducing or stopping the immunosuppression[24].

Passive immunoprophylaxis with CMV-immune plasma or globulin has been used in an attempt to decrease the incidence of primary CMV and its consequences in recipients of bone marrow and renal transplants.

Meyers found significantly less CMV infection in bone marrow transplant recipients treated with immune serum globulin provided the granulocyte transfusion donors were CMV-seronegative[25], while Winston documented no difference in the incidence of CMV infection in either group[26]. Condie treated 52 renal transplant recipients with high titre globulin in an uncontrolled trial and showed some clinical improvement[27]. More recently the same group, in a randomized controlled trial of IV hyperimmune native CMV globulin, prevented CMV infection for 120 days after bone marrow transplantation[28].

Another preventative option against CMV infection is active immunization using CMV vaccine. In a study of 91 renal transplant recipients using the Towne strain of live attentuated cytomegalovirus vaccine and a placebo given eight weeks before renal transplantation, Plotkin showed that although CMV infection occurred in 26 of the 30 (87%) seronegative vaccinees or placebo-treated patients who had received kidneys from seropositive donors, the infection caused by CMV was much less severe in the vaccinees than in the placebo-treated patients[29]. The Towne strain CMV vaccine was well-tolerated in these renal transplant recipients and did not induce vaccine virus excretion. Immunosuppressive therapy after transplantation did not reactivate the vaccine virus from a theoretical latent state, as vaccinated patients who received kidneys from seronegative donors showed no evidence of Towne CMV excretion post-transplantation. In addition renal transplantation from seropositive donors was followed by non-vaccine CMV excretion as shown by restriction endonuclease assays. The use of subunit, non-replicating CMV vaccine is the next phase of this active immunoprophylaxis programme.

The efficacy of acyclovir in the prevention of CMV disease has been assessed mainly in bone marrow transplant recipients. Saral gave IV acyclovir $250 \, \text{mg/m}^2$ or placebo for 18 days, commencing 3 days before bone marrow transplantation: 50% of acyclovir-treated patients and 70% of placebo-treated patients were CMV seropositive and, during the follow-up period, CMV was cultured from four acyclovir recipients and from two placebo recipients[30]. Hann has documented similar lack of effect of acyclovir in preventing CMV infection[31]. Gluckman, on the other hand, using oral acyclovir 200 mg 6-hourly from 8 days before to 35 days after bone marrow transplantation, observed no incidence of CMV infection until acyclovir therapy was stopped[32].

Hirsch used α-interferon 3×10^6 units intramuscularly before renal transplantation, then three times a week for 6 weeks, and twice a week for a further 8 weeks, in CMV positive recipients, and showed less overt CMV disease in the interferon-treated group during the treatment period but no effect on asymptomatic/covert CMV infection as reflected in CMV viraemia and viruria[33].

Acyclovir has been used to treat overt CMV disease in immunocompromized patients. Using IV acyclovir $500 \, \text{mg/m}^2$ 8-hourly for 7 days versus placebo in 16 immunocompromised patients with overt CMV infection, Balfour found that acyclovir recipients improved more quickly with a more rapid defervescence than the control patients[34]. This relative lack of acyclovir effect in CMV disease is not surprising given the *in vitro* resistance of CMV to acyclovir[35].

9-(1,3-Dihydroxy-2-propoxymethyl)-guanine (DHPG) inhibits viral replication *in vitro* of all human herpes viruses including CMV. In CMV-infected cells, DHPG is phosphorylated to DHPG-monophosphate by a cellular deoxyguanosine kinase, then further phosphorylated to the triphosphate by other cellular enzymes. The DHPG-triphosphate competitively inhibits binding of deoxyguanosine triphosphate to DNA polymerase, inhibiting DNA synthesis and also terminating DNA elongation. The collaborative DHPG treatment study group reported their preliminary findings in the treatment of severe CMV infection in severely immunocompromised patients. 84% of those with CMV retinitis and 62% of those with gastrointestinal involvement showed some clinical improvement, while CMV pneumonitis was much less responsive. Neutropenia is the major limiting side effect of this new drug[36].

Trisodium phosphonoformate (foscarnet), a virostatic broad spectrum antiviral drug, has been given to several patients with severe CMV disease. Ringden reported the use of foscarnet in 35 transplant recipients: all nine bone marrow transplant recipients with CMV pneumonitis died but better results were obtained in 19 renal transplant recipients where four out of six with CMV pneumonitis survived[37]. Foscarnet is currently under further investigation.

The major features of overt CMV disease occurring in renal transplant recipients are summarized in Table 12.3.

Skin and wound infection

The skin and subcutaneous tissues of the immunocompromised host have several important functions. Firstly, its major role is as a physical barrier to opportunistic invasion by micro-organisms. Secondly, its rich blood supply makes it a frequent and readily visible site of metastatic spread of infection both from the skin as well as to the skin from internal organs and the blood stream. In this latter respect, the skin can serve as an early warning or alarm for systemic opportunistic infection. Thirdly, skin infection is a common problem and potentially life-threatening in immunosuppressed patients with a frequency of 22–23%[38].

During transplantation surgery the physical barrier of the skin is breached with the potential risk of surgical wound infections, both superficial and deep. However, with improved surgical technique and expertise, superficial wound infections and deep transplant wound infections due to leakage from the urinary tract have become uncommon early complications of renal transplantation. Most of this improvement can be attributed to the skilled surgical techniques, the pre-operative management of lower urinary tract infection, and the careful use of peri-operative antimicrobial chemoprophylaxis[39].

Table 12.3 Overt cytomegalovirus infection in renal transplantation

Clinical complications	Predisposing factors
Fatigue, rigors, headache, arthralgia, myalgia, fever	Seropositive donor
	Seropositive recipient
High fatality rate dissemination: lung gastrointestinal tract with ulceration and haemorrhage pancreas liver	Parent or cadaver kidney donor Inaccurate HLA-matching
Other opportunist infection: gram negative bacilli *Pneumocystis carinii* fungi	
Neutropenia	
Transplant rejection/dysfunction	

Diabetic renal transplant recipients who often have small vessel disease and/or peripheral neuropathy, and whose diabetic control may be upset by concomitant corticosteroid therapy, are prone to mixed aerobic/anaerobic cellulitis and soft tissue infection of the lower limbs. When surgical debridement and antimicrobial chemotherapy fail, then amputation of the ischaemic/ infected extremity is mandatory.

Wolfson and his colleagues, in a retrospective review of the cutaneous infections seen in immunocompromized patients, reported 31 episodes of cutaneous infection over 12 years. Twenty-two of these episodes arose in renal transplant recipients[40]. The results are summarized in Table 12.4. The gross morphology of the skin lesions associated with infection in the immunocompromised host was never pathognomonic and thus early skin biopsy for histological, microbiological and fungal culture is essential if the full benefits of these early warning signs are to be realized. 'Transplant elbow' refers to the *Staphylococcus aureus* cellulitis of the elbow, induced by steroid-associated skin thinning, a profound steroid-induced lower limb myopathy

Table 12.4 Cutaneous infections and the immunocompromised host[40]: breakdown of 31 episodes

Bacterial/atypical mycobacteria (11 episodes)	Fungi (17 episodes)	Viruses/algae (3 episodes)
E. coli	Aspergillus	Papilloma virus
Pseudomonas aeruginosa – ecthyma gangrenosum	Candida tropicalis	Prototheca
Group A Streptococci – cellulitis	Cryptococcus neoformans	
Staphylococcus aureus – 'transplant elbow'	Rhizopus	
Nocardia asteroides	Phycomyces	
Mycobacterium cheloni	Trichophyton spp.	
Mycobacterium marinum		

and the need to push with the elbows when attempting to sit up in bed.

The main viral causes of cutaneous infection in the immunosuppressed are papillomavirus, herpes simplex (HSV) and herpes varicella zoster virus (HVZV). Papillomavirus, the cause of warts in normal people, may produce extensive verrucous lesions in as many as 40% of patients after renal transplantation[38]. Malignant transformation to squamous cell carcinoma has been described[41].

More common than papillomavirus infection are primary and recrudescent HSV and HVZV infections[42]. Renal, cardiac and bone marrow transplant recipients frequently excrete HSV-1 from the oropharynx whilst immunosuppressed, but remain asymptomatic. Localized nasolabial or anogenital infections caused by HSV occur in up to 50% of such immunosuppressed patients. Occasionally HSV-1 may cause bronchopulmonary and oesophageal infection especially when endotracheal intubation or nasogastric intubation has been used.

Large ulcerated lesions around the mouth and anus known as herpes phagenda may interfere with eating and bladder and rectal functions as well as serving as a potential point of entry for secondary bacterial infection. These severe herpes simplex infections may be prevented by[43] or treated with acyclovir[44].

Medical staff must avoid direct contact with potentially infective HSV-1 lesions and are strongly advised to wear gloves and plastic aprons when handling such patients. Patients with disseminated cutaneous HSV infection or eczema herpeticum must be isolated in a single room.

Recrudescent herpes varicella zoster virus (shingles) with or without dissemination to lungs, liver and central nervous system occurs in up to 10% of renal transplant recipients and in about 50% of bone marrow transplant recipients, in whom a third have evidence of disseminated varicella zoster and a quarter a generalized recurrent chickenpox-like illness[45]. Although acyclovir and vidarabine reduce the risk of cutaneous and visceral dissemination in immunosuppressed patients with herpes zoster, a recent study has shown that acyclovir is more effective than vidarabine, not only in the prevention of dissemination of HVZV but also in the promotion of skin healing and pain relief[46]. In that study renal insufficiency developed in three out of eleven acyclovir-treated patients but the contribution of the potentially nephrotoxic agent, cyclosporin A, cannot be excluded.

Passive immunization with zoster immune globulin (ZIG) should be given intramuscularly to prevent primary varicella zoster infection in immunocompromised patients. Varicella zoster is highly contagious and may remain so in immunosuppressed patients as long as crusted lesions are visible. Strict isolation of infected patients is essential if they cannot be safely discharged from hospital.

Urinary tract infection

Bacterial urinary tract infection in renal transplant recipients has been reported with a variable incidence of 35–79% and is frequently the source of Gram negative bacteraemia. The incidence of urinary tract infection after renal transplantation has been reduced by careful treatment of pre-operative infection and considered use of peri-operative antimicrobial chemotherapy. Avoiding and correcting obstructive structural lesions of the kidney drainage has contributed to a reduced incidence of urinary tract infection.

The timing of the post-transplant urinary tract infection must also be considered: infection occurring 6 months or more post-transplantation may be regarded as relatively harmless and may be treated with a 10–14 day course of antimicrobial chemotherapy, these late infections are rarely associated with bacteraemia and have an excellent prognosis. By contrast, urinary tract infection occurring within 3 months of renal transplantation is frequently complicated by symptomatic pyelonephritis, bacteraemia, renal graft dysfunction and an increased incidence of graft rejection. Treatment with bactericidal antimicrobial chemotherapy is essential and should be prolonged for 6 weeks at least[47]. In an attempt to prevent this early and serious form of post-transplant urinary tract infection a recent randomized controlled study of oral co-trimoxazole forte prescribed at the time of catheter removal and continued for the first four months post-transplant proved effective in reducing the risk of Gram negative bacterial urinary tract infection and bacteraemia[48]. In post-transplant patients presenting with recurrent urinary tract infections, the presence of an obstructive structural or functional lesion such as ureteral stricture or ureteral reflux must be excluded.

Urinary excretion of papovavirus, in particular the polyoma virus BK, is common after renal transplantation. Although this may be completely asymptomatic the onset of ureteral stricture or obstruction and renal allograft dysfunction has been associated with these viruses[49]. More recently haemorrhagic cystitis has been attributed to the polyoma BK virus in bone marrow transplantation[50].

Bronchopulmonary infections

Bronchopulmonary infection was identified in the early days of transplantation surgery as a life-threatening cause of inflammatory lung disease. The potential causes of pulmonary inflammation in the immunosuppressed host range from the banal viral and bacterial pathogens to the exotic and unusual fungi and protozoans. This range of named species causing opportunistic lung infection in the immunosuppressed host is shown in Table 12.5. The differential diagnosis of fever and new pulmonary infiltrates in a post-transplant patient includes non-infective causes of lung shadowing such as pulmonary emboli and infarction, pulmonary haemorrhage, pulmonary oedema, radiation pneumonitis, drug-induced pulmonary disease and non-specific interstitial pneumonitis. Many factors influence the likelihood of a specific pathogen being responsible for the pulmonary infiltrate. These incude the duration between transplantation and the onset of pulmonary signs and symptoms; the intensity of current immunosuppression; an exposure history; presence of nosocomial infection; and infection patterns within the institution.

Ramsey reviewed 227 renal transplant recipients and found 54 patients with fever and pulmonary infiltrates, 27 of whom died as a result of their pulmonary infection[51]. In 36 (66%) there was an infection present: 12 of

Table 12.5 Opportunistic pathogens causing bronchopulmonary infection in immunosuppressed patients

Bacteria	Fungi	Protozoa	Viruses
Streptococcus pneumoniae	Aspergillus	Pneumocystis carinii	CMV
Pseudomonas spp.	Candida	Toxoplasma gondii	Herpes simplex
Serratia marcescens	Cryptococcus		Herpes varicella
Nocardia asteroides	neoformans		zoster
Mycobacteria spp.	Phycomycetes		Adenovirus
Listeria monocytogenes	Coccidioidomycosis		
Legionella spp.			

these were bacterial, predominantly Gram negative bacilli; eight *Nocardia asteroides*; five *Aspergillus fumigatus*; one *Cryptococcus neoformans* and one *Pneumocystis carinii*. There were nine viral infections, eight of them CMV. In 28% of patients the primary process was either pulmonary embolism or pulmonary oedema, and in 6% no objective cause was identified. Superinfection with organisms such as gram negative bacilli, *Candida albicans*, *Torulopsis glabrata* and herpes simplex occurred in 42% of patients, many of whom had a coincidental CMV pneumonitis and accompanying leukopenia. The vast majority (96%) of the secondarily infected patients died.

CMV pneumonitis is the most common cause of fever and a major cause of death in renal transplant recipients. It begins 1–4 months after transplantation and presents with fever, unproductive cough, dyspnoea and hypoxia as well as constitutional upset including myalgia and arthralgia. The chest X-ray reveals a diffuse bilateral, symmetrical, interstitial and alveolar infiltrate, although occasional focal consolidation may be seen. CMV viruria and viraemia are variable. The diagnosis can only be made by lung biopsy when large intranuclear inclusion bodies within alveolar epithelial cells are seen. The presence of a severe leukopenia in a patient with CMV pneumonitis indicates a high risk of secondary infection and death. Previously *Pneumocystis carinii* was the major secondary infecting organism but prophylaxis with cotrimoxazole has made this infection less common. Co-trimoxazole has been used as long-term prophylaxis for severe early post-renal transplant pyelonephritis[47], and this use of cotrimoxazole may account for the low incidence of *Pneumocystis carinii* pneumonia in Ramsey's series.

Antiviral chemotherapy with adenosine arabinoside, α-interferon and acyclovir has been shown to be ineffective against cytomegalovirus infection. Although DHPG has been shown to have some clinical effect on CMV retinitis and CMV gastrointestinal disease, it is of little short-term value in CMV pneumonitis[36]. The prophylaxis against CMV infection has been discussed in the section on systemic disease.

Other opportunistic bronchopulmonary infections occurring post-transplantation include Legionnaires' disease caused by *Legionella pneumophila*[6] and *Legionella micdadei*[52]. Legionnaires' disease may arise sporadically but clustering of cases must raise the possibility of nosocomial transmission. When such a nosocomial outbreak of Legionnaires' disease is identified, the prophylactic use of erythromycin may be considered[53].

Mycobacterial infections with *Mycobacterium tuberculosis* and atypical mycobacteria such as *Mycobacterium kansasii* and *Mycobacterium fortuitum* are uncommon opportunistic post-transplantation lung pathogens, but a careful assessment for mycobacterial infection in any immunosuppressed, corticosteroid-treated patient must be undertaken. Coutts described an incidence of five cases in 400 renal transplant recipients. These patients presented with miliary opacification or lower lobe shadowing as well as the more typical upper lobe consolidation. The importance of tuberculosis in these immunosuppressed patients is not so much the high attack rate but, more importantly, that failure to diagnose tuberculosis or late institution of antituberculous chemotherapy carry a high fatality rate[54].

As effective therapy of opportunistic lung infection is highly dependent on an accurate diagnosis, the early use of aggressive investigations such as transtracheal aspiration, fibre optic bronchoscopy with lavage and biopsy is mandatory.

Gastrointestinal tract infections

Reactivation of HSV is common in immunosuppressed patients and most transplant recipients excrete HSV-1 in throat secretions during the first week post-transplant at a time when they are receiving large doses of immunosuppressive therapy to prevent allograft rejection[55] The majority of these reactivated infections are asymptomatic or characterized by oropharyngeal ulceration. Occasionally some of these lesions may become more chronic with destruction of involved perioral skin, herpes phagenda[56]. Extension of the herpetic infection from the mouth to the oesophagus and respiratory tract, either spontaneously or secondary to nasogastric or endotracheal intubation, leads to severe oesophagitis and tracheobronchitis with pneumonia respectively[57,58]. Oesophagitis is characterized by odynophagia and dysphagia and is confirmed by oesophagoscopy. As herpetic oesophagitis is difficult to differentiate from candida oesophagitis, histological examination and tissue cultures are indicated. Dissemination of HSV to viscera is uncommon even in severely immunocompromised patients but herpetic hepatitis has occurred after renal transplantation[59,60]. Herpes hepatitis can progress rapidly to fulminating hepatic failure with disseminated intravascular coagulation and death.

Herpes simplex virus infections after renal transplantation can be prevented by oral acyclovir and actively treated with IV acyclovir. Reduced intensity of immunosuppressive therapy also helps to reduce the severity of herpes infection.

Gastrointestinal fungal infections with candida spp. affect the mouth, oesophagus, stomach and upper small bowel[61]. About 50% of patients with *Candida* oesophagitis do not have concurrent oral candidiasis. The symptoms of candida oesophagitis are indistinguishable from herpetic oesophagitis and endoscopic inspection with biopsy, tissue staining and culture is essential to define the cause of the oesophagitis accurately. HSV and candida may both be present in the same patient. The late complications of candida oesophagitis include bleeding, perforation from the lower third of the oesophagus and irreversible oesophageal stricture. Candidaemia and dissemination to vital organs is uncommon post-transplant, but is more likely at times of severe leukopenia when spread to liver, spleen, lungs, skin, brain, bone, joints, eyes and heart may occur. Diagnosis of disseminated candidiasis is difficult but any superficial skin lesion should be biopsied and appropriately stained. Intravenous amphotericin B is the treatment of choice with additional 5-fluorocytosine if the patient is slow to respond.

Cytomegalovirus disease of the gastrointestinal tract occurs in the presence of disseminated CMV infection[12] and may affect the oesophagus, stomach, duodenum or colon. CMV may be found in the gastrointestinal tract coincidentally at autopsy but it is impossible to ascribe any clinical significance to such an observation. On the other hand, however, CMV has been described as causing gastrointestinal haemorrhage from gastric mucosal ulceration[62] and from the caecum and colon[63].

Strongyloides stercoralis is a nematode helminth found widely in the tropics and which infects the upper gastrointestinal tract. The extent of both the disease and symptoms are related to the intensity and extent of gastrointestinal infestation. Symptoms vary from asymptomatic through dyspepsia to severe diarrhoea and malabsorption. Ova are produced by parthenogenetic females in the upper small bowel, the ova developing into rhabditiform larvae that are usually passed with the stool into the soil where they metamorphose to filariform larvae. The filariform larvae are infective and, having penetrated the human skin, migrate in the blood to the lungs and ultimately to the upper small bowel mucosa. Occasionally rhabditiform larvae metamorphose into filariform larvae in the bowel lumen or on the perianal skin and thus directly reinfect the host. This is known as *auto-infection.*

Under conditions of immunosuppression with impaired cell-mediated immunity, auto-infection is highly probable and larvae migrate from the gut mucosa to disseminate widely to vital organs, in particular the lungs and central nervous system. Gram negative polymicrobial septicaemia and meningitis are frequent accompaniments and clues to hyperinvasive strongyloidiasis. Blood eosinophilia is common in mild strongyloidiasis but is rare in the severe hyperinvasive form of this disease. Treatment is difficult with thiabendazole and therefore screening for this potentially fatal condition by stool and duodenal juice examination is recommended for transplant candidates with a history of prior residence in tropical areas[64].

Bacterial gastroenteritis is uncommon in transplant recipients but can be serious when it occurs. Berk and colleagues described eight cases of severe non-typhoidal salmonellosis occurring amongst 410 renal transplant recipients. The syndrome was characterized by fever, leukopenia, pneumonia, diarrhoea, visceral abscesses, pyelonephritis, venous thromboses and pleural effusion. The need for stool and blood cultures is self-evident, and treatment with parenteral chloramphenicol or co-trimoxazole mandatory[65].

Acute hepatitis in immunosuppressed post-renal-transplant patients is usually viral and caused by type A, type B, non-A non-B, herpes simplex and cytomegalovirus[66]. Biochemical and clinical hepatitis may occur in up to 45% of renal transplant recipients, hepatitis B and cytomegalovirus accounting for 20% each in one series. The incidence of chronic hepatitis in renal transplant patients is 6–16%, with much morbidity and mortality caused by progressive liver damage. With screening of blood and organ donors for HbsAg carriage, the most important cause of both acute and chronic hepatitis in renal transplant recipients is now non-A non-B hepatitis[67].

The major pathogens and associated gastrointestinal syndromes are summarized in Table 12.6.

Central nervous system infections

With increasing numbers of chronically immunosuppressed patients, it has become apparent that the CNS is a major site of infection in these patients. Opportunistic CNS infection now ranks second in frequency to those of the lung. Several features of the opportunistic CNS infections make their identification difficult as the list of potential organisms is large and the clinical manifestations of infection may be subtle and masked by the concomitant suppression of the host's inflammatory response. A high index of suspicion is essential as good quality survival is dependent on early and accurate diagnosis and prompt initiation of effective therapy. An urgent CT brain scan with contrast enhancement to exclude mass lesions such as brain abscess/abscesses and malignancies, especially Epstein–Barr virus-associated lymphoma, can be safely followed by assessment of an adequate volume of CSF.

In a recent ten-year retrospective survey of CNS infection in the chronically immunosuppressed, a total of 49 immunosuppressed patients were found to have 55 infections, 30 (61%) of these patients dying as a direct result of the CNS infection. Three organisms accounted for 58% of the infections:

Table 12.6 Opportunistic infections of the gastrointestinal and hepatic systems in immunosuppressed patients

Syndrome	Opportunistic pathogen
Stomatitis	Herpes simplex Type I *Candida albicans*
Oesophagitis	Herpes simplex Type I *Candida albicans* CMV
Small bowel infection	*Candida albicans*
Diarrhoea	*Strongyloides stercoralis*
Malabsorption	Non-typhoidal salmonella
GI haemorrhage	CMV
Acute hepatitis	Hepatitis virus A
Chronic hepatitis:	{ Hepatitis virus B { Hepatitis virus non-A, non-B CMV Herpes simplex Type I Herpes varicella zoster virus

Cryptococcus neoformans, Listeria monocytogenes and *Aspergillus fumigatus*[68]. Of the 300 patients who underwent renal transplantation, 20 (7%) developed CNS infection, nine of them dying as a result. Although the peak incidence of infection occurred 1–4 months post-renal-transplantation, aspergillus infection occurred exclusively at 1–4 months, cryptococcal infection after 6 months and *Listeria monocytogenes* at any time. Leukopenia, uraemia, acute renal graft rejection, intercurrent CMV infection and high dose prednisolone therapy are strongly associated with opportunistic CNS infection.

Fever and headache were the most common clinical presenting symptoms but less than one third had meningeal irritation and less than half had evidence of altered consciousness. Thus a post-renal-transplant patient with headache and fever of long or short duration must be actively and urgently investigated for central nervous system infection. Other infections documented in this study were toxoplasma encephalitis, rhinocerebral mucormycosis and *Psudomonas aeruginosa* meningitis. The presence of black necrotic lesions on the hard palate or nasal mucous membranes, ophthalmoplegia and proptosis should alert the clinician to the possibility of rhinocerebral mucormycosis.

Patients who have received organ transplants and/or those receiving daily immunosuppressive doses of corticosteroids have a predictable defect in cell-mediated immunity and are thus at risk of infection with intracellular pathogens. A check list of these pathogens and the associated central nervous system symptoms is shown in Table 12.7.

Bacterial infection of the CNS – Listeria monocytogenes is the most common bacterial cause of opportunistic CNS infection and presents in one of three ways: bacteraemia only, meningitis with bacteraemia, or cerebritis/meningoencephalitis. The CSF findings are indicative of a purulent bacterial meningitis rather than a lymphocytic pleocytosis. Combined therapy with an aminoglycoside and high dose ampicillin for 21 days is recommended with close monitoring of serum aminoglycoside levels. Co-trimoxazole and vancomycin may be suitable alternative therapies but insufficient information is available at present to recommend them[69].

Acute pyogenic infections with *Streptococcus pneumoniae*, *Haemophilus influenzae* type B, and aerobic Gram negative bacilli such as *Pseudomonas aeruginosa* and *Klebsiella* spp. arising from the gastrointestinal tract are less less common but treatable causes of acute meningitis in immunosuppressed patients.

Nocardia asteroides, Mycobacterium tuberculosis, Aspergillus spp. and *Cryptococcus neoformans* share certain clinical features such as metastatic spread to various organs especially skin, muscle, kidneys and liver. Clinically these organisms produce indolent disease with fever, headache and malaise. Nocardia has a propensity to produce a single brain abscess with focal CNS signs and occasionally skin abscesses or nodules allowing of biopsy for diagnosis. As *Mycobacterium tuberculosis* is a rather rare cause of CNS infection in immunosuppressed patients, the finding of a lymphocytic pleocytosis in the CSF of such a patient must prompt investigation for fungal

Table 12.7 CNS opportunistic pathogens and clinical syndromes produced

Clinical presentation	Pathogen(s) likely
Acute meningitis	Listeria monocytogenes Aerobic Gram negative bacilli Streptococcus pneumoniae Haemophilus influenzae

Subacute meningitis	Cryptococcus neoformans
	Mycobacterium tuberculosis
	and possibly:
	    Listeria monocytogenes
	    Strongyloides
	    Cryptococcus

Encephalitis	Listeria monocytogenes
	Toxoplasma gondii
	Herpes varicella zoster virus
	and possibly:
	    JC papovavirus (polyoma virus)
	    Strongyloides
	    Cryptococcus

Brain abscess	Aspergillus spp.
	Nocardia asteroides
	Toxoplasma gondii
	and possibly:
	    Cryptococcus
	    Listeria
	    Mucormycosis

CNS infection.

Fungal infections of the CNS – Cryptococcus neoformans commonly causes an indolent subacute meningitis and occasionally an isolated brain abscess. In the post-renal-transplant patient, cryptococcal CNS infection occurs after 6 months or more of continuous immunosuppressive therapy. Clinically, cryptococcal CNS infection is an insidious and subtle disease although it can present as an acute meningitis in the immunosuppressed. Metastatic lung and skin lesions may serve as early warnings of disseminated cryptococcal infection when the diagnosis is confirmed by histology. Diagnosis depends on India ink staining of CSF and on the more sensitive latex agglutination tests for cryptococcal antigen in CSF. Treatment with amphotericin B (0.6–1.0 mg/kg/d) for at least six weeks is essential although it is uncertain whether additional 5-fluorocytosine improves the cure rate of approximately 50%[70].

Aspergillus spp. are the second most common cause of fungal CNS infections in the immunosuppressed patient, occurring between the first and fifth months of renal transplantation when immunosuppression is at its most intense and the concomitant and additional immunosuppressive effect of CMV infection is most likely. Aspergillus infections occurring within the first month of immunosuppression should raise the possibilities of nosocomial transmission and an environmental source such as building material. CNS aspergillus infection is the result of metastatic spread via the blood from the lungs: concomitant spread to the skin may produce non-specific lesions, biopsy of which may reveal the diagnosis. Occasionally aspergillus may spread directly and invasively to the meninges and brain from an infected nasal sinus[71]. The CSF in aspergillus CNS infection may be normal or show a pleocytosis with either lymphocytes or granulocytes. Intravenous amphotericin B is the drug of choice, supplemented by surgical removal of aspergillosis-infected sinus or ear tissue.

Candida infection of the CNS may occur in association with disseminated candidiasis in the immunosuppressed host. Disseminated candidiasis occurs in association with IV catheter-related infection, gastrointestinal candida colonization and, in renal transplant patients, with obstructive uropathy and candidal pyelonephritis. A subacute or chronic meningitis is the most likely clinical presentation although candidal brain abscesses do occur[68].

Rhinocerebral mucormycosis occurs in immunocompromised diabetic patients with keto-acidosis, and in patients on corticosteroids and with leukopenia. It invades the CNS from the adjacent nasal sinuses and palate, spreading through the blood vessels via the orbit and sinuses. A characteristic black eschar may be seen on the palate and nasal mucosa from which purulent black fluid is seen to drain. Ophthalmoplegia and proptosis are seen. Involvement of the brain results in impaired consciousness and focal signs depending on the area of brain involved[72].

Fungal infections of the CNS require prolonged therapy with intravenous amphotericin B with the possible addition of 5-fluorocytosine in cryptoccal and candidal infection. As aspergillosis and mucor both invade and obstruct blood vessels, surgical debridement is essential to promote blood flow to infected areas.

Viral infection of the CNS – HV Z virus, the cause of chickenpox (varicella), causes a severe and potentially fatal infection in immunosuppressed patients. Although zoster-immune globulin (ZIG) may prevent or attenuate varicella infection in at-risk patients, cell-mediated immunity is the crucial factor controlling this infection. In immunosuppressed post-transplant patients visceral dissemination occurs in about one third. Prolonged fever and recurrent crops of herpetic vesicles are indicative of visceral dissemination. Varicella meningo-encephalitis usually begins at the end of the first week of the illness but may begin with the onset of the skin lesions. Acyclovir is the recommended therapy for varicella encephalitis. Herpes zoster (shingles) can occur at any time after a previous attack of varicella (chickenpox) but is more frequent and likely in patients receiving immunosuppressive therapy with a cumulative incidence of nearly 50% in bone marrow transplant recipients[73]. The peak incidence is 4–5 months post-transplantation, most patients presenting as dermatomal classical 'shingles', 30% of whom will have cutaneous dissemination. Of untreated patients, 5–10% may die due to visceral dissemination to lungs, liver and CNS. Recovery is aided by reducing the intensity of immunosuppressive therapy and by giving IV acyclovir[46]. However, prolonged zoster infections lasting as long as 24 weeks have been described[45]. Clinical encephalitis may occur anytime between one and eight weeks following the onset of cutaneous herpes zoster. Long-term complications of herpes varicella zoster infection include intractable post-herpetic neuralgia, granulomatous angiitis of the CNS[74] and a syndrome not dissimilar to progressive multifocal leukoencephalopathy[75].

Herpes simplex encephalitis does not occur any more frequently in the immunosuppressed population. It manifests as fever, headache, altered consciousness and personality. CT brain scan or EEG may reveal localized abnormalities in the temporal lobes and definitive diagnosis is made by brain biopsy. The early and aggressive use of IV acyclovir, 30 mg/kg/d in three divided doses, is recommended to reduce the mortality although serious neurological sequelae are common[76].

Epstein–Barr virus (EBV) is a transforming herpesvirus that infects and replicates in B lymphocytes and has been associated with the development of lympho-proliferative disorders in immunodeficient hosts such as recipients of renal[77] and bone marrow[78] transplants. Some of these EBV-associated lymphomas occur within the central nervous system[79].

J C polyoma virus, one of the papovavirus group, causes progressive multifocal leukoencephalopathy (PML) and is seen in patients with chronically suppressed cell-mediated immunity. There are a few reports of PML in renal transplant recipients[80]. PML presents in two ways: firstly as slowly progressive focal defects such as hemiparesis with or without aphasia – ataxia, dysarthria and eye movement disorders are less common; secondly as progressive confusion and a meningo-encephalitic disease. This condition pursues a rapid progression to death within a few weeks of diagnosis. Firm diagnosis can only be reached by brain biopsy. There is no effective treatment available.

CMV does not appear to involve the brain directly but is a cause of a distinctive retinitis occurring in transplant patients on immunosuppressive therapy[81]. CMV retinitis is a late manifestation of disseminated CMV infection occurring after 6 months of continued immunosuppression. Patients complain of blurred vision, scotoma and impaired visual acuity, and visual impairment can be progressive and irreversible. Ophthalmoscopy reveals small opaque areas of necrosis within the retina which spread centrifugally with patches of flame-like haemorrhage. The recent use of DHPG in patients with CMV retinitis showed some improvement in the retinal appearances[36].

Parasitic infection of the CNS – The protozoan *Toxoplasma gondii* occasionally infects the CNS of chronically immunosuppressed patients causing a diffuse encephalitis or multiple brain abscesses[82]. It is a common CNS pathogen in acquired immunodeficiency syndrome (AIDS). As IgM antibody to toxoplasma is frequently absent in severely compromised patients, a brain biopsy is the only certain way of making a diagnosis of toxoplasma encephalitis. Treatment with pyrimethamine and high dose sulphadiazine is then indicated.

The nematode *Strongyloides stercoralis* can, under conditions of intense immunosuppression, migrate from the upper gastrointestinal tract to invade the bloodstream and metastasise to multiple organs including the lungs and brain. This 'hyperinvasive syndrome' is frequently accompanied by polymicrobial Gram negative bacteraemia and meningitis. Strongyloidiasis must be excluded prior to immunosuppression of patients who have lived in an endemic area, even decades before. Treatment with repeated courses of thiabendazole are unpleasant and rarely eradicative[64].

Bone and joint infections

Osteomyelitis and septic arthritis are uncommon post-transplantation infections, but must be considered in any patient who has been or is bacteraemic and presents with symptoms referable to one or more joints. *Staphylococcus aureus, Staphylococcus epidermidis* and other Gram positive and Gram negative organisms may be found. More unusual causes of opportunistic joint infection include *mycobacteria tuberculosis*, atypical mycobacteria, *Candida* spp. and *Aspergillus* spp. Tuberculous arthritis is uncommon: it occurred in 3 out of 845 renal transplant recipients. Diagnosis requires joint aspiration and occasionally synovial biopsy and appropriate staining[83].

Infections transmitted by donor organ

The transmission of malaria, both vivax and falciparum, is an uncommon occurrence but one with a severe prognosis in the immunosuppressed patient. The absence of a recent travel history delays the diagnosis and thus the initiation of effective antimalarial chemotherapy[84,85]. Other serious but unusual infections thought to have been transmitted with the donor organ include strongyloidiasis[86], toxoplasmosis[87] and tuberculosis[88].

Unusual cause of PUO in transplant recipients

The immunosuppression post-transplantation may reactivate some unusual latent infections. Post-transplantation fever of unknown origin with a pancytopenia should prompt consideration of visceral leishmaniasis, a very rare cause of fever even in immunocompetent non-tropical residents[89,90].

CONCLUSION

Infection will remain a challenging problem for clinicans looking after immunocompromised post-transplantation patients. Lower doses of corticosteroids have already been shown to reduce the risks of severe opportunistic infections[21], although the recent introduction of cyclosporin A remains to be evaluated in terms of opportunistic infection rates. The use of pre-transplantation vaccination with polyvalent pneumococcal vaccine, hepatitis B vaccine and CMV Townes vaccine is currently under evaluation. There are prospects of safer subunit vaccines for cytomegalovirus and Epstein–Barr virus. Antimicrobial chemoprophylaxis with agents such as co-trimoxazole has been shown to reduce early and serious urinary tract infection post-transplantation[48], and may even prevent *pneumocystis carinii* pneumonia, nocardiosis, listeria infection and pneumococcal infection. Awareness of the nosocomial hazards from air conditioning and plumbing systems of aspergillosis and Legionnaires' disease has already directed attention to the importance of safe engineering within hospitals.

References

1. Eickhoff, T. C., Olin, D., Anderson, R. J. et al. (1972). Current problems and approaches to diagnosis of infection in renal transplant recipients. *Transplant Proc.*, **4**, 693–8
2. Meuleman, J. and Katz, P. (1985). The immunologic effects, kinetics and use of glucocorticoids. *Med. Clinics N.A.*, **69**, 805–16
3. Ramsey, P. G., Rubin, R. H., Tolkoff-Rubin, N. E. et al. (1980). The renal transplant patient with fever and pulmonary infiltrates: aetiology, clinical manifestations and management. *Medicine (Baltimore)*, **59**, 202–22
4. Haley, C. E., Cohen, M. L., Halter,, J. and Meyer, R. D. (1979). Nosocomial Legionnaires' disease: a continuing common source epidemic at Wadsworth Memorial Centre. *Ann. Intern. Med.*, **90**, 583–6
5. Cohen, M. L., Broome, C. V., Paris, A. L. et al. (1979). Fatal nosocomial Legionnaires' disease: clinical and epidemiological characteristics. *Ann. Intern. Med.*, **90**, 611–3
6. Tobin, J. O. H., Beare, J., Dunnill, M. S. et al. (1980). Legionnaires' disease in a transplant unit: isolation of the causative agent from shower baths. *Lancet*, **2**, 118–21
7. Kirby, B. K., Snyder, K. M., Meyer, R. D. and Finegold, S. M. (1980). Legionnaires' disease: report of sixty-five nosocomially acquired cases and review of the literature. *Medicine (Baltimore)*, **59**, 118–205
8. Myerowitz, R. L., Pasculle, A. W., Dowling, J. N. et al. (1979). Opportunist lung infection due to 'Pittsburgh Pneumonia Agent'. *N. Engl. J. Med.*, **301**, 953–8
9. Singer, C., Armstrong, D., Rosen, P. P. and Schottenfield, D. (1975). Pneumocystis carinii pneumonia: a cluster of 11 cases. *Am. J. Med.*, **82**, 772–7
10. Arnour, P. M., Anderson, P., Mainous, P. D. and Smith, E. J. (1978). Pulmonary aspergillosis during hospital renovation. *Am. Rev. Resp. Dis.*, **118**, 49–53
11. Aisner, J., Schimpff, S. C., Bennett, J. E. et al. (1976). Aspergillus infections in cancer patients: association with fireproofing materials in a new hospital. *J. Am. Med. Assoc.*, **235**, 411–3
12. Petersin, P. K., Balfour, H. H., Marker, S. C., Fryd, D. S., Howard, R. J. and Symmons, R. L. (1980). Cytomegalovirus disease in renal allograft recipients: a prospective study of the clinical features, risk factors and impact on renal transplantation. *Medicine (Baltimore)*, **59**, 283–300
13. Rubin, R. H., Russell, P. S., Levin, M. et al. (1979). Summary of a workshop on cytomegalovirus infections during organ transplantation. *J. Inf. Dis.*, **139**, 728–9
14. Ho, M., Suwansirikul, Dowling, S. L. et al. (1975). The transplanted kidney as a source of cytomegalovirus infection. *N. Engl. J. Med.*, **293**, 1109–12
15. Betts, R. F., Freeman, R. B., Douglas, R. G. et al. (1975). Transmission of cytomegalovirus infection with renal allograft. *Kidney Int.*, **8**, 385–94
16. Orsi, E. V., Howard, J. L., Baturay, N. et al. (1978). High incidence of virus isolation from donor and recipient tissues associated with renal transplantation. *Nature*, **272**, 372–3
17. Wertheim, P., Buurman, C., Geelen, J. et al. (1983). Transmission of cytomegalovirus by renal allograft demonstrated by restriction enzyme analysis. *Lancet*, **1**, 980–1
18. Schooley, R. T., Hirsch, M. S., Colvin, R. B. et al. (1983). Association of herpes virus infections with T-lymphocyte subset alterations, glomerulopathy and opportunistic infections after renal transplantation. *N. Engl. J. Med.*, **308**, 307–13
19. Cosimi, A. B., Colvin, R. B., Burton, R. C. et al. (1981). Use of monoclonal antibodies to T-cell subsets for immunological monitoring and treatment in recipients of renal allografts. *N. Engl. J. Med.*, **305**, 308–14
20. Richardson, W. P., Colvin, R. B., Cheeseman, S. H. et al. (1981). Glomerulopathy associated with cytomegalovirus viraemia in renal allografts. *N. Engl. J. Med.*, **305**, 57–63
21. Morris, P. J., Chan, L., French, M. E. et al. (1982). Low dose oral prednisolone in renal transplantation. *Lancet*, **1**, 525–7

22. European Multicentre Trial Group. (1983). Cyclosporin in cadaveric renal transplantation: one year follow up of a multicentre trial. *Lancet*, **2**, 986–9
23. Stiller, C. (1983). The requirements for maintenance steroids in cyclosporin treated renal transplant patients. *Transplant. Proc.*, **15**, 2490–4
24. Starzl, T. E., Nalesnik, M. A., Porter, K. A. *et al.* (1984). Reversibility of lymphomas and lymphoproliferative lesions developing under cyclosporin-steroid therapy. *Lancet*, **1**, 583–7
25. Meyers, J. C., Leszczynski, J., Zaia, J. A. *et al.* (1983). Prevention of cytomegalovirus infection by cytomegalovirus immune globulin after bone marrow transplant. *Ann. Intern. Med.*, **98**, 442–6
26. Winston, D. J., Pollard, R. B., Ho, W. G. *et al.* (1982). Cytomegalovirus immune plasma in bone marrow transplant recipients. *Ann. Intern. Med.*, **97**, 11–8
27. Condie, R. M., Hall, B. L., Howard, R. J. *et al.* (1979). Treatment of life threatening infections in renal transplant recipients with high-dose intravenous human IgG. *Transplant. Proc.*, **11**, 66–8
28. Condie, R. M. and O'Reilly, R. J. (1984). Prevention of CMV infection by prophylaxis with an IV hyperimmune, native, unmodified CMV globulin: randomised trial in bone marrow transplant recipients. *Am. J. Med.*, **76**, 134–41
29. Plotkin, S. A., Smiley, M. L. and Friedman, H. M. (1984). Towne vaccine induced prevention of cytomegalovirus disease after renal transplantation. *Lancet*, **1**, 528–30
30. Saral, R., Burns, W. H., Laskin, O. L. *et al.* (1981). Acyclovir prophylaxis of herpes simplex virus infections: a randomised, double-blind, controlled trial in bone marrow transplantation. *N. Engl. J. Med.*, **305**, 63–7
31. Hann, I. M., Prentice, H. G., Blacklock, H. A. *et al.* (1983). Acyclovir prophylaxis against herpes virus infections in severely immunocompromised patients: randomised double blind trial. *Br. Med. J.*, **287**, 384–8
32. Gluckman, E., Lotsberg, J., Devergie, A. *et al.* (1983). Prophylaxis of herpes infection after bone marrow transplantation by oral acyclovir. *Lancet*, **2**, 706–8
33. Hirsch, M. S., Schooley, R. T., Cosimi, A. B. *et al.* (1983). Effects of interferon alpha on cytomegalovirus reactivation symptoms in renal transplant recipients. *N. Engl. J. Med.*, **308**, 1489–93
34. Balfour, H. H., Bean, B., Mitchell, C. D. *et al.* (1982). Acyclovir in immunocompromised patients with cytomegalovirus disease. *Am. J. Med.*, **73**, 1A. 241–8
35. Crumpacker, C. S., Schnipper, L. E., Zaia, J. A. *et al.* (1979). Growth inhibition by acycloguanosine of herpes viruses isolated from human infections. *Antimicrob. Ag. Chemother.*, **15**, 642–5
36. Collaborative DHPG Treatment Study Group. (1986). Treatment of serious cytomegalovirus infections with 9-(1-3-dihydroxy-2-propoxymethyl) guanine in patients with AIDS and other immunodeficiencies. *N. Engl. J. Med.*, **314**, 801–5
37. Ringden, O., Wilczek, H., Lonnqvist, B. *et al.* (1985). Foscarnet for cytomegalovirus infections. *Lancet*, **1**, 1503–4
38. Koranda, F., Dehmel, E. Kahn, G. *et al.* (1974). Cutaneous complications in immunosuppressed renal homograft recipients. *J. Am. Med. Assoc.*, **229**, 419–24
39. Kyriakides, G. K., Simmons, R. L. and Najarian, J. S. (1975). Wound infections in renal transplant wound: pathogenetic and prognostic factors. *Ann. Surg.*, **186**, 770–5
40. Wolfson, J. S., Sober, A. J. and Rubin, R. H. (1985). Dermatologic manifestations of infections in immunocompromised patients. *Medicine (Baltimore)*, **64**, 115–33
41. Mullen, D. L. Silverberg, S. G., Penn, I. *et al.* (1976). Squamous cell carcinoma of the skin and lip in renal homograft recipients. *Cancer*, **37**, 729–34
42. Ho, M. (1977). Virus infections after transplantation in man – Brief review. *Arch. Virol.*, **55**, 1–24
43. Saral, R., Burns, W. H., Laskin, O. L. *et al.* (1981). Acyclovir prophylaxis of Herpes simplex infection. *N. Engl. J. Med.*, **305**, 63–7
44. Meyers, J. D., Wade, J. C., Mitchell, C. D. *et al.* (1982). Multicentre collaborative trial of intravenous acyclovir for treatment of mucocutaneous herpes simplex virus infections in the immunocompromised host. *Am. J. Med.*, **73** (1A), 229–35
45. Gallagher, J. G. and Merigan, T. C. (1979). Prolonged herpes zoster infection associated with immunosuppressive therapy. *Ann. Intern. Med.*, **91**, 842–6

46. Sherp, D. H., Dandlıker, P. S. and Meyers, J. D. (1986). Treatment of Varicella zoster virus infection in severely immunocompromised patients: a randomised comparison of acyclovir and vidarabine. *N. Engl. J. Med.*, **314**, 208–12

47. Rubin, R. H., Fang, L. S. T., Cosimi, A. B. *et al.* (1979). Usefulness of the antibody-control bacteria assay in the management of urinary tract infection in the renal transplant patient. *Transplantation*, **27**, 18–20

48. Tolkoff-Rubin, N. E., Cosimi, A. B. and Russell, P. S. (1982). A controlled study of cotrimoxazole prophylaxis against urinary tract infection in renal transplant recipients. *Rev. Infect. Dis.*, **4**, 614–8

49. Hogan, T. F., Borden, E. C., McBain, J. A. *et al.* (1980). Human polyomavirus infections with JC virus and BK virus in renal transplant patients. *Ann. Intern. Med.*, **92**, 373–8

50. Rice, S. J., Bishop, J. A., Apperley, J. *et al.* (1985). BK virus as a cause of haemorrhagic cystitis after bone marrow transplantation. *Lancet*, **2**, 844–5

51. Ramsey, P. G., Rubin, R. H. and Tolkoff-Rubin, N. E. (1980). The renal transplant patient with fever and pulmonary infiltrates: aetiology, clinical manifestations and management. *Medicine (Baltimore)*, **59**, 206–22

52. Myerowitz, R. L., Pasculle, A. W., Dowling, J. N. *et al.* (1979). Opportunistic lung infection due to 'Pittsburgh Pneumonia Agent'. *N. Engl. J. Med.*, **301**, 953–61

53. Vereerstraeten, P., Stolear, J. C., Schoutens-Serruys, E. *et al.* (1986). Erythromycin prophylaxis for Legionnaires' disease in immunosuppressed patients in a contaminated hospital environment. *Transplantation*, **41**, 52–4

54. Coutts, I. I., Jegarajah, S. and Stark, J. E. (1979). TB in renal transplant recipients. *Br. J. Dis. Chest*, **73**, 141–8

55. Meyers, J. D., Fluornoy, N. and Thomas, E. D. (1980). Infection with herpes simplex virus and cell mediated immunity after marrow transplantation. *J. Infect.*, **142**, 338–46

56. Shneidman, D. W., Barr, R. J. and Graham, J. H. (1979). Chronic cutaneous herpes simplex. *J. Am. Med. Assoc.*, **241**, 592–4

57. Nash, G. and Ross, J. G. (1974). Herpetic oesophagitis: a common cause of oesophageal ulceration. *Hum. Pathol.*, **5**, 339–45

58. Ramsey, P. G., Fife, K. H., Hackman, R. C. *et al.* (1982). Herpes simplex virus pneumonia: clinical, virologic and pathologic features in 20 patients. *Ann. Intern. Med.*, **97**, 813–20

59. Anuras, S. and Summers, R. (1976). Fulminant herpes simplex hepatitis in an adult: report of a case in renal transplant recipient. *Gastroenterology*, **70**, 425–8

60. Elliott, W. C., Houghton, D. C., Bryant, R. E. *et al.* (1980). Herpes simplex type I hepatitis in renal transplantation. *Arch. Intern. Med.*, **140**, 1656–60

61. Joshi, S. N., Garvin, P. J. and Sunwoo, Y. C. (1981). Candidiasis of the duodenum and jejunum. *Gastroenterology*, **80**, 829–33

62. Diethelm, A. G., Gore, I., Ch'ien, L. T. *et al.* (1976). Gastrointestinal haemorrhage secondary to cytomegalovirus after renal transplantation. *Am. J. Surg.*, **131**, 371–4

63. Sutherland, D. E. R., Chan, F. Y., Foucar, E. *et al.* (1979). The bleeding caecal ulcer in transplant patients. *Surgery*, **86**, 386–98

64. Scouden, E. B., Schaffner, W. and Stone, W. J. (1978). Overwhelming strongyloidiasis: an unappreciated opportunistic infection. *Medicine (Baltimore)*, **57**, 527–44

65. Berk, M. R., Meyers, A. M. and Cassal, W. (1984). Non-typhoid salmonella infections after renal transplantation – a serious clinical problem. *Nephron*, **37**, 186–9

66. Sopko, J. and Anuras, S. (1978). Liver disease in renal transplant recipients. *Am. J. Med.*, **64**, 139–46

67. Ware, A. J., Luby, P., Hollinger, B. *et al.* (1979). Aetiology of liver disease in renal transplant patients. *Ann. Intern. Med.*, **91**, 364–71

68. Hooper, D. C., Pruitt, A. A. and Rubin, R. H. (1982). Central nervous system infection in the chronically immunosuppressed. *Medicine (Baltimore)*, **61**, 166–88

69. Nieman, R. E. and Lorber, B. (1980). Listeriosis in adults: a changing pattern. Report of 8 cases and review of the literature 1968–78. *Rev. Infect. Dis.*, **2**, 207–27

70. Sabetta, J. R. and Andriole, V. T. (1985). Cryptococcal infection of the central nervous system. *Med. Clin. N.Am.*, **69**, 333–44

71. Swerdlow, B. and Deresinski, S. (1984). Development of aspergillus sinusitis in a patient receiving amphotericin B. *Am. J. Med.*, **76**, 162–6

72. Lehrer, R. I., Howard, D. H. and Sypherd, P. S. (1980). Mucormycosis. *Ann. Intern. Med.*, **93**, 93–108

73. Atkinson, K., Meyers, J. D., Storb, R. *et al.* (1980). Varicella zoster virus infection after bone marrow transplantation for aplastic anaemia or leukaemia. *Transplantation*, **29**, 47–50

74. Linnemann, C. C. Jr. and Alvira, M. M. (1980). Pathogenesis of varicella zoster angiitis in the CNS. *Arch. Neurol.*, **37**, 239–40

75. Horten, B., Price, R. W., and Jimenez, D. (1981). Multifocal varicella zoster virus leukoencephalitis temporarily remote from herpes zoster. *Ann. Neurol.*, **9**, 251–66

76. Whitley, R. J., Alford, C. A., Hirsch, M. S. *et al.* (1986). Vidarabine versus acyclovir therapy in herpes simplex encephalitis. *N. Engl. J. Med.*, **314**, 144–9

77. Hanto, D. W., Frizzera, G., Gajl-Peczalska, J. *et al.* (1981). The Epstein–Barr virus (EBV) in the pathogenesis of post-transplant lymphoma. *Transplant. Proc.*, **13**, 756–60

78. Schuback, W. H., Hackman, R., Neiman, P. E. *et al.* (1982). A monoclonal immunoblastic sarcoma in donor cells bearing Epstein–Barr virus genomes following allogeneic marrow grafting for acute lymphoblastic leukaemia. *Blood*, **60**, 180–7

79. Hochberg, F. H., Miller, G., Schooley, R. T. *et al.* (1983). Central nervous system lymphoma related to Epstein–Barr virus. *N. Engl. J. Med.*, **309**, 745–8

80. Manz, H. J., Dinsdale, H. B. and Morrin, R. A. F. (1971). Progressive multifocal leukoencephalopathy after renal transplantation. *Ann. Intern. Med.*, **75**, 77–81

81. Egbert, P. R., Pollard, R. B., Gallagher, J. B. *et al.* (1980). Cytomegalovirus retinitis in immunosuppressed hosts II. Ocular manifestations. *Ann. Intern. Med.*, **93**, 664–70

82. Reynolds, E. S., Walls, K. W. and Pfeiffer, R. I. (1966). Generalised toxoplasmosis following renal transplantation. *Arch. Intern. Med.*, **118**, 401–5

83. Ascher, N. L., Simmons, R. L., Marker, S. *et al.* (1978). TB joint disease in transplant patients. *Am. J. Surg.*, **135**, 853–6

84. Holzer, B. R., Gluck, Z., Zambelli, D. *et al.* (1985). Transmission of malaria by renal transplantation. *Transplantation*, **39**, 315–6

85. Johnson, I. D. A. (1981). Possible transmission of malaria by renal transplant. *Br. Med. J.*, **282**, 780

86. Hoy, W. E., Roberts, N. J. and Bryson, M. F. (1981). Transmission of Strongyloides by kidney transplant? *J. Am. Med. Assoc.*, **246**, 1937–9

87. Ryning, F. W., McCleod, R., Maddox, J. C. *et al.* (1979). Probable transmission of T Gondii by organ transplantation (heart). *Ann. Intern. Med.*, **90**, 47–9

88. Peters, T. G., Reiter, C. G. and Boswell, R. L. (1984). Transmission of TB by kidney transplantation. *Transplantation*, **38**, 514–6

89. Ma, D. D. F., Concannon, A. J. and Hayes, J. (1979). Fatal Leishmaniasis in renal transplant patients. *Lancet*, **2**, 311–2

90. Broeckaert-Van Orshoven, A., Michielsen, P. and Vandepitte, J. (1979). Fatal Leishmaniasis in renal transplant patient. *Lancet*, **2**, 740–1

91. Young, L. S. (1983). Infections complicating bone marrow transplantation. In "Proceedings of the second international symposium on the compromised host", (Ed.) Gaya, H. S. and Easmon, C., pp. 27–35. London. Academic Press.

Index

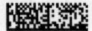